Family Communication, Connections, *and* Health Transitions

Health Communication

Gary L. Kreps, Series Editor

Vol. 1

The Health Communication series is part of the Peter Lang Media and Communication list.
Every volume is peer reviewed and meets the highest quality standards for content and production.

PETER LANG
New York • Washington, D.C./Baltimore • Bern
Frankfurt • Berlin • Brussels • Vienna • Oxford

Family Communication, Connections, *and* Health Transitions

Going Through This Together

Edited by Michelle Miller-Day

PETER LANG
New York • Washington, D.C./Baltimore • Bern
Frankfurt • Berlin • Brussels • Vienna • Oxford

Library of Congress Cataloging-in-Publication Data

Family communication, connections, and health transitions /
edited by Michelle Miller-Day.
p. ; cm. — (Health communication; v. 1)
Includes bibliographical references and index.
1. Sick—Family relationships. 2. Communication in families.
3. Chronically ill—Family relationships. I. Miller-Day, Michelle A.
II. Series: Health communication (New York, N.Y.); v. 1.
[DNLM: 1. Family Relations. 2. Adaptation, Psychological. 3. Caregivers—psychology. 4. Communication. 5. Family Health. WA 308 F1973 2010]
R726.5.F347 610—dc22 2010023507
ISBN 978-1-4331-1069-6 (hardcover)
ISBN 978-1-4331-1068-9 (paperback)
ISSN 2153-1277

Bibliographic information published by **Die Deutsche Nationalbibliothek**.
Die Deutsche Nationalbibliothek lists this publication in the "Deutsche Nationalbibliografie"; detailed bibliographic data is available on the Internet at http://dnb.d-nb.de/.

The paper in this book meets the guidelines for permanence and durability of the Committee on Production Guidelines for Book Longevity of the Council of Library Resources.

29 Broadway, 18th floor, New York, NY 10006
www.peterlang.com

Printed in the United States of America

To my family…

Edward Day
Jordan Rassulo
Joshua Miller-Day
Donna (Miller) Hodan
Bonnie Day
Edward Hodan

In memory of…

Bernard Miller
Leonard Day
Magi Colby

Offering support to…

Magi Colby's family

With special thanks to…

Sophie Appel
Gary Kreps
Allison Kootsikas
Thomas Hipper
Dana Naughton

CONTENTS

LIST OF TABLES AND FIGURES

Health Transitions and Family Communication: An Introduction

Michelle Miller-Day

THE PENNSYLVANIA STATE UNIVERSITY

> I drove Annie to [the hospital] this morning and we got bad news. Her white cell counts and hemoglobin fell dramatically over the last week, indicating that the cancer has not been eradicated sufficiently from her bone marrow to start consolidation therapy. She has to go back to the hospital Wed. morning for a more aggressive round of induction therapy, followed immediately by a stem cell or marrow transplant. He told us the chemo will be worse than last time and there is significant risk with the transplant, even if a suitable donor is found. We will have HLA tissue typing done before admission on Wed. so that there is time to find a donor. Her brothers are the most likely candidates…It has been a really bad Monday. She will likely be inpatient *another* 4-6 weeks and is crushed by this prognosis. I'm mostly scared and really, really angry. This is not the news we went up there to get, and she has been really well and energetic these last few days. I hate this fucking disease. The rest of today and tomorrow we will take care of loose ends, pack for her stay, and eat cookies till we throw up (it's a bonding ritual for us).

This is the text of an e-mail message sent to me while in the process of editing this volume. I share this message with you because it embodies what this book is about—health, families, connection, communication, heartbreak, and eating cookies together as a display of solidarity. The book is about individuals like my friend Annie[1] who seek and need support during times of ill health. But, it is also about family members who not only provide—but require their own—support, comfort, information and hope.

When family members experience a diagnosis of a chronic disease (e.g., cancer) or a health crisis (e.g., postpartum depression), not only the diagnosed individuals, but entire families experience immediate and long-term stress as a consequence (Rolland, 1994a; Roy, 2006). Health conditions can introduce dramatic changes in a family mem-

1 Her name was changed to protect her identity.

ber's behavior or in a family's daily routine. Family members may be uncertain about what to do, how to help, or how the health condition will affect their family life. Indeed, most families enter the world of illness and disability without a psychosocial map.

Families with members dealing with serious health conditions may be confronted with significant challenges posed by treatment regimes, impacts on day-to-day activities, disruption of family roles, possible threat of death, creating meaning of the illness experience, and a host of psychosocial challenges (Roy, 2006). Sociological and psychological research exists that suggests these kinds of challenges affect general family functioning (Martire, Lustig, Schulz, Miller, & Helgeson, 2004) and the health outcomes of patients (Liu & Gallagher-Thompson, 2009). However, there is very little research that examines the ways in which health transitions shape day-to-day communication within families or what the consequences of communication adaptation might have on physical and psychological functioning of all family members. The remainder of this chapter defines health transitions, provides a brief review of the research literature on families and health, and offers a preview of the forthcoming chapters.

Health Transitions

In family life there are developmental transitions that may be expected or even planned for (e.g., such as the birth of a new child) which require all members to adapt to increased stress. For many families, however, there are *unexpected* transitions, such as a member's diagnosis of a serious health condition. Transitions highlight change and adjustment. By definition, a transition is a passage—or change—from one state to another (dictionary.com, n.d). Families confront a variety of transition periods when a member suffers from a serious health condition. There is not one single transition from relative health to ill heath, but countless changes and adjustments that may include the onset of symptoms, diagnosis, prognoses, course of treatment, post-treatment and possibly incapacitation and the transition to end-of-life. During these transition periods, families are sometimes at their most vulnerable because certain health transitions (e.g., intensive treatment regimes) can introduce dramatic changes into the family system that require substantive adaptation and reassessment rather than minor alterations to a family's daily routine (Roy, 2006; Sidhu, Passmore, & Baker, 2005). Health transitions are not navigated by the afflicted individual alone. As people cope with and adjust to myriad health transitions, so too do their family members.

The Interdependence of Families and Health: A Brief Overview

The link between health and family is reciprocal in nature. That is, just as family relationships and processes affect physical and mental health, health conditions influence family relationships and processes. To provide a foundation for understanding this interdependence, I begin by providing some working definitions of family and health.

Families and Health

What is family? In the 21st century defining family is a complex endeavor. As Baxter and colleagues (2009) point out, family is a hotly contested term among scholars. Definitions of this sort ultimately determine who counts as a "family" and who does not, and this may have implications for policy and treatment of family systems. For this reason, a structural definition of family is often employed in scholarly research and by government agencies. Structural definitions such as, "a group of two people or more related by birth, marriage, or adoption and residing together" (U.S. Census Bureau, 2001, p. 4) highlight the role of blood and legal ties as well as co-residence. This book, however, places communication at the core of defining family; therefore, it reflects a constitutive definition of family—privileging the role of communication (Baxter et al.). From a constitutive perspective, family is defined as a group of persons who interact and through their interactions constitute a family identity. The research presented here argues that family is constructed and maintained through communication.

What about health? The World Health Organization defines health as a state of physical and mental well-being, not simply the absence of disease (World Health Organization, 1946). This broad definition of health focuses on the physical and emotional quality of people's lives. As numerous studies have pointed out, physical and mental health correlate highly; they share common causes and they affect each other.

The interdependence of family and health provides the foundation of this volume. When an individual is coping with a health condition, he or she is not just loosely linked to family members who can be of assistance. I, and the authors of the chapters in this book, argue that typically an afflicted individual is embedded within a family system and this has implications for health care (see chapters 11, 13) and family adaptation (see chapters 2, 3, 4, 5, 6, 8, 14). An illness can become a powerful member of the family. Individuals within a family system may be impatient to move past a health crisis so that life can go back to normal. But for many families experiencing health crises, daily life will need to be recalibrated and adjusted to accommodate the illness. Communication is the mechanism through which adjustment occurs. As the information, examples, and personal narratives presented in this book illustrate, effective communication among and between patients, family members, and care providers is essential for successful navigation of health transitions.

Unfortunately, communication scholars have had surprisingly little to contribute to the conversation on families and health. By its very nature, the study of families and health is interdisciplinary and although we are just beginning to explore these topics in the field of communication, our discipline has much to contribute. The following represents a brief interdisciplinary overview of what is known about the impacts of families on health and the impacts of ill health on families.

The Impact of Families on Health and Well-Being

Epidemiological research has demonstrated that being married is protective against chronic health conditions (Ross, Mirowsky, & Goldsteen, 1990). Results of the National Longitudinal Mortality Study reveal that, across all causes of mortality and across different nonmarried populations (never married, divorced/ separated, and widowed), nonmarried individuals had elevated rates of mortality compared to married individuals, with higher incidence of coronary heart disease, stroke, pneumonia, and certain kinds of cancer, (Johnson, Backlund, Sorlie, & Loveless, 2000). Additionally, nonmarried individuals have higher levels of psychological distress such as depression and anxiety (Kiecolt-Glaser & Newton, 2001; Mastekaasa, 1994).

In addition to marital status, marital quality appears to impact health. Several studies reveal a relationship between marital satisfaction or strain and women's health. Troxel (2006) revealed that, for middle-aged women, marital dissatisfaction was associated with high blood pressure, LDL cholesterol levels, and aortic calcification. Levenson, Cartensen, and Gottman (1993) found that wives experiencing marital distress reported more mental and physical health problems than their husbands. Specifically for women, marital strain has been associated with increased symptoms of premenstrual symptoms (Coughlin, 1990), ulcers (Levenstein, Ackerman, Kiecolt-Glaser, & Dubois, 1999), coronary events (Coyne, Rohrbaugh, Shoham, Sonnega, Nicklas, & Cranford, 2001), and increased systolic blood pressure (Jacobson, Gottman, Waltz, Rushe, Bobcock, & Holtzworth-Monroe, 1994; Morell & Apple, 1990). Marital satisfaction, on the other hand, has been associated with better overall health for both genders (Ganong & Coleman, 1991) and having caring, supportive spouses can lead to improved immune function (Carrere & Gottman, 1999). Although satisfying marriages generally protect and improve health, they protect men's well-being more so than women's (Johnson et al., 2000; Mayne, O'Leary, McCrady, Contrada, & Labouvie, 1997).

Parental warmth and support appear to be central to children's heath. Wickrama, Lorenz, and Conger (1997), found that parental warmth and support were significant predictors of changes in a child's physical health complaints over a three-month period (e.g., headaches, sore throat, and allergies) and Varni, Wilcox, Hansen and Brik (1988) reported that family support accounted for 22% of variance in depression and anxiety for kids with juvenile arthritis. Moreover, Compas, Slavin, Wagner, and Vannatta (1986) discovered higher levels of anxiety in adolescence for youth whose parents were perceived as nonsupportive.

Support from family members may improve physical health directly or indirectly. Of the many functions served by families, social support is among the most important. Social support involves communication behavior that is responsive to another's needs with the intention of providing assistance (Burleson & MacGeorge, 2002). Emotional support specifically has been found to decrease depression, anxiety, and other psychological problems for receivers of the support (Scwarzer & Leppin, 1991) and, over time, psychological well-being improves subsequent physical well-being (Canary, 2008). By protecting and improving psychological well-being, social support also improves physical health and survival.

Social support from family members also impacts physical health by encouraging and reinforcing preventative behaviors. Parents and relational partners are more likely to encourage family members to quit smoking, to eat diets low in cholesterol and high in fruits and vegetables, and to eat balanced meals (Hayes & Ross, 1987). Women, in particular, often discourage smoking, drug use, or heavy drinking in the house, cook low-cholesterol meals and keep fattening food out of the house, and schedule checkups.

In addition to impacts on general health, there is also much empirical work that has demonstrated how patients and their support systems cope with health conditions to enhance recovery (Broderick, 1993; Minuchin, Rosman, & Baker, 1978; Rolland, 1994ab; 1989). The family-systems approach to recovery posits that the patient and family members are part of a complex integrated system with established patterns of communicating and interacting and that illness poses a significant challenge to these patterns (McDaniel, Hepworth, & Doherty, 1992; Rolland, 1994b). Substantial evidence points to the benefits of family social support for recovery from a variety of conditions such as stroke (Kwakkel, Wagenaar, Kollen, & Lankhorst, 1996), traumatic brain injury (Maitz & Sachs, 1995), breast cancer (Neuling & Winefield, 1988), and depression (McDaniel et al.).

Impact of Health Challenges on Families

Just as families affect health and well-being, ill health affects families in a variety of ways. Several studies have revealed that patients and their intimate partners experience adverse psychological reactions to the onset of ill health, especially with chronic illness (for a full discussion see Roy, 2006). Illness is typically considered to be a negative life event. Certain health conditions may severely limit the type of activities in which family members can engage, increase family member stress, and increase the "caregiving burden" of families (Cantor, 1980; Zarit, Reever, & Bach-Peterson, 1980). Since family networks are not necessarily trained or prepared to deal with the demands of care for a member suffering from a health condition, this care may create a burden for those providing direct care. Changes in medical practice resulting in shorter inpatient hospital stays and longer survival have substantially increased the numbers of individuals with health conditions being cared for in the home and increased the burdens on carers, as well (Martire et al., 2004).

Health conditions may also affect family members' roles and responsibilities. Family life can become disorganized, household routines upset, and stress increased by uncertainty about how to manage the illness (Zarit et al., 1980). Research finds that family members assume additional responsibilities following the illness of family members, and there is often increased dependency on healthy members of the family (Hummert & Nussbaum, 2001; Vrabec, 1997). Although Michela (1986) demonstrated that patients who increased dependency on spouses initially reported higher levels of marital satisfaction, the spouses reported significantly less marital satisfaction. Since then, a wealth of research has revealed that long-term illness may place a burden on caregivers and adversely affect the quality of their relationships (Adams, 2007). The longer the period of caregiving and dependency, the more ambiguity there may be about role expectations (Scheinkman, 1988). Even the strongest relationships may be strained by role strain and uncertainty in managing illness and other health transitions.

A health condition that is chronic or that lasts for a long period of time can powerfully challenge couples' communication skills. But, sensitive, open, direct communication about a range of issues is essential to living well with chronic disorders (Roy, 2004). Important discussions for couples include understanding the illness and its psychosocial demands over time, beliefs about who or what caused the disorder and what can affect its course; how to live with threatened loss; personal and relationship priorities; the roles of patient and caregiver; how to maintain a balanced, mutual relationship; and wills and advance directives concerning a possible terminal phase (Roy).

While open discussion of these issues is recommended by some, other research suggests that during times of health transitions, privacy and managing boundaries around private information may be important to members with health conditions and their families

(Petronio, 2002). During these transitions family members may need to renegotiate to whom, when, and how much information is shared about the health condition.

To summarize, there is interdependence between health and family relationships. Marital status, marital quality, and family warmth and support appear to impact the health of family members, with supportive relationships linked to, not just general well-being, but recovery from illness. Moreover, health transitions are not navigated by the afflicted individual alone. Patients are embedded within a family system, and as they cope with and adjust to myriad health transitions, so too do their family members.

The research introduced here is elaborated in the forthcoming chapters. The studies reported in this book point to a variety of communication questions that may be pursued when investigating the intersection of family and health. What are the message features of supportive communication? (How are these messages perceived? What are the barriers to messages of support being perceived as supportive?) What communication competencies serve to buffer families from the disabling effects of stressors during health transitions and to promote recovery and successful adaptation? How is information managed and privacy protected during times of transition?

Since there is ample evidence that communication behavior such as providing social support is associated with positive health outcomes for families, perhaps it is time to move to these questions of *how* this communication becomes associated with positive family health outcomes.

This volume seeks to jump into the conversation about families and health in the areas posed above, represent the lived experience of family life during health transitions, and offer an agenda for future studies.

The Chapters

I firmly believe that science is not achieved by distancing itself from the world. So, in this book I endeavor to capture family life as it is lived for those individuals experiencing health transitions and their families. Bochner (1995) challenged communication scholars to de-emphasize studying family in the "largely abstract, cognitive, and objective world" (p. viii) and, instead, seek an understanding of the family in its inherent concreteness, emotionality, and subjectivity. Many of the chapters herein accept this challenge, with the implicit assumption that individuals must be studied in depth to be understood in general. While not all chapters in this book take an interpretivist approach to describing, representing, and interpreting experience; there are a number of chapters that do. As a pragmatist, I agree that, "no perspective of inquiry is privileged over another; all have something to offer in understanding family life" (Stamp, 2004, p. 21). In these pages, surveys are implemented, experiments are conducted, descriptive case studies are presented, and autoethnographic accounts are shared. All these forms of inquiry serve to tell part of the story and provide insight into family communication and family life during times of health transition.

Bringing together veteran communication researchers along with newcomers; and drawing on research, clinical insight, and personal experience to illuminate these issues, this book provides a discussion of communication patterns and processes involved in the day-to-day management of health conditions.

Section one of this volume focuses on *Family interdependence in managing health transitions*. Segrin and Badger (chapter 1) begin the discussion of family interdependence in the context of cancer. This chapter discusses how and why diseases like breast and prostate cancer affect whole family systems. Further, this chapter provides evidence of the profound impacts and communication challenges these diseases pose for the marital subsystem. Readers will learn how social interaction processes such as social support and communal coping can help and hurt the quality of life and adjustment of the patient with breast or prostate cancer and their family members. This chapter also reviews the results of original research conducted by the authors offering stringent tests of emotional contagion in families with cancer, revealing that as patients' physical and psychological condition improved, so too did the emotional state of their partners. This chapter is followed by another look at family interdependence and cancer when Carla Fisher (chapter 2) explores how mothers and daughters partner side-by-side and take on cancer together. Individual life-span interviews with breast cancer patients and their mothers/daughters illuminate how mothers and daughters cope with breast cancer together—how they communicatively share the disease—and, in essence, are each other's strength. Taking a developmental approach, Fisher provides evidence that the communication of social support may be perceived differently at different stages of life development. In chapter 3, Weber and Solomon also examine breast cancer and further hone our understanding of family communication about cancer and coping. Weber and Solomon focus their inquiry on emotional and cognitive reactions to stressors associated with breast cancer and identify unique communication patterns enacted by relational partners. Moving beyond the context of cancer, chapter 4 examines spousal interdependence in managing diabetes. J. Lynne Brown provides a detailed review of the literature available on couple communication patterns and their role in management of type 2 diabetes and reports original findings from a study of couple communication and adjustment during the first year of a type 2 diabetes diagnosis. She reveals patterns of difference among cohesive, enmeshed, and disengaged couples regarding how they manage diabetes in their household. These results suggest that baseline relational cohesion may impact the type and quality of support provided in a marital relationship during the first year of disease management. To conclude this section, Anderson Dearmen (chapter 5) provides an insightful first-hand account of postpartum depression. This chapter is autoethnographic in nature. Autoethnography refers to writing about the personal and its relationship to cultural phenomena. As Ellis (2004) explains, autoethnography is a genre of writing and research that relies on personal narrative, layered within and often in juxtaposition to social scientific evidence. Anderson Dearmen's account provides her readers with a discerning explanation of the barriers women face to diagnosis and treatment of postpartum depression, the ways in which postpartum depression can affect family relationships, and the critical role family members can play in providing support and care for women suffering with postpartum depression.

The second section of this volume addresses *Stigma.* In chapter 6, Rossetto, Smith, and Jones address stigma and taboo. This chapter highlights how politeness and co-ownership of health information provide challenges to families when they discuss taboo or stigmatized health conditions. They explore how people with stigmatized health conditions enact disclosures and examine how these disclosures are interpreted, revealing important findings pertaining to information management. One insight provided by this research is that while disclosure of a health condition provides an access point for obtaining information, support, and treatment, it simultaneously opens the door to potential stigma. Erica Bauer (chapter 7) concludes this section with a discussion of stigma and how it affects disclosure of mental illness within and by families. She offers a model explaining how disclosure of a stigmatized illness is affected by the receiver's orientation to the illness and the receiver's level of intimacy with the person labeled with the stigmatizing condition.

Section three is titled *Living with invisible illness,* and, using techniques of narrative and autoethnography, it uncovers the lived experience of families adapting to members with an invisible illness. Giving voice to the experience of having an invisible illness, Emily Bowlby (chapter 8) provides an autoethnographic examination of invisible illness/disability and the impact of this on her family relationships. The author "layers" alternating voices of herself as a scholar and as a family member living with an invisible disability. Similarly, Pettigrew and Pettigrew (chapter 9) provide a moving autoethnographic account of relationship, transition into marriage, and managing an invisible, unnamed, painful, and sometimes debilitating health condition. This chapter is a love poem; a poem of commitment and endurance. Breanne and Jonathan Pettigrew successfully illustrate how they reframe stress, negotiate privacy rules, and support their relational identity. These authors conclude with a discussion of four communication strategies they implement to cope with Breanne's illness: counseling (informational and emotional guidance), cuddle time (affection and relationship building), crowding (seeking support from others), and confessing commitment (reducing relational uncertainty and reinforcing relational identity). Section four of the book is *Interfacing with others.* This section addresses communication and the interface of patients, families, and other social networks. Petronio and Sweeney-Lewis (chapter 10) begin this section with a comprehensive review of how medical disclosure plays a part in the care of individuals with cancer. Sandra and Shannon explore management of private information across a patient's trajectory of care—from initial diagnosis, discussions of prognosis, and post-treatment, to the end-of-life. This chapter is followed by Steuber and Solomon (chapter 11) who explore how couples disseminate information about infertility to their family and social networks and what the implications are for revealing, or not revealing, this information. The authors report findings from their study of infertile couples and social networks, providing insight into disclosure, negative communication experiences, and privacy management issues related to infertility. This section ends with a chapter by Foster and Cohen-Katz (chapter 12) that offers an applied perspective on medical education, health, and families. A health communication scholar and medical educator (Foster) pairs with a clinical psychologist (Cohen-Katz) to co-author this chapter on ways in which health care professionals can best respond to the complexity of family relationships during times of health transition for a family member. The chapter describes the *family life-cycle model* and the *family meeting,* how these elements fit within the overall philosophy and approach to training physicians, and how the experiences of implementing these elements can inform family and health communication more generally. For health care professionals, this chapter outlines fundamental theory as well as useful practices for working with families.

The final section of the proposed volume—section five—is titled *End-of-Life*. In this last section, Hipper, Catona, and Nussbaum (chapter 13) provide a thorough review of how primary and secondary caregivers in the family manage Alzheimer's disease. This chapter explores how far the "ripple effect" of caregiving changes the familial relational dynamics and argues for the use of the term caregiving networks instead of focusing on a static, singular caregiver. In the next chapter, Pitts (chapter 14) presents an intriguing case study of one family to examine how they co-construct positive end-of-life experiences. Providing rich details about discourse practices in one extended family system, this chapter argues that dying is both an individual and collective experience. Finally, Vande Berg and Trujillo's end-of-life story (chapter 15) is a raw, moving, and incredibly informative account. In this chapter we travel with Leah Vande Berg through her final days, hours, and minutes of her death. We peer over the shoulder of her husband, Nick Trujillo, and struggle along with him as he shares in this communal experience.

Dear reader, I wish for you to be enlightened, moved, and inspired to conduct more communication research at the intersection of family and health. This volume does not provide a definitive conclusion to these matters, but a stepping off point. Happy reading.

References

Adams, K. B. (2007). Specific effects of caring for a spouse with dementia: Differences in depressive symptoms between caregiver and non-caregiver spouses. *International Psychogeriatrics, 20,* 508-520.

Baxter, L. A., Henauw, C., Huisman, D., Livesay, C. B., Norwood, K., Su, H., Wolf, B., & Young, B. (2009). Lay conceptions of family: A replication and extension. *Journal of Family Communication, 9,* 170-189.

Bochner, A. P. (1985). Perspectives on inquiry: Representation, conversation, and reflection: In M. L. Knapp & G. R. Miller (Eds.). *Handbook of interpersonal communication* (pp. 27-58). Beverly Hills, CA: Sage.

Broderick, C. B. (1993). *Understanding family process: Basics of family systems theory.* Newbury Park, CA: Sage.

Burleson, B. R., & MacGeorge, E. L. (2002). Supportive communication. In M. L. Knapp & J. Daly (Eds.), Handbook of interpersonal communication 3rd ed. (pp. 374–424). Thousand Oaks, CA: Sage.

Canary, H. E. (2008) Creating supportive connections: A decade of research on support for families of children with disabilities. *Health Communication, 23,* 13-426.

Cantor, M. (1980). The informal support system: Its relevance in the lives of the elderly. In E. Borgotta & N. McCluskey (Eds.), *Aging and society* (pp.131-144). Beverly Hills, CA: Sage.

Carrere, S., & Gottman, J. (1999). Predicting the future of marriages. In E. M. Hetherington (Ed.) *Coping with divorce, single parenting, and remarriages* (pp. 3-23). Mahwah, NJ: LEA, Publishers.

Compas, B. E., Slavin, L. A., Wagner, B. M., & Vannatta, K. (1986). Relationship of life events and social support with psychological dysfunction among adolescents. *Journal of Youth and Adolescence, 15,* 205-221.

Coughlin, P. C. (1990). Premenstrual syndrome: How marital satisfaction and role choice affect symptom severity. *Social Work, 35,* 351-355.

Coyne, J. C., Rohrbaugh, M. J., Shoham V., Sonnega J. S., Nicklas, J. M., & Cranford, J. A. (2001). Prognostic importance of marital quality for survival of congestive heart failure. *American Journal of Cardiology, 88,* 526-529.

Dictionary.com Unabridged. transition. (n.d.). Retrieved from Dictionary.com website: http://dictionary.reference.com/browse/transition

Ellis, C. (2004). *The ethnographic "I": A methodological novel about ethnography*. Lanham, MD: Altamira Press.

Ganong, L. H., & Coleman, M. (1991). Remarriage and health. *Research in Nursing and Health, 14*, 205-211.

Hayes, D., & Ross, C. E. (1987). Concern with appearance, health beliefs, and eating habits. *Journal of Health and Social Behavior, 28*, 120-130.

Hummert, M. L., & Nussbaum, J. F. (2001). Aging, communication, and health: Linking research and practice for successful aging. Mahwah, NJ: Lawrence Erlbaum Associates, Inc.

Jacobson, N. S., Gottman, J. M., Waltz, J., Rushe, R., Bobcock, J., & Holtzworth-Monroe, A. (1994). Affect, verbal content, and psychophysiology in the arguments of couples with a violent husband. *Journal of Consulting and Clinical Psychology, 62*, 982-988.

Johnson, N. J., Backlund, E., Sorlie, P. D., & Loveless, C. A. (2000). Marital status and mortality: The National Longitudinal Mortality Study. *Annals of Epidemiology, 10*, 224-238.

Kiecolt-Glaser, J. K., & Newton, T. (2001). Marriage and health: His and hers. *Psychological Bulletin, 127*, 472-503.

Kwakkel, G., Wagenaar, R., Kollen, B. J., Lankhorst, G. J. (1996). Predicting disability in stroke: A critical review of the literature. Ageing, 25, 479-489.

Levenson, R. W., Cartensen, L. L., & Gottman, J. M. (1993). Long-term marriage: Age, gender, and satisfaction. *Psychology and Aging, 2*, 301-313.

Levenstein, S., Ackerman, S., Kiecolt-Glaser, J. K., & Dubois, A. (1999). Stress and peptic ulcer disease. *Journal of the American Medical Association, 281*, 10-11.

Liu, W., & Gallagher-Thompson, D. (2009). Impact of dementia caregiving: Risks, strains, and growth. In S. H. Qualls, & S. H. Zarit (Eds.), *Aging families and caregiving* (pp. 85-112). Hoboken: John Wiley & Sons, Inc.

Maitz, E. A., & Sachs, P. (1995). Treating families of individuals with traumatic brain-injury from a family systems perspective. *Journal of Head Trauma Rehabilitation, 10*(2), 1-11.

Martire, L. M., Lustig, A. P., Schulz, R., Miller, G. E., Helgeson, V. S. (2004). Is it beneficial to involve a family member? A meta-analytic review of psychosocial interventions for chronic illness. *Health Psychology, 23*, 599-611.

Mastekaasa, A. (1994). Marital status, distress, and well-being: An international comparison. *Journal of Comparative Family Studies, 25*, 183-206.

Mayne, T. J., O'Leary, A., McCrady, B., Contrada, R., & Labouvie E. (1997). The differential effects of acute marital distress on emotional, physiological and immune functions in maritally distressed men and women. *Psychological Health, 12*, 277-288.

McDaniel, S. H., Hepworth, J., & Doherty, W. J. (1992). *Medical family therapy: A biopsychosocial approach to families with health problems*. New York: Basic Books.

Michela, J. (1986). Interpersonal and individual impacts of a husband's heart attack. In A. Baum & J. E. Singer (Eds.), *Handbook of psychology and health.* Volume 5: *Stress and coping* (pp. 255-301). Hillsdale, NJ: Erlbaum.

Mickelson, K. D. (2001). Perceived stigma, social support, and depression. *Personality and Social Psychology Bulletin, 27,* 1046-1056.

Minuchin, S., Rosman, B. L., & Baker, L. (1978). *Psychosomatic families.* Cambridge, MA: Harvard University Press.

Morell, M. A., & Apple, R. F. (1990). Affect expression, marital satisfaction, and stress reactivity among premenopausal women during a conflictual marital discussion. *Psychology of Women Quarterly, 14,* 387-402.

Neuling, S. J., & Winefield, H. R. (1988). Social support and recovery after surgery for breast cancer: Frequency and correlates of supportive behaviours by family, friends and surgeon. *Social Science and Medicine, 27,* 385-392.

Petronio, S. (2002). *Boundaries of privacy: Dialectics of disclosure.* Albany: State University of New York Press.

Rolland, J. (1989). Chronic illness and the family life-cycle. In B. Carter & M. McGoldrick (Eds.), *The changing family life-cycle* (pp. 433-456). Boston: Allyn & Bacon.

Rolland, J. S. (1994a). In sickness and in health: The impact of illness on couples' relationships. *Journal of Marital and Family Therapy,20,* 327-336.

Rolland, J. S. (1994b). *Families, illness and disability: An integrative treatment model.* New York: Basic Books.

Ross, C. E., Mirowsky, J., & Goldsteen, K. (1990). The impact of the family on health: The decade in review. *Journal of Marriage and Family, 52,* 4, 1059-1078.

Roy, R. (2004). *Chronic pain, loss, and grief.* Toronto, Canada: University of Toronto Press.

Roy, R. (2006). *Chronic pain and family: A clinical perspective.* New York: Springer.

Scheinkman, M. (1988). Graduate student marriages: An organizational/interactional view. *Family Process, 27*(3), 351-368.

Schwarzer, R., & Leppin, A. (1991). Social support and mental health: A conceptual and empirical overview. In L. Montado, S. H. Flipp, & M. J. Lerner (Eds.), *Life crises and the experience of loss in adult life* (pp. 435-458). Hillsdale, NJ: Lawrence Erlbaum.

Sidhu, R., Passmore, A., & Baker, D. (2005). An investigation into parent perceptions of the needs of siblings of children with cancer. *Journal of Pediatric Oncology Nursing, 22,* 276-287.

Stamp, G. (2004). Theories of family relationships and family relationships theoretical model. In A. Vangelisti (Ed.) *Handbook of family communication* (pp.1-30). Mahwah, NJ: LEA, Publishers.

Troxel, W. M. (2006). *Marital quality, communal strength, and physical health* (Doctoral Dissertation). Retrieved from http://etd.library.pitt.edu/ETD/available/etd-4252006-34937/unrestricted/TroxelETD2006.pdf

U.S. Census Bureau. (2001, June). *American's families and living arrangements: Population characteristics* (Current Population Reports, Series P20-537). Retrieved from http://www.census.gov/prod/2001pubs/p20-537.pdf.

Varni, J. W., Wilcox, K. T., Hanson, V., & Brik, R. (1988). Chronic musculoskeletal pain and functional status in juvenile rheumatoid arthritis: An empirical model. *Pain, 32*(1), 1-7.

Vrabec, N. J. (1997). Literature review of social support and caregiver burden, 1980 to 1995. *Journal of Nursing Scholarship, 29,* 383-388.

Wickrama, K., Lorenz, F. O., & Conger, R. D. (1997). Marital quality and physical illness: A latent growth curve analysis. *Journal of Marriage and the Family, 59,* 143-155.

World Health Organization. (1946). Preamble to the Constitution of the World Health Organization as adopted by the International Health Conference, New York, July 1946; signed on 22 of July 1946 by the representatives of 61 States (Official Records of the World Health Organization, no. 2, p. 100).

Zarit, S. H., Reever, K. E., & Bach-Peterson, J. (1980). Relatives of the impaired elderly: Correlates of feeling of burden. *Gerontologist,* 20, 649-655.

PART 1

Family Interdependence in Managing Health Transitions

CHAPTER 1

Interdependence in Family Systems: Adjusting to Breast and Prostate Cancer

Chris Segrin and Terry A. Badger

UNIVERSITY OF ARIZONA

The diagnosis and treatment of cancer, like any major illness, can be extremely challenging and distressing to the person attempting to cope with and adjust to the myriad physical and psychological burdens that accompany these diseases. At the same time, it is abundantly evident that intimate partners and family members are also affected by the cancer experience of someone near to them. In fact, the well-being of the cancer survivor and his or her partners and family can be entwined by processes of mutual influence as we will show in our review of the research on cancer patients and their partners.

The focus of this chapter is on interpersonal processes that link the well-being of cancer patients to the well-being of their partners and family members. This interdependence appears to be the result of several interpersonal processes, two of which we will focus on in particular: social support and emotional contagion. Even though we incorporate data from a variety of different cancer patients into our reasoning and conclusions, special attention is paid to breast and prostate cancer survivors and their spouses and families. People with breast and prostate cancer have fairly unique interpersonal stressors to adjust to, especially in the context of sexuality and intimacy in the marital dyad. For example, breast cancer treatment often entails disfiguring surgery that can damage the body image of the survivor, creating substantial problems with sexuality. Similarly, therapies for breast cancer such as radiation, chemo-therapy, and hormone blocking therapy have substantial side effects that can also make physical intimacy and other pleasant interpersonal experiences a substantial challenge. Like breast cancer, prostate cancer and its treatment can have serious side effects that include urinary incontinence, erectile dysfunction, fatigue, depression, and pain, which contribute to decreased sexual enjoyment and interest and increased social isolation (Burke, Lawrence, & Perczek, 2003; Kornblith, Herr, Ofman, Scher, & Holland, 1994). It is therefore understandable why spouses and intimate partners of breast and prostate cancer survivors can experience distress that is on par with the survivor him- or herself (Kornblith et al., 1994).

Distress in Cancer Survivors and Their Partners

In addition to the obvious threats to current and future physical health, cancer survivors are often afflicted with substantial psychological and interpersonal distress. For example, breast cancer and its treatment can precipitate episodes of depression and anxiety, as well as concerns with body image, sexuality, and mortality (Kunkel & Chen, 2003). Disruptions in sexual functioning following breast or prostate cancer may be a function of both psychological and physiological (e.g., effects of surgery, radiation, chemotherapy) factors (e.g., Wilmoth & Botchway, 1999). Between 10 and 25% of women with breast cancer have a concurrent episode of major depressive disorder (Fann et al., 2008), and among cancer patients more generally, 16-26% experience significant depressive symptomatology (Stommel, Kurtz, Kurtz, Given, & Given, 2004). This is a substantial complicating factor as depression is associated with decreased compliance with adjuvant therapy and a number of cognitive and functional impairments (Fann et al.). Furthermore, depression is associated with potentially detrimental alternations in autonomic regulation in women with breast cancer (Giese-Davis et al., 2006). Fortunately, for many people with cancer, depression and other forms of psychological distress tend to improve over time, with the worst period experienced shortly after diagnosis and during active treatment (Helgeson, Snyder, & Steltman, 2004; Stommel et al.). Along with depression, problems with fatigue and sleep disturbance are also common in breast cancer patients (Payne, Piper, Rabinowitz, & Zimmerman, 2006).

There is also abundant evidence pointing to heightened risk for psychological distress in men with prostate cancer. The incidence of clinically significant levels of depression and anxiety in men with prostate cancer has been estimated at 16% and 12%, respectively (Sharpley & Christie, 2007). For prostate cancer patients on hormone blocking therapy, the risk of major depressive disorder is eight times the national rate of depression in men, and 32 times the rate of depression in men over age 65 (Pirl, Siegel, Goode, & Smith, 2002). It is therefore understandable why the risk of suicide in men with prostate cancer is 4.24 times that of their age- and gender-specific cohorts (Llorente et al., 2005). Northouse and Northouse (1988) identified a core set of tasks confronted by patients as they struggle to adjust and cope with cancer and its treatment. These include maintaining a sense of control, seeking information, disclosing feelings, and searching for meaning. These are monumental tasks that are made all the more challenging by the psychological distress and burden carried by the cancer patient.

Like any major illness, breast and prostate cancer do not affect just the patients, but family, friends, and especially spouses of patients. In a report entitled "Hidden Mortality in Cancer: Spouse Caregivers" Braun, Mikulincer, Rydall, Walsh, and Rodin (2007) showed that close to 40% of cancer patients' spouses scored above the cutoff for clinically significant levels of depression on the Beck Depression Inventory-II. In fact, a greater percentage of spouses had clinically significant levels of depression than the patients themselves (23%). Depression in these spouses was predicted by higher levels of caregiving burden, avoidant or anxious attachment styles, and lower marital satisfaction (Braun et al.). One review of the literature indicated that approximately 20-30% of the partners of cancer patients have significant psychological distress or mood disturbance (Pitceathly & Maguire, 2003).

Research on partners of breast cancer patients reveals a variety of burdens and challenges faced by this population. For example, husbands of women with breast cancer report problems with depression and sleep disturbances, as well as difficulties that arise from missed work (Woloski-Wruble & Kadmon, 2002). In some cases husbands can get preoccupied with the patient's condition and therefore neglect their own well-being, while becoming engulfed in fear and anxiety (Donnelly et al., 2000). Men are often socialized to be problem solvers and generally feel helpless while watching their wives struggle with cancer (Lethborg, Kissane, & Burns, 2003). Husbands of breast cancer patients frequently report problems with intimacy and sexuality (Kadmon, Ganz, Rom, & Woloski-Wruble, 2008), especially if their spouse had a mastectomy as part of the cancer treatment (Wellisch, Jamison, & Pasnau, 1978). Unfortunately, when partners of women with breast cancer experience high levels of distress they tend to be less actively engaged in helping the woman effectively cope with and adjust to the illness and its treatment (Hinnen, Hagedoorn, Sanderman, & Ranchor, 2007). Incidentally, distress in the social network of women with cancer extends well beyond their husbands and partners. First-degree female relatives who are in close contact with and provide care for breast cancer patients also experience significant distress, although this is mitigated by social support provided to these relatives (Zapka, Fisher, Lemon, Clemow, & Fletcher, 2006).

The partners of prostate cancer patients are also a population at risk for psychological distress and adjustment problems. In one sample of wives of prostate cancer patients, a significant portion reported problems with tiredness (56%), worrying (56%), decreased sexual enjoyment (49%), trouble sleeping (37%), tenseness (35%), and depression (25%) (Kornblith et al., 1994). In fact, wives will often experience more psychological distress than patients themselves. Wives of prostate cancer survivors inevitably face many of the same issues and stressors as their husbands, namely, fear of death, the need to make a treatment decision and its attendant implications, and feelings of a loss of control (Heyman & Rosner, 1996). Wives will sometimes experience distress associated with the delicate balance between providing care and support to their ill husband and honoring his need and desire for self-reliance (Gray, Fitch, Phillips, Labrecque, & Fergus, 2000).

Northouse and Northouse (1988) argued that family members of cancer patients must confront a number of communication challenges, most of which reflect the management of their own distress. These include hiding their emotional concerns from each other, obtaining information, and coping with their feelings of helplessness. An empirical investigation of cancer patients' wives indicated remarkable psychological burdens borne by these partners that included loneliness, uncertainty, fear of the husband's death, depression, and hopelessness, along with family and financial difficulties (Kalayjian, 1989). By far, however, emotional difficulties were most overwhelming for the wives in Kalayjian's investigation.

It is abundantly evident that many people with cancer experience substantial psychological distress in conjunction with the diagnosis and treatment of their disease. This distress is also experienced by their intimate partners and immediate family members. In the pages that follow, we highlight two theoretical mechanisms that represent interdependent interpersonal processes that could explain this concordant distress in dyads coping with cancer. These mechanisms are the perception and reception of social support and emotional contagion. However, before examining these two phenomena in detail, it is instructive to briefly examine the research that shows a connection between interpersonal relationships and health outcomes more generally, as this constitutes the empirical foundation on which subsequent theories of close relationships and health have been developed.

Close Relationships and Health Outcomes

Presently, it is a well accepted fact that marriage, family, and other close relationships play an important role in health maintenance as well as health problems. Although the mechanisms by which close relationships impact health are numerous and not always well understood, there is strong evidence to suggest that people with supportive and satisfying relationships enjoy better health than those with distressing and unsupportive relationships. For example, numerous marital communication and relational processes can predispose spouses to health problems. Data from the National Survey of Families and Households show that marital conflict is a significant risk factor for functional health impairments (Choi & Marks, 2008). When spouses express negativity and hostility in their conflicts, exaggerated physiological responses in immune, cardiovascular, and endocrine domains often follow (Robles & Kiecolt-Glaser, 2003; Whitson & El-Sheikh, 2003). Women who are prone to compliance during conflict with their husbands, thus subjugating their own concerns, have a risk of mortality over a 10-year observation that is four times higher than that of women who openly expressed their concerns to their husbands (Eaker, Sullivan, Kelly-Hayes, D'Agostino, & Benjamin, 2007).

Even though it is possible that health problems could lead to marital strain and difficulties, longitudinal analyses with growth curve techniques suggest that negative marital experiences affect health trajectories to a much greater extent than health trajectories affect marital difficulties (Umberson, Williams, Powers, Liu, & Needham, 2006).

Simply being married is associated with better physical health than being unmarried or lacking other immediate forms of social integration (House, Landis, & Umberson, 1988). In fact, House et al. have argued that a lack of social integration represents a health risk every bit as powerful as cigarette smoking, high blood pressure, or obesity. Even though divorce and widowhood represent substantial risks to former spouses' health (Bennett, 2006), remaining in a dissatisfying marriage is associated with poorer health outcomes than divorcing and remaining unmarried (Hawkins & Booth, 2005). Therefore, the quality of the marriage is every bit as important, if not more so, than the mere presence of a marriage.

Several causal mechanisms linking marital (or other close relationship) quality to health and mortality have emerged in the research literature. Umberson (1987) delineated four such paths. First, *individual attributes* that allow people to attract and flourish in social relationships, such as personality characteristics and lack of psychological impairment, also bode well for maintaining a positive health status. One could therefore view such individual attributes as a collection of third variables that cause both positive social relationships as well as good health through such things as performance of beneficial health behaviors, lack of psychological distress, and avoidance of negative health behaviors. Second, *behavioral mechanisms* such as performance of health-promoting behaviors (e.g., exercise, good diet) can also provide an explanation for the health benefits of quality social relationships. Relational partners are often a vital and persuasive source of social influence, encouraging people to avoid risky, health-damaging behaviors, and to perform beneficial and preventative health behaviors such as seeking medical care when symptoms arise. People with better social integration would be expected to be exposed to greater social influence aimed at health promotion from their relational partners. Third, there are a host of *physiological* mechanisms that mediate the social relationship and health association. For example, happily married people have better immune and endocrine functioning than unmarried people or people in distressed marriages (Kiecolt-Glaser, 1999). Fourth, close relationships function to provide *buffering and prevention of stressors*. As we will discuss later in this chapter, marriage and other close relationships can often be a source of social support that can profoundly lessen and mitigate the ill effects of stressful events. In some cases, close relationships can even prevent potential stressors such as economic hardships, unavailable transportation, and loneliness.

Any discussion of marriage/close relationships and health must recognize the key role that psychological distress plays in both marital well-being and physical health. Increasingly scientists are recognizing that the mind-body distinction is a false dichotomy. Psychology clearly affects health and health status has numerous psychological consequences. A quality marriage can contribute to a general sense of well-being, happiness, and life satisfaction. The psychological well-being and orderly lifestyle that goes hand in hand with a satisfying marriage is also beneficial to physical health (Umberson, 1987). Unfortunately, the prophylactic and salutary effects of marriage on health represent but one side of the coin. When marriages become strained and distressed, spouses are at a dramatically higher risk for a host of psychological problems (Whisman, 2007). The very same chronic negative emotions that are experienced as a consequence of marital distress and conflict increase the risk for a variety of health problems such as coronary heart disease for example (Pettit, Grover, & Lewinsohn, 2007). As we will demonstrate later in this chapter, the supposedly intrapersonal phenomena of psychological distress and negative affect have a distinctly interpersonal appearance in the close relationships of people coping with cancer and its treatment.

The Exchange of Social Support with Cancer Survivors

Social support is a multifaceted communication behavior that has received intensive attention in the context of coping, recovery, and quality of life for people with cancer. The various socially supportive behaviors include emotional support (showing care, concern, and trying to help the patient feel good), instrumental support (providing tangible goods or services), and informational support (providing information and help with decision making). There are several theoretical mechanisms by which social support has salutary effects on well-being (Cohen & Wills, 1985). In what is known as the *main effect model,* social support is hypothesized to be associated with better well-being because it provides a sense of positive affect, social connection, self-worth, and stability in one's life. Consistent with the main effect model, social support from a spouse has been found to predict higher marital satisfaction and lower levels of depressive symptoms and perceived stress (Dehle, Larsen, & Landers, 2001). People who feel good about themselves and their marriage are hypothesized to be more diligent about engaging in health-protective behaviors and avoiding health-damaging behaviors, thus experiencing better health. A related, but different, model known as the *buffering model* holds that social support can effectively interfere with, or buffer, the psychological processes that connect stress to poor health. For example, social support can help people to appraise potentially stressful events as less stressful, inhibit maladaptive responses to stressful events, and facilitate beneficial counter-responses to stressful events, thereby leading to better health and well-being (Cohen & Wills).

Social Support and Psychological Distress in Cancer Patients

Supportive communication from spouses and other family members can play a crucial role in adjusting to cancer. However, its effects are not entirely straightforward. At a general level, a great deal of evidence points to the conclusion that available social support is associated with lower levels of psychological distress and mood disturbance and higher quality of life among women with breast cancer (e.g., Koopman, Hermanson, Diamond, Angell, & Spiegel, 1998; Mellon & Northouse, 2001; Neuling & Winefield, 1988; Northouse, 1988). Social support from family members tends to be associated with lower psychological distress for both breast and prostate cancer patients (Baider, Ever-Hadani, Goldzweig, Wygoda, & Peretz, 2003). Conversely, breast cancer patients with the greatest levels of depression tend to be those with the lowest-quality social support provided by their social networks (Badger, Braden, Longman, & Mishel, 1999). Social support may help to alleviate psychological distress in cancer patients through its beneficial effects on cognitive processing (Roberts, Lepore, & Helgeson, 2006). The prostate cancer patients in the Roberts et al. study with most social support appeared to enjoy better mental functioning because of lower levels of intrusive thoughts and searching for meaning (e.g., "Why me?"). Therefore, as supportive communication is exchanged, people with cancer have an opportunity to discuss their concerns, expectations, and uncertainties with a sympathetic partner. This, in turn, lessens the sort of intrusive cognitions that can otherwise create a significant psychological burden for people coping with cancer.

The provision of emotional support has proven to be particularly beneficial to health-related quality of life among women with breast cancer (Arora, Rutten, Gustafson, Moser, & Hawkins, 2007; Helgeson & Cohen, 1996). Arora et al. found that over 80% of the women in their investigation found family and friends to be an important source of emotional support. Perhaps it is because the management, experience, and expression of emotion plays such a major role in adjustment to cancer that this particular type of social support is so beneficial to cancer patients. An investigation of breast and prostate cancer patients found that emotional support provided by family members was associated with reduced anxiety, depression, and hostility (Gotcher, 1992). These same families in Gotcher's study that provided high levels of emotional support had higher levels of communication in general with the patient. Among several different family communication variables, Gotcher (1993) found that emotional support was by far the best predictor of cancer patients' psychological distress and global adjustment.

The desire for emotional support is especially pronounced in cancer patients who have a high affiliative need (Manne, Alfieri, Taylor, & Dougherty, 1999a). People with a high affiliative need seek stimulation from and emotional connection with others. It is interesting to note that the cancer patients with high affiliative needs had a preference for emotional but not instrumental support (Manne et al.). What is more, these investigators found no association between physical impairment and desire for instrumental support, but there was a positive association between impairment and desire for emotional support, at least among female cancer patients. Cancer patients with physical impairments do not necessarily want practical assistance from their support networks, but they often seem to be looking instead for expressions of caring and concern. Finally, there appear to be some cultural variations in the association between emotional support and good health with, Asians apparently benefiting more than European Americans (Uchida, Kitayama, Mesquita, Reyes, & Morling, 2008), although Anglo-Americans express a greater need for social support than Asian-Americans (Wellisch et al., 1999).

Social Support and Health Outcomes in Cancer Patients

The benefits of social support from spouses and other family members extend far beyond psychological well-being. Among women with breast cancer, high levels of available social support are associated with lower levels of salivary cortisol (Turner-Cobb, Sephton, Koopman, Blake-Mortimer, & Spiegel, 2000). Lower cortisol concentrations are indicative of healthier neuroendocrine functioning, leading Turner et al. to speculate that tumor progression could be accelerated by higher levels of cortisol among those patients with lower levels of available social support. Among women with breast cancer, emotional support from social network members significantly lowers the risk for mortality (Ell, Nishimoto, Mediansky, Mantell, & Hamovitch, 1992; Maunsell, Brisson, & Deschenes, 1995). The ability to confide in a spouse and having dependable network members who provided social support and help has been associated with both decreased risk of mortality and recurrence for women with breast cancer (Weihs, Enright, & Simmens, 2008). Krongrad, Lai, Burke, Goodkin, and Lai (1996) studied the survival of 146,979 men with prostate cancer who were married, divorced, single, widowed, or separated. They found that the men who were married, suggesting higher social integration and availability of support from an intimate partner, had significantly longer mean survival.

Notwithstanding the favorable evidence for social support, its status as a protective factor in reducing mortality risk is questioned by recent findings suggesting that availability of social support is associated with an *increased* risk for mortality (Cousson-Gelie, Bruchon-Schweitzer, Dilhuydy, & Jutand, 2007). This research team followed 75 breast cancer patients over the course of 10 years, during which 43

(57.3%) had died. The women's satisfaction with their social support was unrelated to mortality risk, but availability of social support had a hazard ratio of 1.04 which was statistically significant, and indicated that risk of mortality was higher for those with more social support. How is it possible that women with breast cancer who have more available social support are at increased risk for mortality? Even though this is a longitudinal investigation, causal inferences about the effects of social support are not possible because social support was only measured at one point in time and could easily be confounded with women's overall physical health. In other words, it is possible that at the initiation of the study, women in the poorest health reported most social support, possibly reflecting the fact that their social network was responding to their ill health. These findings are comparable to those of Neuling and Winefield (1988) who found social support from friends to be positively associated with anxiety, depression, and physical problems among women with breast cancer. Again, it is at least possible that those in most distress were perceived by friends as having the most need for social support.

Dynamics and Variations in the Experience of Social Support

As beneficial as social support can be for some cancer patients, it is a form of communication that tends to diminish over time. Women who were followed from breast cancer diagnosis to 60 days and then one year reported a gradual decrease in social support from their spouse, family, and friends (Northouse, Templin, Mood, & Oberst, 1998). Arora et al. (2007) also found that the availability and quality of social support for women with breast cancer decreased over time, especially social support associated with problem solving, but less so with emotional support. An interesting aspect of their findings is that women with the most intensive cancer treatments had the highest levels of helpful support, lending some credence to the idea that those in most peril who have the greatest support needs will often be the recipients of high levels of support from their social networks (see also Bloom, Stewart, Johnston, Banks, & Fobair, 2001).

Although it would be premature to conclude that marital communication and support differ for breast and prostate cancer survivors, at least some evidence points to the difficulties experienced by spouses of prostate cancer patients as they try to help their partners. In one sample of men with advanced-stage prostate cancer and their spouses, there appeared to be little marital communication about the implication of prostate cancer on their lives (Boehmer & Clark, 2000). Even though some couples with breast cancer are classifiable as "non-talkers," many more openly share their feelings with each other and fewer than 30% express concern about their communication and inability to share feelings with their partner (Hilton, 1994). When wives try to exercise some social influence and get their husbands with prostate cancer to engage in health-enhancing behaviors (e.g., diet, sleep, exercises to counteract some of the treatment side effects, relaxation), their efforts are often to no avail (Helgeson, Novak, Lepore, & Eton, 2004). It is certainly possible that some of the different dynamics in the marital communication of couples with breast vs. prostate cancer reflect gender differences in preferences for communication by the patient.

In an ideal world, the communication behavior exchanged between cancer patients and their family members would be helpful and supportive. Naturally, this is not always the case, and the unsupportive behaviors of social network members can be as problematic as the supportive behaviors are for the well-being of people with cancer. Manne and her colleagues examined two common unsupportive communication behaviors, critical responses and avoidant responses, exchanged between women with breast cancer and their significant others, most of whom were husbands (Manne, Ostroff, Winkel, Grana, & Fox, 2005). Understandably, women who perceived higher levels of unsupportive partner behaviors were at increased risk for psychological distress both concurrently and prospectively. Two notoriously detrimental communication behaviors from the marital communication literature, demand-withdraw and mutual avoidance, are equally corrosive to the marital well-being and psychological distress of women with breast cancer (Manne et al., 2006). In contrast, constructive communication behaviors such as mutual discussion of issues, expression of feelings, understanding of views, and feeling that issues are resolved through discussion can be beneficial to both relationship satisfaction and psychological well-being (Manne et al., 2006). Unsupportive behaviors from a partner tend to increase the psychological distress of women with breast cancer, in part, because they undermine the women's perceived coping ability (Manne et al., 2003). In other words, women whose partners expressed unsupportive behaviors had lowered coping efficacy, feeling that they were not handling the emotional stress of the cancer or adjusting to the changes and disruptions that it posed. This, in turn, contributed to higher psychological distress. Fortunately, the detrimental effects of partner unsupportive behaviors on the coping efficacy of women with breast cancer can be buffered by emotional support from other family and friends (Manne et al., 2003). So long as women have emotional support available from these other sources, they are able to feel that they are coping well, despite the presence of unsupportive behaviors from their partners.

For the most part, the exchange of negative and unhelpful communication behaviors (e.g., expressing anger, criticism, complaining) with cancer patients is relatively rare, but relationship scientists are beginning to develop a good understanding of when and why this happens. It appears that as the ill partner becomes more impaired, the healthy spouse has to make increasing personal sacrifices in order to provide care to the patient (Manne, Alfieri, Taylor, & Dougherty, 1999b). This engenders negative affect and resentment in the healthy partner that can culminate in complaining to and criticizing the patient. Fortunately, this process appears to be arrested by high levels of marital satisfaction (Manne et al). In other words, the pattern of patient impairment, partner restrictions, negative affect, and the attendant negative communication behaviors is a phenomenon that is largely confined to marriages on the lower half of the satisfaction continuum. Research on marital interactions of cancer patients has revealed an effect that is otherwise well-documented in family science: The ill effects of negative and unsupportive spousal behaviors are more detrimental to the psychological well-being of spouses than positive and supportive behaviors are beneficial (Manne, Taylor, Dougherty, & Kemeny, 1997). Findings such as these show that not all communication behavior directed at cancer patients is supportive, and when this communication from significant others takes on a negative or unhelpful tone, an already bad situation can be made worse in terms of patients' psychological distress.

Social Support and Quality of Life in Breast and Prostate Cancer Survivors and Their Partners

Our research team has been testing the effectiveness of a psychosocial intervention to improve the quality of life of cancer patients and their partners (e.g., Badger, Segrin, Meek, Lopez, & Bonham, 2004, 2005; Badger et al., 2005; Badger, Segrin, Dorros, Meek, & Lopez, 2007). In our research with breast cancer suvivors, we examined social support, relationship satisfaction, and several quality-of-life indicators (e.g., symptoms of depression, negative affect, positive affect) over a period of 12 weeks in 96 dyads. All women were asked to nominate a partner who would participate with them in the investigation. In most cases (74%), the women selected a husband or significant other to participate. However, because not all women are in a committed relationship, we allowed them to participate with other members of their social network, and 17% selected an adult daughter, 4% some other family member (i.e., son, cousin, sister), and 3% participated with a friend. All participants completed the Index of Socially Supportive Behaviors (Barrera, Sandler, & Ramsay, 1981), the Relationship Assessment Scale (Hendrick, 1988), and several quality-of-life measures (depression, negative affect, positive affect) at time 1, before the intervention started, and then again at 6 weeks and 10 weeks from the baseline. The results in Table 1.1 show that relationship satisfaction was negatively associated with negative affect at time 1 and depression at time 2, and it was positively associated with positive affect at time 1. Although not depicted in the table, the social support received by women with breast cancer was significantly related to higher relationship satisfaction at time 1, $r = .33$, $p < .01$, and time 2, $r = .22$, $p < .05$, but not time 3, $r = .14$, *ns*. In contrast, the correlations for social support when measured as a global index are not suggestive of any substantial associations with quality of life at any points in time with the exception of *higher* negative affect at time 1.

Table 1.1 Correlations between Social Support, Relationship Satisfaction, and Quality-of-Life Indicators at T1-T3

	Depression T_n	Negative Affect T_n	Positive Affect T_n
social support *T1*	.16	.21*	.16
relationship satisfaction *T1*	-.19	-.20*	.21*
social support *T2*	.04	.14	.07
relationship satisfaction *T2*	-.22*	-.15	.11
social support *T3*	.03	.10	.14
relationship satisfaction *T3*	-.11	-.13	.08

Note: T_n = measurement time corresponding to variable in row. * $p < .05$.

To digress momentarily, it is evident from past research that not all socially supportive behaviors, or behaviors intended to be socially supportive, have the same effect on people coping with serious illness. To illustrate, Manne and her colleagues had women with breast cancer discuss a cancer related issue for which they needed support with their partners (Manne et al., 2004). The patients with the lowest distress were those whose partners responded to their self-disclosures with humor or with a self-disclosure of their own. In contrast, women with the highest levels of distress had partners who responded to their self-disclosures with proposed solutions. These results suggest that women with breast cancer might benefit from socially supportive behaviors that reflect intimacy, emotional connection, and at times, light-heartedness. However, advice and proposed solutions are not what they are looking for. The measure of social support that we used in our investigation had specific items that reflected many of these concepts. Upon closer inspection of the individual social support items, a pattern of associations with relationship satisfaction and the quality-of-life indicators became apparent (see Table 1.2).

Table 1.2 Correlations between Selected Social Support Items, Relationship Satisfaction, and Quality-of-Life Indicators

Social Support Item	Relationship Satisfaction	Depression	Negative Affect	Positive Affect
1. Gave you some information on how to do something	.08	.13	.20*	.04
2. Checked back with you to see if you followed the advice you were given	.10	.31**	.30**	-.03
3. Told you who you should see for assistance	.07	.26*	.35**	-.09
4. Assisted you in setting a goal for yourself	.16	.10	.23*	.10
5. Told you that he/she feels very close to you	.31**	-.12	.01	.18
6. Let you know that he/she will always be around if you need assistance	.31**	-.11	.03	.19
7. Told you that you are OK just the way you are	.37***	-.10	.01	.30**
8. Comforted you by showing some physical affection	.36***	-.22*	-.07	.24*
9. Expressed esteem or respect for a competency or personal quality of yours	.27	-.08	-.04	.21*
10. Listened to you talk about your private feelings	.32**	.01	.04	.20*
11. Agreed that what you wanted to do was right	.35**	-.09	-.06	.26*
12. Let you know that you did something well	.23*	-.06	-.05	.18
13. Talked with you about some interests of yours	.42***	.01	.05	.28**
14. Joked and kidded to cheer you up	.25*	.08	.12	.14

Note: * $p < .05$. ** $p < .01$. *** $p < .001$.

Items 1-4 on this scale reflect provision of advice and proposed solutions to problems. Receiving this type of social support had no association with relationship satisfaction, but it was in many cases associated with *higher* psychological distress. In contrast, items 5-14 reflect acceptance, agreement, a positive emotional connection, and humor. These types of socially supportive behaviors were uniformly associated with higher relationship satisfaction for women with breast cancer. Although they were generally unrelated to the negative indicators of quality of life (i.e., symptoms of depression and negative affect) they were more consistently associated with greater positive affect among the women. It should be noted that all of the correlations presented in Table 1.2 are based on time 1 data, before any potential influence of the psychosocial intervention could have impacted these variables. The distinction in this pattern of correlations is rather clear: Women with breast cancer are happy to the extent that their intimate partners and family members are providing social supportive behaviors that affirm their relationship and show acceptance, but there appears to be no benefit in providing advice and solutions to the women.

Because the correlations presented in Table 1.2 are entirely cross-sectional, it is not possible to infer that offering advice and problem solutions to women with breast cancer worsens their negative affect and symptoms of depression or that affirmation and acceptance improves their quality of life. Therefore we explored associations between these variables longitudinally. The advice (items 1-4) and agreement/affirmation (items 5-14) items each formed an internally consistent composite index (α = .75 and .90 respectively). We used these scales to predict time1-time 3 changes in the quality-of-life indicators with hierarchical multiple regression analyses that treated the time 3 quality-of-life indicator as the dependent variable, with the corresponding time 1 quality-of-life indicator entered on the first step and the social support variable on the second. Neither social support variable was predictive of time 1-time 3 changes in depression, negative affect, or positive affect. However, women who received more of the agreement/affirmation support at time 1 had reported levels of relationship satisfaction that increased from time 1 to time 3 ($\beta = .17, p < .05$). However, the advice/problem solution support at time 1 was unrelated to changes in their relationship satisfaction over the 12-week time 1-time 3 interval ($\beta = .02$, *ns*).

As noted previously, the experience of breast and prostate cancer can be as detrimental to the psychological well-being of spouses and intimate partners as it is to the person afflicted with the disease. We investigated the mental health of 63 male partners (primarily husbands) of women with breast cancer (Segrin, Badger, Sieger, Meek, & Lopez, 2006). As with the women, we measured social support, relationship satisfaction, and several quality-of-life indicators. Tests of concurrent associations indicated that men who received more social support had higher levels of positive affect, as would be expected. However, it was also the case that the social support received by these male partners was positively associated with their negative affect, and at some times, higher levels of depression. Longitudinal analyses examining data collected over a 10-week interval showed that time 1 social support significantly predicted lower perceptions of stress and higher levels of positive affect at time 3, controlling for time 1 stress and positive affect, respectively. There was also a marginal trend suggestive of lower symptoms of depression at time 3, controlling for time 1 depression, as a function of higher social support at time 1. These results indicate that male partners of breast cancer patients benefit from social support in terms of lessening their perceptions of stress and perhaps symptoms of depression, and increasing their positive affect as they adjust to this stressor. However, we were still puzzled by the concurrent associations suggesting that social support is sometimes positively correlated with indicators of distress such as negative affect and depression.

To explore the possibility that men's social support networks provide greater support to the extent that the men experienced distress, we conducted a series of regression analyses predicting changes in *social support* over time, using time 1 indicators of distress. Results showed that men's depression, negative affect, and perceptions of stress at time 1 significantly predicted increases in social support provided to them over the 10-week study. These additional findings explain why social support might be negatively correlated with men's distress concurrently, but beneficial to their mental health over time. To the extent that the men are distressed at any point in time, their social networks appear to provide increased social support, and in the long run, this support is beneficial to their well-being (see also Morse & Fife, 1998; Wagner, Bigatti, & Storniolo, 2006).

We are presently testing the effectiveness of a psychosocial intervention to improve quality of life for prostate cancer survivors and their partners. Thus far we have 35 dyads enrolled in the investigation. The average prostate cancer survivor in this study is 68 years old, and 60% have stage III or IV prostate cancer indicating an advanced disease state. We measured social support from both family and friends with the Perceived Social Support scales (Procidano & Heller, 1983) and several indicators of physical, psychological, and social well-being. These included symptom distress, prostate cancer specific problems (e.g., urinary problems, sexual dysfunction), perceived stress, positive affect, negative affect, depression, fatigue, social well-being (e.g., illness interfering with personal relationships or employment), and anxiety. Despite the small sample, measures taken at baseline, before the intervention commenced, are clearly suggestive of manifold benefits from social support on these patients' quality of life, with particularly strong associations with lower depression, anxiety, and fatigue (see Table 1.3).

Table 1.3 Correlations between Social Support Sources and Quality-of-Life Indicators

Quality-of-Life Measure	Social Support from Friends	Social Support from Family
General Symptom Distress	-.32$_a$	-.37*
Fatigue	-.36*	-.45**
Prostate Cancer Problems	-.35*	-.16
Positive Affect	.30$_a$	.37*
Negative Affect	-.30$_a$	-.10
Depression	-.39*	-.44**
Perceived Stress	-.32$_a$	-.38*
Anxiety	-.48**	-.53**
Social Well-Being	.22	.45**

Note: * $p < .05$. ** $p < .01$. *** $p < .001$. $_a$ $p = .06$-$.09$

Summary

Social support can be highly beneficial to people who are adjusting to cancer and its treatment. Couples who engage in relationship-focused coping or communal coping (Coyne & Smith, 1991; Lyons, Sullivan, Ritvo, & Coyne, 1995) take a "team approach" to coping with life's stressors, viewing them as relationship problems more than individual problems. This appears to pay substantial dividends to both patient and partner. It is becoming apparent that, at least to the person with cancer, the effects of different forms of supportive communication are not homogeneous. Emotional support, including acceptance and affirmation, appears to reign supreme among the various incarnations of social support. However, not all communication behavior exchanged with cancer patients has a supportive element, and unsupportive behaviors can be particularly deleterious to the well-being of people coping with cancer. Our own research with breast and prostate cancer survivors and their partners illustrates a number of beneficial correlates of social support for the psychological, physical, and relational well-being of survivors and their partners.

Emotional Contagion in Dyads Adjusting to Cancer

The diagnosis and treatment of cancer is a highly emotional experience for patients and their loved ones. A diagnosis of cancer can trigger myriad feelings such as fear, anxiety, uncertainty, anger, and sadness that stem from questions and concerns about one's own mortality, long-term physical capability, care of children, finances, employment, and health care needs to name but a few of the psychological burdens borne by cancer patients. However, the experience of these emotions is by no means confined to the person with cancer. Intimate partners and family members also experience distress pursuant to many of these same concerns. In the case of breast and prostate cancer, the disease and its treatment have side effects and implications that are highly consequential to sexuality and relational intimacy. This provides all the more reason for spouses and intimate partners to experience distress in conjunction with the cancer diagnosis and treatment.

Understanding the process of emotional expression and management among cancer patients and their partners is now recognized as a vital pursuit in health, affective, and relationship sciences. Substantial evidence is accumulating to suggest that the experience of depression predicts a shorter time until recurrence and shorter survival for women with breast cancer (Giese-Davis & Spiegel, 2003). However, it is not just the experience of negative affect, but its management and expression (or lack thereof) that is influential to health outcomes for people with cancer. Cancer patients who self-report higher levels of emotional suppression tend to have more mood disturbance and lower efficacy for managing their emotions (Owen et al., 2006). The use of protective buffering, in which people hide their worries and deny their concerns, is associated with increased psychological distress in both breast cancer survivors and their partners (Manne et al., 2007). It is particularly noteworthy that this effect was documented both intrapersonally (e.g., patient protective buffering → patient distress) and interpersonally (partner protective buffering → patient distress) in the Manne et al. investigation. Women with recurrent breast cancer who are emotionally constrained, whereby emotional self-control and stoicism are significant elements of their self-concepts, are at elevated risk of mortality in contrast to women with low emotional constraint (Weihs, Enright, Simmens, & Reiss, 2000). Women in the Weihs et al. investigation with high chronic anxiety also had higher mortality than those with low chronic anxiety. This pattern of findings may be deconstructed by additional data in which emotional repression and high anxiety in women with breast cancer have been linked with aberrations in diurnal cortisol rhythms (Giese-Davis, Sephton, Abercrombie, Duran, & Spiegel, 2004). Giese-Davis et al., observe that this dysregulation may be an expression of more fundamental problems with appraising threat, enacting effective coping with the stress, and appropriately expressing its attendant negative affect.

Theoretical Models of Shared Affective Experience

The idea that people's cancer-related emotional experiences also affect their families and networks can be understood from the perspective of *family systems theory*. The systems theory concepts of interdependence and mutual influence predict that major events such as serious illness affect the larger family or social network, not just the individual (Bertalanffy, 1975; Broderick, 1993). Family systems theory would predict that family and social network members experience distress themselves as a family member with cancer becomes more distressed with the illness. Consequently, affective states and other quality-of-life indicators should be interdependent among cancer patients and their immediate social network members. For such relationships, this is a both a blessing and a curse, as noted by DeVellis, Lewis, and Sterba (2003). On the positive side, the interdependence reflected in a communal coping perspective redistributes responsibility for support and coping as a shared phenomenon. However, at the same time, the heightened interdependence of a close relationship can increase expectations for support and enhance the transmission of negative affect from one partner to the other.

Moving from the macroscopic systems theory level to perspectives of greater specificity, there are at least two major lines of theorizing that explain the similarity, concordance, and interdependence of emotional experiences between people with cancer and their spouses/significant others. The first perspective is based on the experience of *shared stressors* (e.g., Westman, Keinan, Roziner, & Benyamini, 2008). Many of the ill-effects of cancer do not just happen to the person diagnosed with the illness. Spouses and other family members also experience the attendant worry, disruption of daily routines, need for time away from work, financial burdens, etc. that often accompany cancer diagnosis and treatment, just as with other major illnesses (Turner-Cobb, Steptoe, Perry, & Axford, 1998; Weihs, Fisher, & Baird, 2002). As both members of the dyad adjust to these secondary stressors, they often go through the same emotional experiences.

A second and related line of theorizing specifies shared affect as a function of *emotional contagion*. The emotional contagion effect has considerable explanatory power in terms of understanding why there would be interdependence in affect and quality-of-life indicators among breast cancer patients and their partners (Hatfield, Cacioppo, & Rapson, 1992, 1994). According to the emotional contagion hypothesis, people "catch" the emotional states of those with whom they interact through largely unconscious interpersonal processes. Emotional contagion theorists observe that people will mimic and synchronize their nonverbal behaviors with those of the people around them. This similarity in behavior is theorized to provide feedback that generates the same emotional experience as those people whose behaviors are being observed and matched.

Emotional contagion figures prominently in Coyne's (1976a, 1976b) *interactional theory of depression* for explaining how people in close relationships can come to share the same emotional state. According to Coyne, the interpersonal behavior of people with depression induces a negative affective state in others. This is due in part to the fact that the behavior of people with depression (e.g., excessive reassurance seeking, complaining, being pessimistic) is aversive to others. This transmission of negative affect is assumed to have lasting implications for interpersonal relationships, prompting other people to reject their depressed partner. In theory, this cycle of interaction sends the affective state of both partners on a downward cascade. This process can explain why spouses often have comparable levels of depression (e.g., Butterworth & Rodgers, 2006; Goodman & Shippy, 2002).

Concordant Affect in Cancer Patients and Their Partners

Research that has assessed the affective state of both cancer survivors and their spouses or intimate partners strongly suggests that they experience many of the same emotions. What is more, the affective state of one partner can have a direct effect on the affective state of the other. For instance, physical distress experienced by women with breast cancer is associated not only with their own emotional distress but with that of their husbands as well (Northouse, Dorris, & Charron-Moore, 1995). Husbands of breast cancer patients report that helping their wives manage the emotional impact of the illness is one of the greatest difficulties they face, and the depth of the wives' adjustment problems tends to be positively correlated with those of their husbands (Northouse, 1994). In one investigation of people with breast or prostate cancer and their spouses, the intradyadic correlation for psychological distress was $r = .48$ for male patients and $r = .44$ for female patients (Baider et al., 2003). In another sample comprised of breast, colorectal, and lung cancer patients and their spouses, intradyadic correlations for psychological distress for three waves of assessment over 6 months were r = .27, .32, and .37, all of which were statistically significant (Fang, Manne, & Pape, 2001).

Northouse, Templin, Mood, and Oberst (1998) followed breast cancer survivors and their husbands for a period of one year and tracked four groups of couples based on patient and spouse median splits on psychological distress (i.e., patient low/husband low, patient high/husband low, etc.). Their findings revealed that 56% of the couples who were in the patient high/husband high distress group at the time of diagnosis, remained in that group 60 days later, and 50% of these couples were still in that group one year later. This remarkable stability in high levels of distress within the dyad is a potential expression of mutual influence processes between spouses. Over time, the mood of breast cancer patients and their husband tends to improve in concert, with no significant husband-wife differences (Northouse & Swann, 1987). In a related investigation, this same research team followed breast cancer survivors and their husbands for a period of one year and used structural equation modeling to test for dyadic effects on emotional distress (Northouse, Templin, & Mood, 2001). Their results documented a significant path from spouse's emotional distress to women's emotional distress and from women's emotional distress to spouse's emotional distress at the one-year follow-up assessment. This investigation provided compelling evidence of mutual influence processes in the affective state of breast cancer survivors and their partners.

Data on concordant affective states in dyads with a prostate cancer survivor are not as abundant as those with a breast cancer survivor, but the evidence that exists points to a comparable conclusion. Kornblith et al. (2001) followed prostate cancer patients and their partners for six months and documented statistically significant improvements in men's emotional well-being over the course of the investigation. At the same time, their spouses' anxiety scores decreased by almost 50%, which marked a statistically significant improvement in spouses' emotional state as well. Two months into the investigation, partners' level of psychological distress was correlated r = .44 with patients' psychological distress. Over time, partners' psychological distress appeared to fluctuate in accord with the patients' clinical response; so as patients' physical and psychological condition improved, so too did the emotional state of their partners. Equally suggestive findings were presented by Northouse et al. (2007) who investigated patients and their spouses in three different groups defined by the phase of prostate cancer: newly diagnosed, biochemical recurrence, and advanced stage. For most indicators of quality of life (e.g., physical, social, emotional) in the various groups, patients and their spouses were far more similar than different. The group that had the lowest quality of life, which was typically the advanced stage group, had the lowest scores for both husband and wife compared to those in the other cancer phase groups.

A recent meta-analysis of 43 studies of couples coping with cancer, with a combined sample of over 7,000, revealed an association between patient and partner distress of $r = .29$ (Hagedoorn, Sanderman, Bolks, Tuinstra, & Coyne, 2008). This meta-analysis also revealed that patients and partners exhibited indistinguishable levels of psychological distress. However, Hagedoorn et al. found that women reported higher psychological distress, regardless of whether they were patient or partner, than men did. The ultimate conclusion of this synthesis of the research literature is that gender is a more discriminating factor in the experience of distress than one's role in the dyad, i.e., patient or partner.

Concurrent and Longitudinal Associations in the Affective States of Breast and Prostate Cancer Survivors and Their Partners

In one of our earlier studies of couples with breast cancer, we used the actor-partner interdependence model (APIM; Kenny & Cook, 1999) to analyze the emotional experiences of breast cancer survivors and their partners before they started participating in our psychosocial intervention (Segrin et al., 2005). The advantage of the APIM is that it tests associations between independent and dependent variables within the person (actor effect) and across persons (partner effects) within dyads, while simultaneously controlling for the partners' initial correlation on the independent variable. The results of these analyses showed that breast cancer survivors with higher levels of negative affect had partners who had more symptoms of depression at the same time. However, the complimentary path (partner negative affect → survivor depression) was not significant. In terms of positive affect, we found that partners' positive affect was significantly and negatively predictive of survivors' symptoms of depression. However, the complimentary path (survivor positive affect → partner depression) was not significant. We also used individual regression analyses to calculate slopes representing changes over time for six quality-of-life indicators in women with breast cancer: depression, positive affect, negative affect, stress, symptom management, and symptoms distress. When we correlated these with the regression slopes for partners' negative affect, we found that all six of the correlations were statistically significant. In other words, partners' negative affect changed over time in concert with all six indicators of the survivors' quality of life. Partners' regression slopes for negative affect were positively correlated with the survivors' negative indicators of quality of life (e.g., depression) and negatively correlated with the positive indicators of quality of life (e.g., symptom management). Therefore, as survivors' depression, stress, etc. worsened over 10 weeks, so too did their partners' negative affect. If the woman's positive affect and symptom management were on an upward trajectory, indicating improvement over time, her partner's negative affect was on a downward trajectory indicating a decrease in negative affect.

With three waves of data from 96 dyads with breast cancer, we sought to further test for emotional contagion effects with the APIM, focusing on contagion of negative affective experiences (i.e., symptoms of depression, negative affect, and perceptions of stress). Results of these analyses appear in Figures 1.1-1.3. Values in the figures are standardized regression coefficients for ease of interpretation and comparison, although tests of significance were based on unstandardized coefficients.

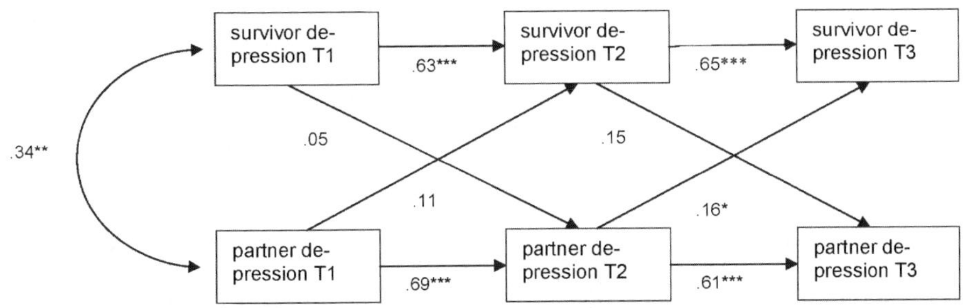

Figure 1.1 Actor-Partner Interdependence for Symptoms of Depression over Times 1-3

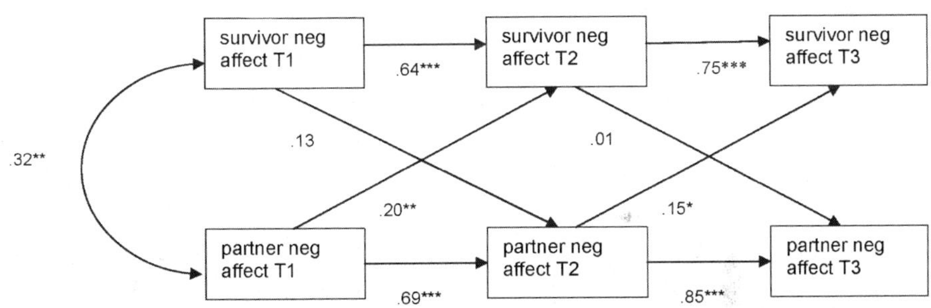

Figure 1.2 Actor-Partner Interdependence for Negative Affect over Times 1-3

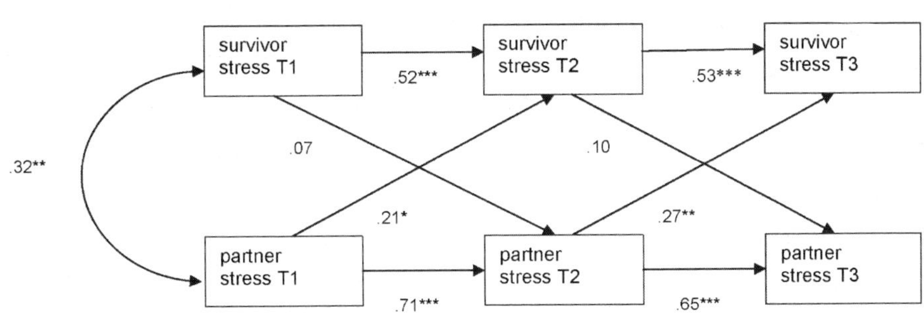

Figure 1.3 Actor-Partner Interdependence for Perceptions of Stress over Times 1-3

There is obvious consistency in the results that appear in Figures 1.1-1.3. To the extent that partners experience negative emotional states at T_n, women with breast cancer exhibit increases in their negative emotional states at T_{n+1}. However, the negative emotional states of the women with breast cancer were not predictive of their partners' subsequent negative emotions. These results represent rather stringent tests of emotional contagion, as they control the significant correlation on the emotion measures at time 1, and because there is such extensive construct stability in all of these variables. Because, T1→T2→T3 depression, etc. scores were so consistent over the 10-week observation, there was little variance in these scores left to be explained by other variables in the model. This makes the significant partner→survivor effects all the more remarkable.

A recently published analysis of survivors' and their partners' experience of anxiety from these same subjects yielded a conclusion that is identical to what is depicted in Figures 1.1-1.3 (Segrin, Badger, Dorros, Meek, & Lopez, 2007). Partner anxiety at time 1 predicted increases in survivor anxiety at time 2, and partner anxiety at time 2 predicted increases in survivor anxiety at time 3. However, there were no significant survivor→partner paths. We argue that women with breast cancer benefit emotionally to the extent that their partners are less anxious and able to keep their negative emotions at reasonable levels.

In our research with prostate cancer patients and their partners, we assessed a number of affective states (e.g., depression, anxiety) three times over a period of four months. Thus far we have enrolled 35 dyads in the study and have complete time 1 to time 3 data for 20 dyads. Intradyadic correlations on four key indicators of emotional distress (depression, anxiety, negative affect, and perceived stress) are presented in Table 1.4.

Table 1.4 Intradyadic Correlations for Emotional Distress between Prostate Cancer Survivors and Their Partners

Emotional Distress Indicator	**@ T1**	**@T2**	**@T3**
depression	.23	.27	.46*
anxiety	.20	.27	.50*
negative affect	.37*	.09	$.42_a$
perceived stress	.29	.23	.23

Note: * $p < .05$. a $p = .07$. T1 $n = 35$. T2 $n = 25$. T3 $n = 20$.

With such a small sample thus far, it is difficult to precisely evaluate the extent to which these data demonstrate the emotional contagion effect. However, several tentative conclusions are already apparent. First, the within-dyad correlations on emotional distress are relatively consistent in showing at least modest associations between survivor and partner, even though many are not statistically significant because of the very small sample size. Second, all of the correlations are positive in direction suggesting that the emotional state of survivor and partner covary in a similar fashion. Third, there is at least a suggestion that over the four-month interval between time 1 to time 3, the within-dyad correlations become stronger. This is consistent with the emotional contagion effect, in that the emotional states of dyad members should become more consistent over time (Segrin, 2004). Naturally, it will be necessary to await additional data before firm conclusions can be made. However, we are already seeing evidence that the emotional states of survivors and their partners over time are not randomly patterned.

Summary

Research on the emotional experiences of people with cancer shows how the ability to openly express emotions can be beneficial to well-being and how detrimental restricted emotional expression can be. Several theoretical models including shared stressors and emotional contagion explain how and why cancer survivors and their partners can share similar emotional experiences. A variety of studies with differing indicators of emotional distress and well-being suggest that partners experience similar levels of psychological distress when coping with cancer. Our research on the transmission of affective states within dyads similarly documents what appear to be emotional contagion effects. However, the bulk of the evidence points to transmission from partner to survivor, rather than vice versa. We interpret this as additional evidence for the importance of a partner in facilitating or complicating cancer survivors' adjustment and recovery.

Conclusion

For many individuals, the experience of cancer represents a major life transition. It is now abundantly clear, however, that this transition is not made solely by the cancer survivor. As people cope with and adjust to cancer and all of its attendant treatments and side effects, so too do their partners and family cope with many of the same issues. As family systems theory postulates, that which affects one member of the family affects the whole family. There are numerous communicative, social psychological, and perhaps even physiological processes by which people with cancer and their partners experience this interdependence. One is through the exchange of social support. The well-being of people with cancer can be affected by the social support that they receive from family and friends. Emotional support appears to be particularly valuable to women with breast cancer. On the other hand, it is also clear that not all forms of social support are equally desired by people adjusting to cancer and some dyads may exchange unhelpful behaviors that only exacerbate their psychological distress. Another process, emotional contagion, involves the shared affective experienced of cancer survivors and their partners. Partners often have levels of psychological distress that are on par with those of the patient. Longitudinal analyses now show that emotional contagion does not merely happen by partners "catching" the emotional distress of the cancer survivor. Rather, there is evidence to suggest that the emotional distress of the cancer survivor is often significantly impacted by the emotional state of his or her partner. This clearly illustrates how cancer, like other family transitions, is deeply embedded in an interpersonal system that both affects and is affected by this major change in health status.

References

Arora, N. K., Rutten, L. J. F., Gustafson, D. H., Moser, R., & Hawkins, R. P. (2007). Perceived helpfulness and impact of social support provided by family, friends, and health care providers to women newly diagnosed with breast cancer. *Psycho-Oncology, 16,* 474-486.

Badger, T. A., Braden, C. J., Longman, A. J., & Mishel, M. M. (1999). Depression burden, self-help interventions, and social support in women receiving treatment for breast cancer. *Journal of Psychosocial Oncology, 17,* 17-35.

Badger, T., Segrin, C., Dorros, S. M., Meek, P., & Lopez, A. M. (2007). Depression and anxiety in women with breast cancer and their partners. *Nursing Research, 56,* 44-53.

Badger, T., Segrin, C., Meek, P., Lopez, A. M., & Bonham, E. (2004). A case study of telephone interpersonal counseling for women with breast cancer and their partners. *Oncology Nursing Forum, 31,* 997-1003.

Badger, T., Segrin, C., Meek, P., Lopez, A. M., & Bonham, E. (2005). Profiles of women with breast cancer: Who responds to a telephone interpersonal counseling intervention? *Journal of Psychosocial Oncology, 23,* 79-100.

Badger, T., Segrin, C., Meek, P., Lopez, A. M., Bonham, E., & Sieger, A. (2005). Telephone interpersonal counseling with women with breast cancer: Symptom management and quality of life. *Oncology Nursing Forum, 32,* 273-279.

Baider, L., Ever-Hadani, P., Goldzweig, G., Wygoda, M. R., Peretz, T. (2003). Is perceived family support a relevant variable in psychological distress? A sample of prostate and breast cancer couples. *Journal of Psychosomatic Research, 55,* 453-460.

Barrera, M., Sandler, I. N., & Ramsay, T. B. (1981). Preliminary development of a scale of social support: Studies on college students. *American Journal of Community Psychiatry, 9,* 435-447.

Bennett, K. M. (2006). Does marital status and marital status change predict physical health in older adults? *Psychological Medicine, 36,* 1313-1320.

Bertalanffy, L., von. (1975). *Perspectives on general systems theory: Scientific-philosophical studies.* New York: George Braziller.

Broderick, C. B. (1993). *Understanding family processes: Basics of family systems theory.* Newbury Park, CA: Sage.

Bloom, J. R., Stewart, S. L., Johnston, M., Banks, P., & Fobair, P. (2001). Sources of support and the physical well-being of young women with breast cancer. *Social Science and Medicine, 53,* 1513-1524.

Boehmer, U., & Clark, J. A. (2000). Communication about prostate cancer between men and their wives. *Journal of Family Practice, 50,* 226-231.

Braun, M., Mikulincer, M., Rydall, A., Walsh, A., & Rodin, G. (2007). Hidden morbidity in cancer: Spouse caregivers. *Journal of Clinical Oncology, 25,* 4829-4834.

Burke, M. A., Lowrance, W., & Perczek, R. (2003). Emotional and cognitive burden of prostate cancer. *Urological Clinics of North America, 30,* 295-304.

Butterworth, P., & Rodgers, B. (2006). Concordance in mental health of spouses: Analysis of a large national household panel survey. *Psychological Medicine, 36,* 685-697.

Choi, H., & Marks, N. F. (2008). Marital conflict, depressive symptoms, and functional impairment. *Journal of Marriage and Family, 70,* 377-390.

Cohen, S., & Wills, T. A. (1985). Stress, social support, and the buffering hypothesis. *Psychological Bulletin, 98,* 310-357.

Cousson-Gelie, F., Bruchon-Schweitzer, M., Dilhuydy, J. M., & Jutand, M. A. (2007). Do anxiety, body image, social support and coping strategies predict survival in breast cancer? A ten-year follow-up study. *Psychosomatics, 48,* 211-216.

Coyne, J. C. (1976a). Toward an interactional description of depression. *Psychiatry, 39,* 28-40.

Coyne, J. C. (1976b). Depression and the response of others. *Journal of Abnormal Psychology, 85,* 186-193.

Coyne, J. C., & Smith, D. A. F. (1991). Couples coping with a myocardial infarction: A contextual perspective on wives' distress. *Journal of Personality and Social Psychology, 61,* 404-412.

Dehle, C., Larsen, D., & Landers, J. E. (2001). Social support and marriage. *The American Journal of Family Therapy, 29,* 307-324.

DeVellis, R. F., Lewis, M. A., & Sterba, K. R. (2003). Interpersonal emotional processes in adjustment to chronic illness. In J. Suls & K. A. Wallston (Eds.), *Social psychological foundations of health and illness* (pp. 256-287). Malden, MA: Blackwell Publishing.

Donnelly, J. M., Kornblith, A. B., Fleishman, S., Zuckerman, E., Raptis, G., Hudis, C. A.,...Holland, J.C. (2000). A pilot study of interpersonal psychotherapy by telephone with cancer patients and their partners. *Psycho-Oncology, 9,* 44-56.

Eaker, E. D., Sullivan, L. M., Kelly-Hayes, M., D'Agostino, R. B., & Benjamin, E. J. (2007). Marital status, marital strain, and risk of coronary heart disease or total mortality: The Farmington Offspring Study. *Psychosomatic Medicine, 69,* 509-513.

Ell, K., Nishimoto, R., Mediansky, L., Mantell, J., & Hamovitch, M. (1992). Social relations, social support and survival among patients with cancer. *Journal of Psychosomatic Research, 36,* 531-541.

Fang, C. Y., Manne, S. L., Pape, S. J. (2001). Functional impairment, marital quality, and patient psychological distress as predictors of psychological distress among cancer patients' spouses. *Health Psychology, 20,* 452-457.

Fann, J. R., Thomas-Rich, A. M., Katon, W. J., Cowley, D., Pepping, M., McGregor, B. A., & Gralow, J. (2008). Major depression after breast cancer: A review of epidemiology and treatment. *General Hospital Psychiatry, 30,* 112-126.

Giese-Davis, J., Sephton, S. E., Abercrombie, H. C., Duran, R. E. F., & Spiegel, D. (2004). Repression and high anxiety are associated with aberrant diurnal cortisol rhythms in women with metastatic breast cancer. *Health Psychology, 23,* 645-650.

Giese-Davis, J., & Spiegel, D. (2003). Emotional expression and cancer progression. In R. J. Davidson, K. R. Scherer, & H. H. Goldsmith (Eds.), *Handbook of affective sciences* (pp. 1053-1082). New York: Oxford University Press.

Giese-Davis, J., Wilhelm, F. H., Conrad, A., Abercrombie, H. C., Sephton, S., Yutsis, M.,... Spiegel, D. (2006). Depression and stress reactivity in metastatic breast cancer. *Psychosomatic Medicine, 68,* 675-683.

Goodman, C. R., & Shippy, R. A. (2002). Is it contagious? Affect similarity among spouses. *Aging and Mental Health, 6,* 266-274.

Gotcher, J. M. (1992). Interpersonal communication and psychosocial adjustment. *Journal of Psychosocial Oncology, 10,* 21-39.

Gotcher, J. M. (1993). The effects of family communication on psychosocial adjustment of cancer patients. *Journal of Applied Communication Research, 21,* 176-188.

Gray, R. E., Fitch, M., Phillips, C., Labrecque, M., & Fergus, K. (2000). Managing the impact of illness: The experiences of men with prostate cancer and their spouses. *Journal of Health Psychology, 5,* 531-548.

Hagedoorn, M., Sanderman, R., Bolks, H. N., Tuinstra, J., & Coyne, J. C. (2008). Distress in couples coping with cacner: A meta-analysis and critical review of role and gender effects. *Psychological Bulletin, 134,* 1-30.

Hatfield, E., Cacioppo, J. T., & Rapson, R. L. (1992). Primitive emotional contagion. In M. S. Clark (Eds.), *Emotion and social behavior* (pp. 151-177). Newbury Park, CA: Sage.

Hatfield, E., Cacioppo, J. T., & Rapson, R. L. (1994). *Emotional contagion.* Paris: Cambridge University Press.

Hawkins, D. N., & Booth, A. (2005). Unhappily ever after: Effects of long-term, low-quality marriages on well-being. *Social Forces, 84,* 445-465.

Helgeson, V. S., & Cohen, S. (1996). Social support and adjustment to cancer: Reconciling descriptive, correlational, and intervention research. *Health Psychology, 15,* 135-148.

Helgeson, V. S., Novak, S. A., Lepore, S., & Eton, D. T. (2004). Spouse social control efforts: Relations to health behavior and well-being among men with prostate cancer. *Journal of Social and Personal Relationships, 21,* 53-68.

Helgeson, V. S., Snyder, P., & Seltman, H. (2004). Psychological and physical adjustment to breast cancer over 4 years: Identifying distinct trajectories of change. *Health Psychology, 23,* 3-15.

Hendrick, S. S. (1988). A generic measure of relationship satisfaction. *Journal of Marriage and the Family, 50,* 93-98.

Heyman, E. N., & Rosner, T. T. (1996). Prostate cancer: An intimate view from patients and wives. *Urologic Nursing, 16,* 37-44.

Hilton, B. A. (1994). Family communication patterns in coping with early breast cancer. *Western Journal of Nursing Research, 16,* 366-391.

Hinnen, C., Hagedoorn, M., Sanderman, R., & Ranchor, A. V. (2007). The role of distress, neuroticism and time since diagnosis in explaining support behaviors in partners of women with breast cancer: Results of a longitudinal analysis. *Psycho-Oncology, 16,* 913-919.

House, J. S., Landis, K. R., & Umberson, D. (1988). Social relationships and health. *Science, 241,* 540-545.

Kadmon, I., Ganz, F. D., Rom, M., & Woloski-Wruble, A. C. (2008). Social, marital, and sexual adjustment of Israeli men whose wives were diagnosed with breast cancer. *Oncology Nursing Forum, 35,* 131-135.

Kalayjian, A. S. (1989). Coping with cancer: The spouse's perspective. *Archives of Psychiatric Nursing, 3,* 166-172.

Kenny, D. A., & Cook, W. L. (1999). Partner effects in relationship research: Conceptual issues, analytic difficulties, and illustrations. *Personal Relationships, 6,* 433-448.

Kiecolt-Glaser, J. K. (1999). Stress, personal relationships, and immune function: Health implications. *Brain, Behavior, and Immunity, 13,* 61-72.

Koopman, C., Hermanson, K., Diamond, S., Angell, K., & Spiegel, D. (1998). Social support, life stress, pain and emotional adjustment to advanced breast cancer. *Psycho-oncology, 7,* 101-111.

Kornblith, A. D., Herdon, J. E., Zuckerman, E., Goodley, P. A., Savarese, D., Vogelzang, N. J., & Holland, J. C. (2001). The impact of docetaxel, estramustine, and low-dose hydrocortisone on quality of life of men with hormone refractory prostate cancer and their partners: A feasibility study. *Annals of Oncology, 12,* 633-641.

Kornblith, A. B., Herr, H. W., Ofman, U. S., Scher, H. I., & Holland, J. C. (1994). Quality of life of patients with prostate cancer and their spouses. *Cancer, 73,* 791-802.

Krongrad, A., Lai, H., Burke, M. A., Goodkin, K., & Lai, S. (1996). Marriage and mortality in prostate cancer. *The Journal of Urology, 156,* 1696-1700.

Kunkel, E. J. S., & Chen, E. I. (2003). Psychiatric aspects of women with breast cancer. *Psychiatric Clinics of North America, 26,* 713-724.

Lethborg, C. E., Kissane, D., & Burns, W. I. (2003). 'It's not the easy part': The experiences of significant others of women with early stage breast cancer, at treatment completion. *Social Work in Health Care, 37,* 63-85.

Llorente, M. D., Burke, M., Gregory, G. R., Bosworth, H. B., Grambow, S. C., Homer, R. D., & Golden, A. (2005). Prostate cancer: A significant risk factor for late-life suicide. *American Journal of Geriatric Psychiatry, 13,* 195-201.

Lyons, R., Sullivan, M. J. L., Ritvo, P., & Coyne, J. C. (Eds.). (1995). *Relationships in chronic illness and disability.* Thousand Oaks, CA: Sage.

Manne, S. L., Alfieri, T., Taylor, K. L., & Dougherty, J. (1999a). Preference for spousal support among individuals with cancer. *Journal of Applied Social Psychology, 29,* 722-749.

Manne, S. L., Alfieri, T., Taylor, K. L., & Dougherty, J. (1999b). Spousal negative responses to cancer patients: The role of social restriction, spouse mood, and relationship satisfaction. *Journal of Consulting and Clinical Psychology, 67,* 352-361.

Manne, S. L., Norton, T. R., Ostroff, J. S., Winkel, G., Fox, K., & Grana, G. (2007). Protective buffering and psychological distress among couples coping with breast cancer: The moderating role of relationship satisfaction. *Journal of Family Psychology, 21,* 380-388.

Manne, S. L., Ostroff, J. S., Norton, T. R., Fox, K., Goldstein, L., & Grana, G. (2006). Cancer-related relationship communication in couples coping with early-stage breast cancer. *Psycho-Oncology, 15,* 234-247.

Manne, S., Ostroff, J., Sherman, M., Heyman, R. E., Ross, S., & Fox, K. (2004). Couples' support-related communication, psychological distress, and relationship satisfaction among women with early stage breast cancer. *Journal of Consulting and Clinical Psychology, 72,* 660-670.

Manne, S., Ostroff, J., Sherman, M., Glassman, M., Ross, S., Goldstein, L., & Fox, K. (2003). Buffering effects of family and friend support on associations between partner unsupportive behaviors and coping among women with breast cancer. *Journal of Social and Personal Relationships, 20,* 771-792.

Manne, S. L., Ostroff, J., Winkel, G., Grana, G., Fox, K. (2005). Partner unsupportive responses, avoidant coping, and distress among women with early stage breast cancer: Patient and partner perspectives. *Heath Psychology, 24,* 635-641.

Manne, S. L., Taylor, K. L., Dougherty, J., & Kemeny, N. (1997). Supportive and negative responses in the partner relationship: Their association with psychological adjustment among individuals with cancer. *Journal of Behavioral Medicine, 20,* 101-125.

Maunsell, E., Brisson, J., & Deschenes, L. (1995). Social support and survival among women with breast cancer. *Cancer, 76,* 631-637.

Mellon, S., & Northouse, L. L. (2001). Family survivorship and quality of life following a cancer diagnosis. *Research in Nursing and Health, 24,* 446-459.

Morse, S. R., & Fife, B. (1998). Coping with a partner's cancer: Adjustment at four stages of the illness trajectory. *Oncology Nursing Forum, 25,* 751-760.

Neuling, S. J., & Winefield, H. R. (1988). Social support and recovery after surgery for breast cancer: Frequency and correlates of supportive behaviours by family, friends and surgeon. *Social Science and Medicine, 27,* 385-392.

Northouse, L. L. (1988). Social support in patients' and husbands' adjustment to breast cancer. *Nursing Research, 37,* 91-95.

Northouse, L. L. (1994). Breast cancer in younger women: Effects on interpersonal and family relations. *Journal of the National Cancer Institute Monographs, 16,* 183-190.

Northouse, L. L., Dorris, G., & Charron-Moore, C. (1995). Factors affecting couples' adjustment to recurrent breast cancer. *Social Science and Medicine, 41,* 69-76.

Northouse, L. L., Mood, D. W., Montie, J. E., Sandler, H. M., Forman, J. D., Hussain, M., ...Kershaw, T. (2007). Living with prostate cancer: Patients' and spouses' psychological status and quality of life. *Journal of Clinical Oncology, 25,* 4171-4177.

Northouse, P. G., & Northouse, L. L. (1988). Communication and cancer: Issues confronting patients, health professionals, and family members. *Journal of Psychosocial Oncology, 5,* 17-46.

Northouse, L. L., & Swan, M. A. (1987). Adjustment of patients and husbands to the initial impact of breast cancer. *Nursing Research, 36,* 221-225.

Northouse, L., Templin, T., & Mood, D. (2001). Couples' adjustment to breast disease during the first year following diagnosis. *Journal of Behavioral Medicine, 24,* 115-135.

Northouse, L. L., Templin, T., Mood, D., & Oberst, M. (1998). Couples' adjustment to breast cancer and benign breast disease: A longitudinal analysis. *Psycho-Oncology, 7,* 37-48.

Owen, J. E., Giese-Davis, J., Cordova, M., Kronenwetter, C., Golant, M., & Spiegel, D. (2006). Self-report and linguistic indicators of emotional expression in narratives as predictors of adjustment to cancer. *Journal of Behavioral Medicine, 29,* 335-345.

Payne, J. K., Piper, B. F., Rabinowitz, I., & Zimmerman, M. B. (2006). Biomarkers, fatigue, sleep, and depressive symptoms in women with breast cancer: A pilot study. *Oncology Nursing Forum, 33,* 775-783.

Pettit, J. W., Grover, K. E., & Lewinsohn, P. M. (2007). Interrelations between psychopathology, psychosocial functioning, and physical health: An integrative perspective. *International Journal of Clinical and Health Psychology, 7,* 453-476.

Pirl, W. F., Siegel, G. I., Goode, M. J., & Smith, M. R. (2002). Depression in men receiving androgen deprivation therapy for prostate cancer: A pilot study. *Psycho-Oncology, 11,* 518-523.

Pitceathly, C., & Maguire, P. (2003). The psychological impact of cancer on patients' partners and other key relatives: A review. *European Journal of Cancer, 39,* 1517-1524.

Procidano, M. E., & Heller, K. (1983). Measures of perceived social support from friends and from family: Three validation studies. *American Journal of Community Psychiatry, 11,* 1-24.

Roberts, K. J., Lepore, S. J., & Helgeson, V. (2006). Social-cognitive correlates of adjustment to prostate cancer. *Psycho-Oncology, 15,* 183-192.

Robles, T. F., & Kiecolt-Glaser, J. K. (2003). The physiology of marriage: Pathways to health. *Physiology and Behavior, 79,* 409-416.

Segrin, C. (2004). Concordance on negative emotion in close relationships: Emotional contagion or assortative mating? *Journal of Social and Clinical Psychology, 23,* 815-835.

Segrin, C., Badger, T., Dorros, S. M., Meek, P., & Lopez, A. M. (2007). Interdependent anxiety and psychological distress in women with breast cancer and their partners. *Psycho-Oncology, 16,* 634-643.

Segrin, C., Badger, T., Meek, P., Lopez, A. M., Bonham, E., & Sieger, A. (2005). Dyadic interdependence on affect and quality-of-life trajectories among women with breast cancer and their partners. *Journal of Social and Personal Relationships, 22,* 673-689.

Segrin, C., Badger, T., Sieger, A., Meek, P., & Lopez, A. M. (2006). Interpersonal well-being and mental health among male partners of women with breast cancer. *Issues in Mental Health Nursing, 27,* 371-389.

Sharpley, C. F., & Christie, D. R. H. (2007). An analysis of the psychometric profile and frequency of anxiety and depression in Australian men with prostate cancer. *Psycho-Oncology, 16,* 660-667.

Stommel, M., Kurtz, M. E., Kurtz, J. C., Given, C. W., & Given, B. A. (2004). A longitudinal analysis of the course of depressive symptomatology in geriatric patients with cancer of the breast, colon, lung, or prostate. *Health Psychology, 23,* 564-573.

Turner-Cobb, J. M., Sephton, S. E., Koopman, C., Blake-Mortimer, S., & Spiegel, D. (2000). Social support and salivary cortisol in women with metastatic breast cancer. *Psychosomatic Medicine, 62,* 337-345.

Turner-Cobb, J. M., Steptoe, A., Perry, L., & Axford, J. (1998). Adjustment in patients with rheumatoid arthritis and their children. *Journal of Rheumatology, 25,* 565-571.

Uchida, Y., Kitayama, S., Mesquita, B., Reyes, J. A. S., & Morling, B. (2008). Is perceived emotional support beneficial? Well-being and health independent and interdependent cultures. *Personality and Social Psychology Bulletin, 34,* 741-754.

Umberson, D. (1987). Family status and health behaviors: Social control as a dimension of social integration. *Journal of Health and Social Behavior, 28,* 306-319.

Umberson, D., Williams, K., Powers, D. A., Lui, H., & Needham, B. (2006). You make me sick: Marital quality and health over the life course. *Journal of Health and Social Behavior, 47,* 1-16.

Wagner, C. D., Bigatti, S. M., & Storniolo, M. (2006). Quality of life of husbands of women with breast cancer. *Psycho-Oncology, 15,* 109-120.

Weihs, K. L., Enright, T. M., & Simmens, S. J. (2008). Close relationships and emotional processing predict decreased mortality in women with breast cancer: Preliminary evidence. *Psychosomatic Medicine, 70,* 117-124.

Weihs, K., Enright, T. M., Simmens, S. J., & Reiss, D. (2000). Negative affectivity, restriction of emotions, and site of metastases predict mortality in recurrent breast cancer. *Journal of Psychosomatic Research, 49,* 59-68.

Weihs, K., Fisher, L., & Baird, M. (2002). Families, health, and behavior. *Family Systems and Health, 20,* 7-46.

Wellisch, D. K., Jamison, K. R., & Pasnau, R. (1978). Psychological aspects of mastectomy: II. The man's perspective. *American Journal of Psychiatry, 135,* 543-546.

Wellisch, D., Kagawa-Singer, M., Reid, S. L., Lin, Y. J., Nishikawa-Lee, S., & Wellish, M. (1999). An exploratory study of social support: A cross-cultural comparison of Chinese-, Japanese-, and Anglo-American breast cancer patients. *Psycho-Oncology, 8,* 207-219.

Westman, M., Keinan, G., Roziner, I., & Benyamini, Y. (2008). The crossover of perceived health between spouses. *Journal of Occupational Health Psychology, 13,* 168-180.

Whisman, M. A. (2007). Marital distress and DSM-IV psychiatric disorders in a population-based national survey. *Journal of Abnormal Psychology, 116,* 638-643.

Whitson, S., & El-Sheikh, M. (2003). Marital conflict and health: Processes and protective factors. *Aggression of Violent Behavior, 8,* 283-312.

Wilmoth, M. C., & Botchway, P. (1999). Psychosexual implications of breast and gynecologic cancer. *Cancer Investigation, 17,* 631-636.

Woloski-Wruble, A., & Kadmon, I. (2002). Breast cancer: Reactions of Israeli men to their wives' diagnosis. *European Journal of Oncology Nursing, 6,* 93-99.

Zapka, J., Fisher, G., Lemon, S., Clemow, L., & Fletcher, K. (2006). Relationship and distress in relatives of breast cancer patients. *Families, Systems, and Health, 24,* 198-212.

CHAPTER 2

"Her Pain Was My Pain" Mothers and Daughters Sharing the Breast Cancer Journey

Carla L. Fisher

ARIZONA STATE UNIVERSITY

She was by my side. My mother was by my side…

—A diagnosed daughter

You've got me, and I've got you…

—A mother to her diagnosed daughter

Cancer is one of the most difficult challenges facing our families today. Breast cancer is the second most common type of cancer diagnosed after prostate cancer and the most common cancer diagnosis for women (American Cancer Society, 2008). The American Cancer Society (ACS) estimates that each year more than 250,000 women are diagnosed with the disease. While the risk of developing the disease increases with age, women can be diagnosed with cancer at any point in their adulthood and diagnosed young-adult women, particularly those in their thirties, tend to have a more aggressive form of the disease (ACS).

Once diagnosed, women experience traumatic changes they must learn to manage that greatly impact their psychological, physical, and relational health. For instance, diagnosed women endure bodily changes, an altered self-image and identity, relational renegotiations, psychological distress, and physiological stress responses (Boyer et al., 2002; Burles, 2006; Cohen, Klein, Kuten, Fried, Zinder, & Pollack, 2002; Cohen & Pollack, 2005; Oktay, 2005; Oktay & Walter, 1991; Spira & Kenemore, 2000). Their ability to cope with breast cancer and emerge resilient is enormously tied to the communicative support they receive in their family relationships. A plethora of studies demonstrate that family communication is a critical component of cancer patients' ability to adjust to the disease, maintain well-being, and manage the various challenges they face (Ell, 1996; Hagedoorn et al., 2000; Helgeson & Cohen, 1999; Pistrang, Barker, & Rutter, 1997). A strong family support network enhances patients' quality of life (Suinn & VandenBos, 1999).

Women diagnosed with breast cancer often seek help in coping with extreme changes in their kin network. Across ages, women describe one particular family bond as a significant part of their breast cancer experience: the mother-daughter relationship (Oktay & Walter, 1991). The mother-daughter relationship is often the longest, most emotionally connected bond a woman will experience in her lifetime and, as such, mothers and daughters are often described as having "linked lives" though they are not without tensions across the life span (Fingerman, 2003; Fischer, 1986). Although research on this bond in a cancer context is scarce, scholars have found that mothers and daughters do share the transition psychologically, physically, and socially (Burles, 2006; Cohen et al., 2002; Cohen & Pollack, 2005; Oktay & Walter, 1991; Spira & Kenemore, 2000). Yet, scholars have mostly ignored the communicative nature of how mothers and daughters share this traumatic health transition.

This chapter centers on the communicative nature of how developmentally diverse diagnosed women partner with their mothers and adult daughters to beat cancer together. A brief review of scholarship is presented, centering on research that has captured the shared nature of breast cancer in this kin bond, including a synopsis of a recently conducted study on developmentally diverse mothers and adult daughters communicatively coping with the disease. The utility of incorporating Baxter's (2006) relational dialectics theory is proposed to better understand how mothers and daughters must communicatively negotiate sharing the breast cancer transition.

Breast Cancer: A Shared Mother-Daughter Transition

Breast cancer greatly alters women's personal lives psychologically, physically, and socially. Still, Spira and Kenemore (2000) have observed that, "The closer others are to the patient, the more likely they are to feel that their life is changed" (p. 174). After a breast cancer diagnosis, this effect seems to greatly apply to diagnosed women's mothers and daughters. In essence, research demonstrates that breast cancer is a shared mother-daughter health crisis.

To begin, scholarship shows that after a woman is diagnosed, her mother-daughter relational bond is inevitably altered. For instance, at times mothers and daughters experience a role reversal as they take on new roles and responsibilities. Daughters sometimes assume maternal responsibilities for their diagnosed mother, including childcare of younger siblings and housework (Burles, 2006). Some daughters also provide social support to their mothers and, for the first time in their relational history, engage in "mothering." While some women welcome these changes, others describe struggling with relational issues of perceived control and power (Oktay & Walter, 1991). In addition to their shared social aspects of the disease, mothers and daughters also share psychological effects of breast cancer. For example, many daughters of diagnosed women ultimately live with a psychological "chronic risk" of developing the disease, the psychological burden their mothers also have (i.e., fear of recurrence) (Kenen, Ardern-Jones, & Eeles, 2003). In addition, daughters of diagnosed women exhibit symptoms of posttraumatic stress disorder (PTSD) when their mothers experience such emotional distress (Boyer et al., 2002). These psychological effects can even extend further and result in physiological changes (e.g., impaired immunological functioning and increased stress hormones) for both diagnosed mothers and their daughters (Cohen & Pollack, 2005).

Mothers and daughters also communicatively share the breast cancer transition. A recent study (see Fisher, 2008) examined how women communicatively adapt to the disease in their mother-daughter relationship. Women's stories, captured in 78 interviews with 40 women diagnosed in one of three age groups (young, middle, and later adulthood) and 38 of their mothers and adult daughters, further demonstrated mothers' and daughters' mirrored breast cancer experiences. In other words, the daughters and mothers of diagnosed women often described their feelings and behavior in direct connection with their diagnosed mother/daughter's emotions and communication. As one mother put it, "When she is strong, I am strong" (later-life mother of diagnosed midlife daughter, 11a).

In one part of the study, diagnosed women (and their mother/daughter) were asked to describe how they coped with the disease by specifically addressing how their mother or daughter emotionally supported them (see Fisher, 2008). Women were also asked to illustrate what forms of communicative adjustment were actually helpful and supportive, hence adaptive, in enabling them to adjust to this disease. A notable theme that emerged in situ across all age groups, "being there," was identified as a primary, helpful form of communicated support. As one diagnosed mother described about her daughter's support, "It's just that she's there and she's concerned, and she's there no matter what" (diagnosed midlife mother of young-adult daughter, 8a). Similarly, a daughter of a diagnosed mother expressed how this support was conveyed:

> It is just being there, letting her know that anything you need or want to talk about, I am here. So just making yourself accessible to her. So I think that was definitely the big thing. Just having her aware that you are there for her because there is not one thing. I do not think there is one thing that you can do as a whole to help the situation ... just having her know that I was there... (Young-adult daughter of diagnosed midlife mother, 28b)

Women communicatively enacted this support in various manners, all of which conveyed a crucial way mothers and daughters share the challenges of breast cancer by coping together. All women discussed "being there" as a verbal expression, in that they would tell one another they were "there" for them. Yet, developmental differences also were present. Women diagnosed in young adulthood and their mothers also explained "being there" as being an advocate at medical appointments or as a companion during down time at home. In opposition, diagnosed midlife women and their mothers and adult daughters expressed this form of support more often as a nonverbal, unspoken sense of presence rather than actual physical or verbalized presence (as many were geographically distant) or as a means of instrumental assistance with children or housework. Additionally, diagnosed later-life women and their daughters talked about both nonverbal and physical presence. Their reported forms of support included shopping for wigs together, celebrating events, and helping out at home. Still, across ages, both diagnosed women and their mothers and daughters felt this form of support was *mutually* beneficial, not just helpful for diagnosed women's adjustment. As one daughter of a diagnosed women stated, "I felt good being around" (young-adult daughter of diagnosed midlife mother, 39b). Similarly, a diagnosed daughter stated about her mother, "I think she appreciates the fact that I've made her a part of it" (diagnosed midlife mother of young-adult daughter, 8a).

Interestingly, however, even though across ages these women collectively expressed this support as "being there," age differences also emerged in whether this form of communicative support was perceived to be helpful or not in diagnosed women's cancer adjustment. For instance, diagnosed women in young adulthood (and their mothers) more frequently perceived this support as invasive, disruptive, or unwanted. As one diagnosed daughter explained, "Sometimes you want to be left alone" (diagnosed young-adult daughter with later-life mother, 21b). Mothers were also aware of such tensions as the following mother of a diagnosed daughter shared:

> The trouble is I think, we're a lot alike and you know how that is. You can just go at each other. And then I'll tell her, "I think it's time for me to go home and are you feeling okay and good enough? If not I'll stay." (Later-life mother of diagnosed young-adult daughter, 34a)

In essence, "being there" seemed to be an important way mothers and daughters communicatively coped with breast cancer together. Still, this form of enacted support was not without strained feelings at times or tensions that emerged in their dialogue. Such tensions demonstrate that how mothers and daughters are communicatively "there" for one another is likely a point of negotiation in their relationship. Baxter's (2006) relational dialectics theory has been widely cited as useful in "rending intelligible the communication processes of relating" (p. 131, see also Baxter & Montgomery, 1996). Grounded in Mikhail Bakhtin's (1981, 1984, 1986, 1990) work on dialogism, relational dialectics theory enables scholars to examine family interaction as a "both/and" experience in that dialogue is characterized by multivocality (many opposed voices coming together) (Baxter, 2006). From this theoretical approach, the inherent struggles that likely accompany sharing the breast cancer transition in the mother-daughter bond could be revealed.

A Dialectical Perspective of Sharing the Breast Cancer Journey

According to Baxter (2006), "to engage in dialogue, participants must fuse their perspectives to some extent while sustaining the uniqueness of their individual perspectives" (p. 132). During interaction, individuals experience ongoing social tensions or dialectical contradictions that characterize the changing nature of their relationship and can also indicate points for negotiation in the relationship. While research demonstrates that mothers and daughters must learn to manage relational dialectics in their bond across the life span (Fisher & Miller-Day, 2006), these contradictions are also points of negotiation when families and individuals cope with various health changes (Kvigne & Kirkevold, 2003; Pawlowski, 2007). Hence, a closer examination of such phenomena can clarify how mothers and daughters must negotiate sharing the breast cancer transition.

Scholars focus on various dialectical contradictions in family contexts, and three of these are often highlighted (Baxter, 2006). First, the integration-separation dialectic addresses one's desire for relational connection as well as personal distance. Second, the expression-privacy dialectic deals with managing the need to share information while at the same time attending to one's desire for privacy. Finally, the stability-change dialectic focuses on how individuals deal with maintaining constancy in a simultaneously dynamic family environment.

Scholars have focused on dialectics to better understand family communication, both in health transitions as well as the mother-daughter bond across time. When families are faced with adjusting to health transitions or managing chronic diseases, they are also challenged with managing relational dialectics in their shared coping. For example, following a stroke, families are often faced with long-term rehabilitation in which family members frequently share in the health care responsibilities and must adjust to the stroke survivor's new condition and needs. Pawlowski (2007) found that families must communicatively manage tensions like fear (of having another stroke) and content (acceptance of health change) as well as interdependence and dependence. Thus, dialectical contradictions can highlight the struggles families encounter in their negotiation of sharing health transitions. In addition, dialectics inform the communicative nature of the mother-daughter bond. For instance, across their relational history, mothers and daughters must manage what to share and what to keep private from one another. Hence, mothers and daughters often "edit" what they tell one another (Kraus, 1989). Withholding information may actually serve a function (Vangelisti, 1994). Miller-Day (2004) found that when mothers and daughters keep secrets they may be engaging in relational maintenance (withholding information to maintain stability in the bond) or to protect each other (withholding information to not hurt the other person). Mothers and daughters also must manage their ever-changing bond while, at the same time, maintaining a sense of familiarity. Even though change can lead to enhanced closeness in their bond, transitions sometimes result in increased distance (Fisher & Miller-Day, 2006). In light of this, how mothers and daughters negotiate their shared experience of a particularly difficult change, a diagnosis of breast cancer, ultimately likely affects them individually and relationally.

Relational dialectics theory provides a lens to examine breast cancer as a both/and experience, hence, a mother-daughter health transition. From this perspective, it is possible to highlight how mothers and daughters communicatively cope with the disease together, how they fuse and differentiate and, ultimately, how they must negotiate the shared nature of this disease experience. As such, the following research focus was proposed.

Research Focus

As was previously mentioned, "being there" is commonly reported by diagnosed women and their mothers and adult daughters as a primary means of adjusting to breast cancer together. Yet, this form of communicated support is not without struggle, which is indicative that sharing the breast cancer transition by "being there" is likely a point of negotiation for mothers and daughters. To investigate this further, the following research question was proposed:

RQ1: What relational dialectics emerge in developmentally diagnosed women's and their mothers' and daughters' descriptions of "being there" during the breast cancer transition?

Method

Sample

As noted, the original study sampled diagnosed women and their mothers and adult daughters. Sampling was purposive since predefined groups of women were needed and proportionality was not the primary concern. Following IRB approval, women were recruited in numerous ways, including a university newswire and database of speech communication students, rural hospitals, cancer clinics, and cancer support groups. To qualify, women had to have been diagnosed with breast cancer and received treatment (surgery, radiation, or chemotherapy) within the last 36 months. They were also asked to recruit their mother or adult daughter to participate. Each participant received $25 compensation and research credit, if enrolled in the university.

Forty recruited women diagnosed with breast cancer represented three age groups: 1) 8 young adults (M_{age} = 34.62, SD = 3.34, Age Range 30-39); 2) 20 midlife adults (13 as mothers: M_{age} = 49.42, SD = 2.50, Age Range 44-52; 7 as daughters: M_{age} = 46.00, SD = 3.00, Age Range 42-51); and 3) 12 later-life adults (M_{age} = 61.92, SD = 4.48, Age Range 57-69).

Thirty-eight women represented their mothers and adult daughters: 25 young adults (M_{age} = 24.74, SD = 6.94, Age Range 18-37), 5 midlife adults (M_{age} = 54.00, SD = 2.35, Age Range 51-56), and 8 later-life adults (M_{age} = 69.86, SD = 7.59, Age Range 58-83). A total of 35 mother-daughter dyads took part. Three dyads had an additional daughter participate whereas five diagnosed women participated without a dyadic partner. Most were Caucasian (98.7%) and from the East Coast (85.3%). Half were married and most had a college-level education.

Procedures

As participants were also taking part in a larger study, only the specific procedures for the findings presented in this chapter are explained. All 78 women participated in an individual, in-depth interview, which was approached using a life-span method in that women described their mother-daughter communication experiences beginning before the diagnosis of cancer and up to the present day. The interview was semi-structured and guided by a script. Women were asked to describe communication enacted to provide emotional support as well as their receipt of this support. Interviews were transcribed in full with a basic transcription, which resulted in 2,434 single-spaced transcribed pages of data.

Analyses

For the purposes of this chapter, the transcripts were re-reviewed. The analyses generated for the form of emotional support termed "being there" were also further analyzed for the presence of dialectical tensions. Analyses were conducted using Glaser and Strauss's (1967) and Strauss and Corbin's (1998) grounded theory approach. Illuminating the participants' communicative experiences required repeated examination until saturation occurred; that is, no new patterns were evident. Data were then analyzed using the qualitative management computer program ATLAS.ti.5.2. Diagnosed women and their mothers' and daughters' perspectives were combined. The analytical process involved the three steps Strauss and Corbin have identified: discovery of concepts through open coding, discovery of categories via thematic salience, and developing and refining the categories by identifying each category's properties and dimensions. According to Owen (1984), thematic salience is reflected in recurrence, repetition, and forcefulness. In the last analytical step, the categories were reviewed again to identify similar descriptions, quotations, and ideas while making a note of these for descriptive purposes. A verification strategy that ensured transferability involved using thick, rich description in the presentation of analyses (Creswell, 2007).

Results

The following findings represented the most common dialectical contradiction to emerge in each age group of diagnosed women's and their mothers' and daughters' descriptions of how they communicatively shared the breast cancer transition by "being there." The most common emergent tension in each age group's experiences is presented below.

Young-Adult Diagnosed Daughters and Their Mothers

Women diagnosed in young adulthood and their mothers most frequently expressed the dialectical tension of *connection/autonomy* in their descriptions of "being there" during breast cancer. Diagnosed daughters often expressed a need for their mother's nurturance but struggled simultaneously with a desire for independence. For instance, daughters described wanting their mothers "there" with them during cancer, as one daughter stated: "I would say it made it easier—the fact that she was by my side ... My mother was by my side" (diagnosed young-adult daughter with midlife mother, 22b). At the same time, many of these women also recognized their mother's need to "be there" or mother them. However, young-adult diagnosed women seemed to also have a strong need for autonomy in their medical decisions and care maintenance, as well as personal space. One daughter described this tension saying:

> She sort of left it up to me and I liked that ... So I asked her [to come] and she was really happy! She wanted to be "wanted" that way but didn't want to impose on me and ask ... But by the time she was going to go, I was ready ... I'm ready to have my space back! (Diagnosed young-adult daughter of midlife mother, 15b)

At times, when mothers and daughters did not effectively negotiate "being there," problems arose as was evident in this daughter's experience: "I understand that I am her daughter, but you still shouldn't be having conversations with my doctor about me ... And again, *I* was wrong for thinking there was anything wrong with that!" (diagnosed young-adult daughter with midlife mother, 33b). Yet, oftentimes mothers were not naïve about their daughters' need for independence and recognized the value of ensuring each woman had personal time, as this mother expressed:

> I didn't want to go anywhere without her … because for all these past months, she's been right there beside me. And I feel like if she's with me, then everything is okay because I know she's okay … It did me good [to leave her daughter alone] and it did her good. Gave her some, you know, a little bit of alone time and it gave me some. (Later-life mother of diagnosed young-adult daughter, 13a)

Middle-Adult Diagnosed Women and Their Mothers and Adult Daughters

Women diagnosed in middle adulthood and their daughters/mothers most frequently expressed the dialectical tension of *protection/expression* in their descriptions of "being there" during breast cancer. Regardless of reporting as a mother *or* daughter, these diagnosed women expressed extreme concern for their daughter/mother's well-being. Their daughters were young adults, sometimes having been late adolescents when they were diagnosed, and their mothers were typically in later adulthood. For diagnosed daughters with aging mothers, they often described grappling with the need for support from their mother and, hence, wanting to express in detail their experiences and, at the same time, these daughters recognized that their mother seemed particularly worried about them. Consequently, daughters were concerned their disclosures would increase their mothers' anxiety related to the disease, particularly when their mothers already had pre-existing struggles with sadness or anxiety. One diagnosed daughter explained, "Sometimes you do not want to lay that much on, you know what I mean?" (diagnosed midlife daughter with later-life mother, 7a).

Diagnosed midlife mothers experienced the same tension with their young-adult daughters, many of whom communicatively withdrew soon after they were told about the diagnosis. These mothers felt their daughters were too young and, therefore, especially vulnerable to any cancer-related information. These mothers worried that sharing too much would only increase their daughters' distress. As a result and as the following mother described, some mothers changed how much they told their daughters during their cancer experience.

> She had a bad time with it. So now I'm not too honest with her unless I'm sure ... If it's serious then I'll tell her. In the beginning I tried to tell everything. Now I think it's too much for her emotionally. (Diagnosed midlife mother of young-adult daughter, 30a)

Interestingly, diagnosed women's daughters and mothers seemed aware of their desire or need to *not* "be there" for all of their mother/daughter's breast cancer experiences. One daughter described avoiding "being there" as a coping mechanism saying, "That's like the only thing I knew that I could do to help myself through it because I'd be a mental wreck" (young-adult daughter of midlife-diagnosed mother, 16b).

Yet, while middle-adulthood diagnosed women expressed a strong desire to protect both their aging mothers and young-adult daughters, they also struggled with a need to express their concerns, feelings, and experiences to receive the support they needed to adjust. Moreover, some diagnosed women felt that when their mother/daughter did not allow them to disclose, they worried more about how their mother/daughter was doing rather than about themselves. Some also expressed feeling uncared for. One diagnosed mother explained this dialectical tension saying:

> I didn't want her more upset than me, you know. The fact that you worry about your daughter when you are like going through this ... You worry about the effects [of this on her] ... But it's funny. I mean if they weren't upset you felt like they didn't care ... I think a little bit you needed to know that this affected [her]. (Diagnosed midlife mother or young-adult daughter, 12a)

Later-Adult Diagnosed Women and Their Adult Daughters

Women diagnosed in later adulthood and their adult daughters most frequently expressed the dialectical tension of *privacy/expression* in their descriptions of "being there" during breast cancer. Like midlife diagnosed women, women in later adulthood described a need to express their experiences. However, unlike women in the younger age groups, these diagnosed women were the only participants to describe a tension to express with a need to maintain privacy. Moreover, these women also described the struggle between privacy and expression in relation to their daughters' need for them to express (rather than just their need). Daughters admitted wanting to "be there" for the mothers in any way possible. They wanted all the details to support their mothers but also for their own ability to cope with the transition. Hence, daughters often had a strong desire for their mothers to express their experiences, whether the mothers wanted to or not. As one daughter stated:

> I remember really feeling the change from when it was just this big nebulous scary thing to okay. This is how it's being dealt with. These are the treatments. These are the steps ... I wanted to know all the details and she had been reluctant to tell me. (Young-adult daughter of diagnosed later-life mother, 9b)

These diagnosed women's daughters were primarily young adults. Both relational partners often described breast cancer as a turning point that changed how they related. Breast cancer led to daughters mothering their mothers. These mothers and daughters now communicated support on a more equal level and both parties described wanting this evolution in their bond. However, sharing the transition by being there for one another also seemed to cause tension in relation to what mothers disclosed or how much daughters wanted to know. For instance, one mother expressed this relational contradiction saying:

> I don't want everybody to know how I feel. You know sometimes you want to hide your emotions. Sometimes like I say—if I'm too down, you know, if I'm down I don't want to [answer] "What's wrong?" I don't always want to tell what I'm thinking ... You know maybe I have an ache or pain somewhere that I'm concerned about ... But I don't always tell them that so—She doesn't need to know everything. Sometimes she thinks she should. (Diagnosed later-life mother of young-adult daughter, 4a)

Discussion

Although breast cancer is a shared mother-daughter transition, their shared experience is not without tension. Baxter's (2006) relational dialectics theory provides an insightful lens to better examine how mothers and daughters need to negotiate being there for one another throughout this health transition. This theoretical perspective highlights the fusion and differentiation mothers and daughters must negotiate as they take on cancer together. Moreover, this perspective has the potential to highlight developmental differences in intergenerational communication. The aforementioned dialectical contradictions, or points of negotiation, in mothers' and daughters' experiences with breast cancer are further reviewed below by considering the impact developmental diversity can have on mothers' and daughters' communicative needs and preferences.

Points of Negotiation: A Need to Consider Developmental Diversity

The struggle for connection and autonomy emerged as a defining point of negotiation for diagnosed young-adult daughters and their mothers. As young adults, these diagnosed women were the closest to the mother-daughter transition that occurs during a daughter's adolescence. This time period is knowingly fraught with issues of autonomy (La Sorsa & Fodor, 1990). During this period of their relationship, daughters encounter a dialectical struggle between wanting their mother's nurturing presence and needing independence and a separate sense of self (Hershberg, 2006; Kaufman, 1999). At the same time, the mother must learn how to accept her daughter's desire for separation from her and may even feel threatened as she sees her daughter becoming independent and needing her less (Hershberg, 2006). Even in emerging and young adulthood, women struggle for independence and a sense of self separate from their mothers. As they become adults, daughters are just beginning to stand on their own. Interestingly, these diagnosed daughters made reference to this dynamic in their mother-daughter bond, and they also seemed aware of their mothers' need to "mother" them. Yet, this understanding competed with daughters' desire to be independent at times. The findings suggest that mothers' support of "being there" can encroach upon daughters' need for independence. These findings not only demonstrate how human development can influence diagnosed women's communication support preferences during breast cancer but illuminate a point of negotiation for mothers and diagnosed young-adult daughters coping together.

For midlife-diagnosed women, protection versus expression defined their dilemmas of jointly coping with cancer. Whether a midlife mother or daughter, these women perceived the need to protect their daughter/mother from additional distress. As such, this concern affected how mothers and daughters could be there for midlife-diagnosed women. A plethora of research on human development suggests that communication during midlife is distinctively a juggling act (for a review see Fingerman, Nussbaum, & Birditt, 2004). At this point in the life span, women have the most relationships in the family and, therefore, the most diverse responsibilities and needs to attend to. They are sandwiched between generations as they maintain relationships with kin members in generations above them (e.g., their mother), below them (e.g., their daughter), as well as within their same generational cohort (e.g., siblings and spouses). At the same time, they are blending their family of origin with their family of procreation, all while assuming greater responsibilities and authority in the collective family. Women in midlife face the most complex communicative tasks in managing multiple roles and relational demands, in addition to their own needs. It is not surprising then that during breast cancer, they perceive their role in much the same way—protecting and ultimately attending to generations above and below them. As such, though, diagnosed midlife women's own needs may become secondary, which may become problematic in their ability to cope with the disease. As Fingerman et al. note, "Middle-aged adults may be forced to focus so much on other people ... their ability to communicate their own needs may become stifled" (p. 145). Hence, for diagnosed midlife women the ability to express and prioritize *their* needs may be a particularly salient point of negotiation for mothers and daughters coping with cancer at this point in the life span.

Finally, later-life diagnosed women were the only participants to describe a contradictory desire for privacy in managing their need for expression. Women in later life explained that they valued their privacy and felt that some things should be kept personal. This difference is likely tied to generational differences in communication preferences. Communication preferences vary across the life span and human development, though often ignored, can play a prominent role in differences that emerge in intergenerational communication (Pecchioni, Wright, & Nussbaum, 2005). Zietlow and Sillars (1988) explain that because individuals in different generations grew up in contrasting sociocultural contexts, they exhibit different communication preferences. Later-life diagnosed mothers' motivation may have been a product of the more closed environment in which they grew to adulthood, as they experienced a social time in which emotional expression was not actively encouraged as is more commonly done today (Segrin, 2003; Zietlow & Sillars). Vangelisti's (1994) work on family secrets may also provide insight, as privacy is often a reason given for keeping secrets. Secrets involve information kept private within certain boundaries (see Communication Privacy Management Theory (CPM), Caughlin & Petronio, 2004; Petronio, 2002). In these diagnosed women's experiences, they may perceive their cancer-related experiences as "conventional secrets," meaning the topic is not wrong to discuss but an individual perceives it to be inappropriate to discuss it. In other words, women diagnosed in later life may perceive some breast cancer related information as conventional secrets as opposed to women diagnosed in earlier generations. As such, sharing information is a particularly poignant issue later-life-diagnosed mothers and their adult daughters should negotiate when taking on cancer together.

These findings demonstrate that human development undoubtedly plays an important role in understanding diversity in communicative experiences within the context of coping with breast cancer as well as managing tensions in intergenerational bonds. Clearly, mothers and daughters share the experience of breast cancer. They mirror each other's emotional changes, social alterations, as well as some of their physiological transformations. Just as importantly, mothers and daughters communicatively cope with breast cancer together. They are concerned for one another, have a strong desire to be there to help each other cope and, ultimately, become partners in fighting breast cancer. Still, sharing this transition is not without difficulties. The presented emergent dialectical tensions heighten areas mothers and daughters should communicatively negotiate so that they can jointly cope with breast cancer in an adaptive, unified manner. Doing so will not only augment their ability to cope effectively but also enhance their unique relational connection.

Future Directions

As was noted, the findings presented herein are brief in that they only reflect the most common dialectical tension that emerged in the descriptions from each age group's experiences. Moreover, diagnosed women's perspectives were combined with their mothers/daughters'. Mothers and daughters experience multiple dialectical contradictions across the life span of their relationship. In addition, as families encounter health crises, they undoubtedly face a multitude of tensions they must learn to manage as they communicatively negotiate *how* they share these transitions. Therefore, a more thorough examination of emergent tensions in mothers' and daughters' experiences as they cope with breast cancer is clearly warranted.

Limitations

Despite rigorous efforts, the sample recruited for this study was somewhat limiting. These findings apply largely to rural Caucasian women's breast cancer experiences. Mothers' and daughters' communicative experiences and relational expectations are influenced by ethnicity and culture (Rastogi & Wampler, 1999). As such, a culturally diverse sample of mothers and daughters would have been preferable and should be recruited in future studies.

Diversity in women's cancer experiences should also be sought. The tensions mothers and daughters face early in the cancer trajectory may vary greatly in comparison to post-treatment or during the transition to survival. Women also experience great variance in their treatment regimens and stage at diagnosis. As such, these factors of influences should be considered in exploring how mothers and daughters cope with breast cancer together.

References

American Cancer Society. (2008). *Cancer facts & figures 2008*. Atlanta: American Cancer Society.

Bakhtin, M. M. (1981). *The dialogic imagination: Four essays by M. M. Bakhtin* (M. Holquist, Ed.; C. Emerson & M. Holquist, Trans.). Austin: University of Texas Press.

Bakhtin, M. M. (1984). *Problems of Dostoevsky's poetics* (C. Emerson, Ed. and Trans.). Minneapolis: University of Minnesota Press.

Bakhtin, M. M. (1986). *Speech genres and other late essays* (C. Emerson & M. Holquist, Eds.; V. McGee, Trans.). Austin: University of Texas Press.

Bakhtin, M. M. (1990). *Art and answerability: Early philosophical essays by M. M. Bakhtin* (M. Holquist & V. Liapunov, Eds.; V. Liapunov & K. Brostrom, Trans.). Austin: University of Texas Press.

Baxter, L. A. (2006). Relational dialectics theory: Multivocal dialogues in family communication. In D. O. Braithwaite & L. A. Baxter (Eds.), *Engaging theories in family communication: Multiple perspectives* (pp. 130-145). Thousand Oaks, CA: Sage.

Baxter, L. A., & Montgomery, B. M. (1996). *Relating: Dialogues & dialectics*. New York: Guilford Press.

Boyer, B. A., Bubel, D., Jacobs, S. R., Knolls, M. L., Harwell, V. D., Magdalena, G.,...Keegan, A. (2002). Posttraumatic stress in women with breast cancer and their daughters. *The American Journal of Family Therapy, 30*, 323-338.

Burles, M. C. (2006). *Mothers and daughters' experiences of breast cancer: Family roles, responsibilities, and relationships.* (Unpublished doctoral dissertation). University of Saskatchewan, Canada.

Caughlin, J. P., & Petronio, S. (2004). Privacy in families. In A. L. Vangelisti (Ed.), *Handbook of family communication* (pp. 379-412). Mahwah, NJ: Erlbaum.

Cohen, M., Klein, E., Kuten, A., Fried, G., Zinder, O., & Pollack, S. (2002). Increased emotional distress in daughters of breast cancer patients is associated with decreased natural cytotoxic activity, elevated levels of stress hormones and decreased secretion of Th1 cytokines. *International Journal of Cancer, 100*, 347-354.

Cohen, M., & Pollack, S. (2005). Mothers with breast cancer and their adult daughters: The relationship between mothers' reaction to breast cancer and their daughters' emotional and neuroimmune status. *Psychosomatic Medicine, 67*, 64-71.

Creswell, J. W. (2007). *Qualitative inquiry and research design.* Thousand Oaks, CA: Sage.

Ell, K. (1996). Social networks, social support and coping with serious illness: The family connection. *Social Science & Medicine, 42*, 173-183.

Fingerman, K. L. (2003). *Mothers and their adult daughters: Mixed emotions, enduring bonds.* New York: Prometheus Books.

Fingerman, K. L., Nussbaum, J. F., & Birditt, K. S. (2004). Keeping all five balls in the air: Juggling family communication at midlife. In A. Vangelisti (Ed.), *Handbook of family communication* (pp. 135-152). Mahwah, NJ: L. Erlbaum Associates.

Fischer, L. R. (1986). *Linked lives.* New York: Harper and Row.

Fisher, C. L. (2008). *Adaptive communicative behavior of mothers and their adult daughters after a breast cancer diagnosis.* (Unpublished doctoral dissertation). The Pennsylvania State University, University Park.

Fisher, C. L., & Miller-Day, M. (2006). Communicating over the life span: The mother-adult daughter relationship. In K. Floyd & M. T. Morman (Eds.), *Widening the family circle: New research on family communication* (pp. 3-20). Thousand Oaks, CA: Sage.

Glaser, B. G., & Strauss, A. L. (1967). *The discovery of grounded theory: Strategies for qualitative research*. New York: Aldine de Gruyter.

Hagedoorn, M., Kuijer, R., Buunk, B. P., DeJong, G., Wobbes, T., & Sanderman, R. (2000). Marital satisfaction in patients with cancer: Does support from intimate partners benefit those who need it most? *Health Psychology, 19,* 274-282.

Helgeson, V. S., & Cohen, S. (1999). Social support and adjustment to cancer: Reconciling descriptive, correlational, and intervention research. In R. M. Suinn & G. R. VandenBos (Eds.), *Cancer patients and their families: Readings on disease course, coping, and psychological interventions* (pp. 53-79). Washington, DC: American Psychological Association.

Hershberg, S. G. (2006). Pathways of growth in the mother-daughter relationship. *Psychoanalytic Inquiry, 26,* 56-69.

Kaufman, J. (1999). Adolescent females' perception of autonomy and control. In M. B. Nadien & F. L. Denmark (Eds.), *Females and autonomy: A life-span perspective* (pp. 43-72). Needham Heights, MA: Allyn & Bacon.

Kenen, R., Ardern-Jones, A., & Eeles, R. (2003). Living with chronic risk: Healthy women with a family history of breast/ovarian cancer. *Health, Risk & Society, 5,* 315-331.

Kraus, S. J. (1989). On adult daughters and their mothers: A peripatetic consideration of developmental tasks. *Journal of Feminist Family Therapy, 1,* 27-35.

Kvigne, K., & Kirkevold, M. (2003). Living with bodily strangeness: Women's experiences of their changing and unpredictable body following a stroke. *Qualitative Health Research, 13,* 1291-1310.

La Sorsa, V. A., & Fodor, I. G. (1990). Adolescent daughter/midlife mother dyad: A new look at separation and self-definition. *Psychology of Women Quarterly, 14,* 593-606.

Miller-Day, M. (2004). *Communication among grandmothers, mothers, and adult daughters: A qualitative study of maternal relationships*. Mahwah, NJ: Erlbaum.

Oktay, J. S. (2005). *Breast cancer: Daughters tell their stories*. New York: Routledge.

Oktay, J. S., & Walter, C. A. (1991). *Breast cancer in the life course: Women's experiences*. New York: Springer.

Owen, W. F. (1984). Interpretive themes in relational communication. *Quarterly Journal of Speech, 70,* 274-287.

Pawlowski, D. R. (2007). Dialectical tensions in families experiencing acute health issues: Stroke survivors' perceptions. In L. H. Turner & R. West (Eds.), *The family communication sourcebook* (pp. 469-490). Thousand Oaks, CA: Sage.

Pecchioni, L. L., Wright, K., & Nussbaum, J. F. (2005). *Life-span communication*. Mahwah, NJ: Erlbaum.

Petronio, S. (2002). *Boundaries of privacy: Dialectics of disclosure*. Albany: SUNY Press.

Pistrang, N., Barker, C., & Rutter, C. (1997). Social support as conversation: Analyzing breast cancer patients' interactions with their partners. *Social Science and Medicine, 45,* 773-782.

Rastogi, M., & Wampler, K. S. (1999). Adult daughters' perception of the mother-daughter relationship: A cross-cultural comparison. *Family Relations, 48,* 327-336.

Segrin, C. (2003). Age moderates the relationship between social support and psychosocial problems. *Human Communication Research, 29,* 317-342.

Spira, M., & Kenemore, E. (2000). Adolescent daughters of mothers with breast cancer: Impact and implications. *Clinical Social Work Journal, 28,* 183-195.

Strauss, A., & Corbin, J. (1998). *Basics of qualitative research: Techniques and procedures for developing grounded theory.* Thousand Oaks, CA: Sage.

Suinn, R. M., & VandenBos, G. R. (1999). *Cancer patients and their families: Readings on disease course, coping, and psychological interventions.* Washington, DC: American Psychological Association.

Vangelisti, A. L. (1994). Family secrets: Forms, functions, and correlates. *Journal of Social and Personal Relationships, 11,* 113-135.

Zietlow, P. H., & Sillars, A. L. (1988). Life-stage differences in communication during marital conflicts. *Journal of Social and Personal Relationships, 5,* 223-245.

CHAPTER 3

Understanding Challenges Associated with Breast Cancer: A Cluster Analysis of Intrapersonal and Interpersonal Stressors

Kirsten M. Weber

THE UNIVERSITY OF GEORGIA

Denise Haunani Solomon

PENNSYLVANIA STATE UNIVERSITY

According to the American Cancer Society (2009), roughly 192,370 women will be diagnosed with invasive breast cancer and about 40,170 women will die from breast cancer in 2009 in the United States alone. In light of the high incidence of breast cancer, medical research has focused on improving methods for early breast cancer detection and producing higher-quality treatments. Research in the social sciences has focused on issues that impact the quality of life for those who are diagnosed; for example, studies have reviewed the stressors that breast cancer patients face throughout the trajectory of their disease (Ashing, Padilla, Tejero, & Kagawa-Singer, 2003; Hilton, 1988; Ohaeri, Campbell, Ilesanmil, & Ohaeri, 1998). Stressors associated with breast cancer can compromise immune functioning among those who are diagnosed; in contrast, adjustment to having breast cancer is linked to enhanced immunological activity (Carlson, Speca, Patel, & Goodey, 2003), cellular immune functioning (McGregor, Antoni, Boyers, Alferi, Blomberg, & Carver, 2004), and decreased rates of metastasis (La Raja et al., 1997).

Given the consequential immunological outcomes associated with adjustment to breast cancer, researchers have developed interventions aimed at addressing problematic issues that patients, couples, and families face following a breast cancer diagnosis. In general, the emphasis of interventions for women diagnosed with breast cancer is to identify effective coping strategies (e.g. Chow, Tsao, & Harth, 2004; Helgeson, Cohen, Schulz, & Yasko, 2000; Okamura, Fukui, Nagasaka, Koike, & Uchitomi, 2003). When partners are invited to participate in these interventions, the focus shifts to how couples can provide support to one another in ways that promote effective coping (e.g., Manne, Ostroff, & Winkel, 2007; Scott, Halford, & Ward, 2004). Similarly, interventions that include breast cancer patients and their family caregivers aim to enhance quality of life for both individuals (Northouse, Kershaw, Mood, & Schafenacker, 2005). Although there are a variety of interventions aimed at decreasing stress among those affected by breast cancer, the effect sizes of these interventions are relatively small and are often short lived (see Scott, Halford, & Ward, 2004). One reason that these interventions may yield minimal effects is that most of the interventions treat all stressors the same. For example, couples may simply be trained to use supportive communication when talking with one another (e.g., Donnelly et al., 2000; Manne et al., 2005; Scott et al., 2004). This approach overlooks how different stressors may involve distinct emotional, cognitive, or communicative reactions.

The aim of this paper is to clarify how stressors associated with breast cancer might vary, and how those differences may impact interactions between relational partners. In doing so, we hope to shed light on how a more nuanced understanding of breast cancer experiences can help couples and families weather this health transition together. In the following section, we review interventions aimed at helping patients and couples to cope with a diagnosis of breast cancer. Then, we discuss stressors associated with a diagnosis of breast cancer and highlight how stressors associated with breast cancer may be differentially experienced. Finally, we report a study of breast cancer survivors to shed light on differences among stressors experienced by women who have been diagnosed with breast cancer and the implication of those differences for couple communication.

Interventions Aimed at Facilitating Adjustment to Breast Cancer

Researchers have developed interventions aimed at helping patients and their partners cope with a breast cancer diagnosis. One approach some interventions have taken is to train patients, partners, or couples as a unit to communicate about issues that arise because of a breast cancer diagnosis. In general, these interventions tend to promote open communication between partners or train couples to provide supportive communication to one another.

The intensity of training associated with teaching open communication skills varies from intervention to intervention. Bultz, Speca, Brasher, Geggie, and Page (2000) provided partners of breast cancer patients with four unstructured sessions in which they could discuss their fears and challenges, including issues associated with communicating with the patient about cancer. Donnelly et al. (2000) adapted the interpersonal psychotherapy approach, which had patients talk face-to-face with a psychologist for roughly 16 sessions and had their partners engage in roughly 11 similar sessions on the phone; one goal of these interactions was to "encourage communication in all relationships" (Donnelly et al., 2000, p. 47). Northouse et al. (2005) had patients and their family caregivers participate in five training sessions focused on addressing, among other things, family involvement, which was aimed at promoting open communication.

Training people to provide social support is both more and less developed than training related to open communication. Manne et al. (2005) and Manne, Ostroff, and Winkel (2007) dedicated an entire 90-minute couple's session to communication concepts and skills with a focus on constructive and destructive communication, and in a follow- up session couples identified constructive ways to communicate support needs. Using the CanCOPE method, Scott, Halford, and Ward (2004) taught couples supportive communication and partner support, which was defined as speaker-listener skills of validation, self-disclosure of thoughts and feelings, and empathic listening. Although Lewis et al. (2008) had the goal of using five educational counseling sessions to enhance communication skills with the specific aim of increasing spousal support to the breast cancer patient, none of the sessions involved training on communication techniques. Similarly, Kuijer, Buunk, De Jong, Ybema, and Sanderman (2004) focused on enhancing social support between partners, but couples were not trained how to communicate with one another.

The focus of many interventions for couples facing breast cancer is to enhance open and supportive communication. Of the studies reviewed, only two assessed communication post-intervention. Lewis et al. (2008) included anecdotal quotes from women to show how their partners had improved in communicating about the breast cancer. Scott, Halford, and Ward (2004) found a significant increase in supportive communication between partners. More generally, the consistency of effects across measures, duration of effects, and effects sizes are typically problematic. For example, Bultz, Speca, Brasher, Geggie, and Page (2000) found that no meaningful shifts occurred on any scale of the MAC, which assessed patient's adjustment to the breast cancer, for either the intervention or the control patients; however, TMD and POMS scores, which assess mood disturbance, decreased for both groups. Northouse et al. (2005) found adjustment effects at a three-month follow-up, but these effects were not sustained at a six-month follow-up. Also, Scott, Halford, and Ward (2004) found that women in the CanCOPE condition were significantly less psychologically distressed than women in the control conditions, but the effect size was small ($d = 0.22$).

One reason these efforts may lack effectiveness is because they have taken a one-size-fits-all approach to using communication; specifically, they suggest that more open or more supportive communication about any aspect of a breast cancer experience will enhance coping. In the following section, we consider how a closer look at stressors associated with breast cancer calls this approach into question.

Stressors Associated with Breast Cancer

Past research has noted a variety of stressors that breast cancer patients and their families face. Some studies have explored the numerous distressing circumstances that breast cancer patients themselves experience (e.g., Cowan & Hoskins, 2007; Kangas, Henry, & Bryant, 2002). Other research has focused on how couples cope with a diagnosis of breast cancer and how cancer impacts the dyad's relationship (e.g., Hodgkinson, Butow, Hunt, Wyse, Hobbs, & Wain, 2007; Shands,

Lewis, Sinsheimer, & Cochrane, 2006). Concerns that children or others in the patient's social network face have also received attention (Edwards & Clarke, 2004). In the following paragraphs, we review literature on stressors that breast cancer patients face individually, with their romantic partner, and within a family unit more generally.

As a breast cancer patient, a woman is confronted with a severe medical illness that she must contextualize within her life. Not surprisingly, many women indicate that being diagnosed with breast cancer is a distressing experience (Compas et al., 1994; Given & Given, 1993; Keitel, Zevon, Rounds, Petrelli, & Karakousis, 1990; Northouse, Laten, & Reddy, 1995; Northouse & Swain, 1987; Omne-Ponten, Holmberg, Bergstrom, Sjoden, & Burns, 1993). Moreover, as many as 35% of women experience posttraumatic stress disorder following a diagnosis of breast cancer (Kangas, Henry, & Bryant, 2002). One concern that women have is about their level of knowledge about treatments (Cowan & Hoskins, 2007; Ravdin, Siminoff, & Harvey, 1998). Treatment decision making is another source of stress for women diagnosed with breast cancer (Stafford, Szczys, Becker, Anderson, & Bushfield, 1998). Concern about treatment side effects (Partridge et al., 2004) and body image (Mandelblatt et al., 2000) are also prevalent among those who have been diagnosed. In addition, many women continue to have fear about recurrence of breast cancer (Gil et al., 2004). Thus, women face myriad stressors following a diagnosis of breast cancer.

In much the same way that women who are diagnosed with breast cancer face stressors associated with their disease, couples also must cope with challenges following a breast cancer diagnosis. Couples confront a variety of concerns, including mounting tension in their relationship, needing to spend time together as a couple, and wondering about how their children are coping (Shands, Lewis, Sinsheimer, & Cochrane, 2006). Couples also contemplate reasons for the cancer (Manne, Ostroff, Winkel, Goldstein, Fox, & Grana, 2004), as well as wonder how they will manage the threat posed by breast cancer (Shands et al., 2006). Not surprisingly, then, couples often have questions about how to support one another (Hodgkinson, Butow, Hunt, Wyse, Hobbs, & Wain, 2007). In some cases, tensions arise as couples negotiate when and how to share the diagnosis with other members of their social network (Weber & Solomon, 2008). Taken together, this literature suggests that couples are faced with a host of stressors following a breast cancer diagnosis.

If we consider the impact of breast cancer on the entire family, a diversity of stressors associated with a diagnosis of breast cancer are revealed. For example, a diagnosis of breast cancer can sometimes be associated with a loss of wages, which has implications for a family's financial stability (Lauzier et al., 2008). Being diagnosed with breast cancer also evokes questions about a family history of the disease (Kash, Holland, Halper, & Miller, 1992) or the need for genetic testing (Meijers-Heijboer et al., 2003), as well as how this information will be shared with children (Bradbury et al., 2007). Family functioning and the distress levels of all members of a family are impacted by a diagnosis of breast cancer (Edwards & Clarke, 2004), and children are especially likely to face emotional and behavioral adjustment following their mother's breast cancer diagnosis (Watson et al., 2006). Relatedly, many women simply worry whether they will be around for their children in the future (Avis, Crawford, & Manuel, 2004). Thus, families must cope with a variety of stressors when one member is diagnosed with breast cancer.

Across this body of literature, then, women diagnosed with breast cancer, their partners, and their families struggle with stressors associated with the disease. Although stressors that women face individually are by no means insignificant, concerns and worries seem to be exacerbated when partners and family members are considered. Because coping with a breast cancer diagnosis is often not an individual undertaking, efforts to improve the effectiveness of interventions that target couple or family communication about stressors are well-placed.

A Phenomenological Approach to Distinguishing Types of Stressors

Thus far in this paper, we have reviewed literature on interventions aimed at reducing stress among breast cancer patients and their partners; in particular, these interventions often train couples to talk more openly with one another and teach couples to use more supportive communication. In addition, we highlighted some of the many stressors that breast cancer patients and their partners face throughout the trajectory of a breast cancer diagnosis. Given the immunological implications for adjustment to having breast cancer (Carlson, Speca, Patel, & Goodey, 2003; La Raja et al., 1997; McGregor, Antoni, Boyers, Alferi, Blomberg, & Carver, 2004), interventions need to maximize their effectiveness. Unfortunately, as noted previously, many interventions are fraught with small effect sizes or short-lived effects (Scott, Halford, & Ward, 2004). In this section, we take a phenomenological approach to understanding stressors associated with breast cancer, with the goal of highlighting variability in breast cancer stressors that can inform more effective couple communication interventions.

Previous categorizations of stressors include individual (Bloom, Stewart, Johnston, & Banks, 1998) or family concerns (Shands, Lewis, Sinsheimer, & Cochrane, 2006), disease (Northouse, Dorris, & Charron-Moore, 1995) or concurrent life event stress (Koopman, Hermanson, Diamond, Angell, & Spiegel 1998), or chronologies of distress that unfold throughout the trajectory of a breast cancer diagnosis (Lebel, Rosberger, Edgar, & Devins, 2007). Although these categorizations of stressors provide useful insight into breast cancer experiences, they neglect the ways in which stressors are experienced by women who are coping with breast cancer. As an alternative, we propose differentiating among stressors based on women's phenomenological experiences of the challenges that coincide with being a breast cancer patient or survivor.

One aspect of phenomenological experience encompasses people's emotions. Appraisal theories of emotion highlight how people's evaluations of environmental stimulus shape emotional experiences (Lazarus, 1991). Appraisals are theorized to occur continuously, automatically, and unconsciously (e.g., Arnold, 1960; Lazarus, 1968; Leventhal & Scherer, 1987; Smith & Lazarus, 1990). As individuals encounter different environmental factors, they evaluate the impact those conditions have on their well-being. In particular, individuals seek to avoid actual or potential harm, and they aim to maximize actual or potential benefits (Smith & Ellsworth, 1987; Smith & Lazarus, 1990). Emotional responses serve to alert individuals when they are confronted by relevant circumstances or environmental stimulus.

Typically, circumstances that align with a person's goals are followed by positive emotions, but situations that create obstacles to goals elicit negative emotions. In these ways, emotions serve as an index of people's phenomenological experience of their circumstances. A second facet of phenomenological experience is the cognitive evaluations people make. As noted, appraisal theories of emotions locate cognitions that occur automatically and unconsciously at the root of distinct emotional experiences (Lazarus, 1991). Judgments that are made more consciously also affect phenomenological experiences. For example, attribution theories highlight how the judgments that people make about themselves and others around them shape their interpretation of behavior (Graham & Folkes, 1990). Specifically, attribution theories suggest that once a person observes a behavior, they then make a judgment about the intended purpose of that behavior. Following, people draw conclusions about the person and their behavior. Importantly, appraising a situation differently can produce different cognitive reactions (see Feldman, 2007). In fact, a main goal of cognitive-behavioral therapy is to help patients appraise situations in ways that create more positive, and less negative, cognitive reactivity (Ma & Teasdale, 2004). Thus, people's cognitive assessments of particular situations are a fundamental aspect of their phenomenological experience.

By applying the logic of appraisal theories of emotions and attribution theories of cognition to stressors associated with breast cancer, we propose that emotions and judgments associated with specific experiences provides a meaningful framework for distinguishing among types of stressors. To evaluate this claim, we pose the following research question about stressors associated with breast cancer.

RQ1: How are stressors associated with breast cancer grouped based on the reactions they generate?

Appraisal theories of emotion and attribution theories of cognition suggest, respectively, that experiences of emotions and cognitions shape behavior. According to appraisal theories of emotion (Lazarus & Folkman, 1984) emotions serve to motivate actions. In particular, specific emotions may prompt actions that have different aims. Moreover, different emotions can alter current and future interactions with one's environment (Scherer, 1982). Therefore, to the extent that a person experiences different emotions, they should engage in different behavioral patterns. Similarly, the ways in which people cognitively define phenomena or events, shapes how people react to those events. For example, Fincham, Bradbury, and Grych (1990) theorized that how relational partners define a conflict episode influences how partners interact during the conflict. To the extent that people perceive events in similar ways, they should react to those events in similar ways. Thus, we propose the following research question:

RQ2: Do the categories of stressors based on reactions evoked correspond with different communication behaviors?

Next, we report a study of breast cancer survivors designed to evaluate these research questions.

Method

We employed a cross-sectional web-based survey that included questions about stressors associated with a breast cancer diagnosis, distress and emotional reactions to those stressors, and characteristics of communication with a spouse about those stressors. Breast cancer patients and survivors were recruited from a variety of breast cancer discussion boards, a statewide newsletter aimed at serving people who have been touched by breast cancer, a listserv distributed to faculty and staff at a large east coast university, and via a snowball sample of breast cancer patients and survivors who participated in a different study. In the following sections, we describe the sample, procedures, and measures that were used in this study.

Participants

Eighty female breast cancer patients completed the survey, 65 participants were reporting on an initial breast cancer diagnosis, and 13 women were reporting on a recurrence of breast cancer (2 individuals did not respond). Participants ranged in age from 32 to 67 with a mean age of 48.10. The sample included 75 Caucasian individuals. The time since diagnosis (initial or recurrent) ranged from only a few months to 20 years, with a mean of 2.8 years (*SD* = 3.4, *median* = 2).

Procedures

The questionnaire was administered through an Internet website. Recruitment postings were placed on a variety of discussion boards designated for breast cancer patients and survivors; additionally, a recruitment statement was included in an online newsletter for a statewide breast cancer coalition and another recruitment statement was listed in a large east coast university listserv for faculty and staff. Individuals who were interested in participating in the study opened a link that directed them to the homepage of the study or emailed the investigator in order to receive the link that directed them to the study homepage. Once at the homepage, participants were instructed to create an individual username and password to access the survey. Because all participants created a username and password, participants could finish the survey in multiple sessions; specifically, the participant could return to the website, log in using her username and password, and continue the survey where she had stopped previously. After completing the questionnaire, responses were submitted online and data were stored on a secure server. Forty-five of the respondents completed the survey in one sitting, and the time to complete the full survey ranged from 6 minutes to 293 minutes (M = 36.70, SD = 37.23, *median* = 26.00).

Participants were presented with a list of stressors that were developed based on the results of a theme analysis of discourse posted in online forums for discussions among breast cancer survivors (Weber & Solomon, 2008). That study identified five stressors associated with the breast cancer diagnosis and treatment: (a) waiting for results, (b) coming to terms with having breast cancer, (c) making a treatment decision, (d) dealing with the logistics of getting treatment, and (e) experiencing the side effects of treatments. Seven other themes identified challenges that occurred throughout the breast cancer experience: (a) coping with body image, (b) coping with feelings about sexuality, (c) getting social support from others, (d) feeling isolated or alone in this experience, (e) managing information sharing and privacy issues, (f) managing other life events, and (g) addressing financial problems. The category of managing other life events was divided into two separate stressors including circumstances that were relatively mundane (i.e., buying groceries, transporting children to and from school) and the management of larger life events (i.e., death in the family, illness in the family, loss of job), which yielded a total of 13 potential stressors.

Respondents indicated that they had experienced 0 to 13 stressors within the past two weeks (*median* = 5, *M* = 5.09, *SD* = 3.72). Those participants who did not identify any recent stressors (*n* = 9) or did not complete follow up questions on any of the stressors they reported (*n* = 14) were dropped from further analyses. Thus, our resulting sample included 66 women who provided data on recent stressors (*M* = 5.05, *SD* = 3.09). Because our goal was to identify patterns associated with the different stressors that women reported, our unit of analysis was each stressor (*N* = 334), and our measures focus on respondents' descriptions of the emotions, cognitions, and communication experiences that characterized each of the stressors they had experienced in the preceding two weeks.

Measures

A variety of closed-ended Likert type scales were used to operationalize the variables in the study. The majority of measures were assessed as single-item ratings; this strategy allowed us to collect several measures of each stressor without overburdening women who were responding to these scales with respect to several different stressors. For some variables (i.e., directness of communication, encouraging conversational communication, and distressing conversational communication), multiple items were used to measure responses to each stressor; in these cases, we averaged responses to the individual scale items (within stressor as the unit of analysis). The measures that we obtained with respect to each stressor are detailed in the following sections.

Intensity of distress. Respondents were asked to indicate on a 5-point Likert scale (1 = *strongly disagree*, 5 = *strongly agree*) their agreement with two statements: (a) "I have been very stressed out about [the stressor]," and (b) "I have spent a lot of time worrying about [the stressor]." The grand mean for these variables, across the full set of

334 stressors was as follows: *stressed* (M = 3.83, SD = 0.86) and *worried* (M = 3.55, SD = 0.89).

Intensity of emotions. Respondents reported their emotional reactions to each of the stressors they identified using 10 single-item measures of specific emotions. Participants were asked to indicate their feelings about [the stressor] using a 5-point Likert scale (1 = *not at all*, 5 = *a lot*). The specific emotion terms presented in the survey and the grand means for the 334 stressors were as follows: *scared* (M = 3.05, SD = 1.12), *angry* (M = 3.06, SD = 1.14), *irritated* (M = 3.39, SD = 0.98), *happy* (M = 2.07, SD = 0.90), *sad* (M = 3.12, SD = 1.07), *shocked* (M = 1.76, SD = 0.81), *surprised* (M = 1.88, SD = 0.87), *guilty* (M = 1.94, SD = 0.89), *embarrassed* (M = 2.06, SD = 1.00), and *hopeful* (M = 3.13, SD = 1.19). Again, the final scores represent the reaction that was reported in association with each stressor within the past two weeks.

The directness and valence of communication. Follow-up questions for each stressor asked participants to indicate if they had discussed the concern with their romantic partner. A total of 110 of the stressors reported on were not communicated to a partner and 221 of the stressors were discussed between relational partners; the mean proportion of stressors discussed with the partner was .62 (SD = .28). Respondents who indicated that they had communicated with their partner were asked to rate statements describing their communication behavior.

The *directness of communication* was assessed by two items: (a) "I was direct in my conversation with my partner about my stress related to [the stressor]," and (b) "I openly told my partner how I felt about [the stressor]." Responses to the two items were recorded using a 5-point Likert scale (1 = *strongly disagree*, 5 = *strongly agree*), and the two variables were averaged to form a single measure of communicative directness (α = .96). The grand mean, reflecting the average score for *directness of communication* across the 334 stressors, indicated a high degree of open communication, on average (M = 4.38, SD = 0.65).

To assess the *encouraging* nature of the communication episode, we asked respondents who had communicated with partners about specific stressors to rate those conversations using several adjectives; responses were recorded on a 5-point scale (1 = *not at all*, 5 = *extremely*). The encouraging nature of communication was indexed by four adjectives: (a) satisfying, (b) open, (c) comfortable, and (d) hopeful. The final measure averaged across all four measures of encouraging communication (α = .88, *M* = 3.64, *SD* = 0.85).

To assess the *distressing* nature of the communication episode, we asked respondents who had communicated with partners about specific stressors to rate those conversations using several adjectives; responses were recorded on a 5-point scale (1 = *not at all*, 5 = *extremely*). The distressing nature of communication was indexed by three adjectives: (a) guarded, (b) upsetting, and (c) tense. Again, responses to items averaged to form a composite measure (α = .85, *M* = 2.36, *SD* = 0.99).

Two single-item measures were used to assess the *positivity* (*M* = 3.53, *SD* = 1.07) and *negativity* of communication (*M* = 2.69, *SD* = 1.13): (a) "I focused on being positive when talking with my partner about finding out that I have breast cancer," and (b) "I had a negative tone when talking with my partner about finding out that I have breast cancer." Responses to the two items were recorded using a 5-point Likert scale (1 = *strongly disagree*, 5 = *strongly agree*).

Supportive communication was assessed by asking participants to rate their conversations with relational partners about specific stressors; responses were recorded on a 5-point scale (1 = *not at all*, 5 = *extremely*). A single-item measure was used to assess *supportive communication* (*M* = 4.14, *SD* = 0.80).

Results

We performed two sets of analyses to shed light on our research questions. First, we conducted a hierarchical cluster analysis (RQ1). Then, we performed an ANOVA to evaluate the associations between the clusters and communication behaviors (RQ2). The results of each analysis are described in turn.

Cluster Analysis

Cluster analysis is an exploratory statistical method that is used to identify naturally occurring groups or patterns of responses that follow from a specific measure (Henry et al., 2005; Taylor et al., 2001). Responses are sorted into groups based on their relative similarities and differences to one another on the measure (Hair et al., 1998; Henry et al., 2005). Specifically, we used emotional reactivity and distress measures to form clusters of stressors associated with breast cancer. To maximize flexibility in determining the appropriate number of clusters, we employed a hierarchical cluster analysis with Ward's linkage clusters using minimized squared Euclidean distances. This particular method allowed us to identify the number of clusters that occurs when the differences between clusters are maximized, but the within-group differences are minimized. We conducted the cluster analysis on a subset of the data (n = 272 stressors; Weber, Solomon, & Goodwin, 2008). Because the full data set is used to evaluate differences between clusters, using only a subset of the data to form the clusters provides a more stringent test of our framework.

Changes that are relatively small in the agglomeration coefficient from one stage to the next suggest that homogeneous clusters were combined in the previous stage, whereas larger changes suggest that heterogeneous clusters were combined (Hair et al., 1998). In our analysis, comparatively small changes in the agglomeration coefficients occurred until four clusters were collapsed into a three-cluster solution. The larger agglomeration coefficients at stage five indicated that the three-cluster solution would be combining relatively distinct groups. Thus, we adopted a four-cluster solution: (a) *finding out,* (b) *fitting the cancer into one's life,* (c) *intrapersonal and identity concerns,* and (d) *life's other nuisances.* Table 3.1 indicates which stressors were grouped into the respective clusters and identifies *N*s and proportions for each stressor category.

Table 3.1 Clusters of Stressors Associated with Breast Cancer

Cluster Name	Stressors Included in Cluster	Subset		Full data set	
		N	Proportion	*N*	Proportion
Fitting the cancer into one's life	Feeling alone Co-occurrence of large life events Making treatment decisions Receiving support Facing financial burden	91	33.5%	113	33.7%
Intrapersonal and identity concerns	Waiting for test results Coming to terms with the diagnosis Coping with treatment side effects Dealing with bodily changes	108	39.7%	137	41.1%
Finding out	Being diagnosed with breast cancer	12	4.4%	11	3.3%
Life's other nuisances	Coping with changes to sexual intimacy Telling others about the diagnosis Facing everyday tasks	61	22.4%	74	22.0%

The profiles of reactions associated with each cluster were relatively distinct (Table 3.2). For *finding out,* women reported being significantly more shocked and surprised than *fitting the cancer into one's life, intrapersonal and identity concerns,* and *life's other nuisances.* Women reported that *fitting the cancer into one's life* was significantly more stressful and irritating than *life's other nuisances,* and provokes significantly more anger and guilt than *intrapersonal and identity concerns* and *life's other nuisances.* Consistent with this pattern, women indicated that they felt less hopeful about *fitting the cancer into one's life* than *intrapersonal and identity concerns. Finding out* and *fitting the cancer into one's life* were reported to be more scary and sad than *life's other nuisances.* Also, women rated *intrapersonal and identity concerns* as significantly more scary than *life's other nuisances,* but they indicated that *life's other nuisances* provoked more guilt than *intrapersonal and identity concerns,* although the latter association merely approached significance.

Table 3.2 Reactivity Profile for Clusters

	Finding out	Fitting cancer into life	Life's other nuisances	Intrapersonal identity concerns
Stressed	*M* = 3.73	*M* = 4.21a	*M* = 3.77b	*M* = 3.99
Scared	*M* = 4.00a	*M* = 3.70a	*M* = 2.36b	*M* = 3.39a
Angry	*M* = 3.36	*M* = 3.70a	*M* = 2.84b	*M* = 3.18b
Irritated	*M* = 3.73	*M* = 3.75a	*M* = 3.21b	*M* = 3.58
Sad	*M* = 4.18a	*M* = 3.57a	*M* = 2.85b	*M* = 3.20
Shocked	*M* = 3.73b	*M* = 1.99a	*M* = 1.68a	*M* = 1.76a
Surprised	*M* = 3.73b	*M* = 2.03a	*M* = 1.78a	*M* = 1.99a
Guilty	*M* = 2.09	*M* = 2.12b	*M* = 2.40*	*M* = 1.69a*
Hopeful	*M* = 3.55	*M* = 2.83a	*M* = 2.97	*M* = 3.36b

Note: Means in the same row that do not share subscripts differ at $p < .05$.
* Indicates the means who share this demarcation differ at p < .10.

One-Way ANOVA

Using the cluster groups that were formed by the hierarchical cluster analyses, an ANOVA was used to determine if communication with a spouse varied by stressor cluster. Although dependence in the data was ignored, the results of the ANOVA indicated that communication did significantly vary by stressor cluster; specifically, the differences among cluster was statistically significant for encouraging communication, F (3, 198) = 3.07, $p < .05$, supportive communication, F (3, 196) = 3.80, $p < .01$, direct communication, F (3, 203) = 2.37, $p < .10$, and distressing communication, F (3, 200) = 2.22, $p < .10$.

Using Bonferroni post hoc comparisons, we were able to determine more specific communication patterns associated with the stressor clusters. In particular, conversations were rated as more encouraging when couples were discussing *intrapersonal and identity concerns* (M = 3.91, SD = 0.84) than when they were talking about stressors associated with *fitting cancer into one's life* (M = 3.49, SD = 1.02). Conversations were also rated as more supportive when couples were discussing *intrapersonal and identity concerns* (M = 4.31, SD = 0.82) compared with conversations about distress associated with *fitting the cancer into one's life* (M = 3.82, SD = 1.16). Women were more direct in their communication when discussing *intrapersonal and identity concerns* (M = 4.48, SD = 0.66) than when communicating about *life's other nuisances* (M = 4.09, SD = 1.04). Additionally, conversations about stress associated *fitting the cancer into one's life* (M = 2.75, SD = 1.33) contained more distressing communication than discussions about *intrapersonal and identity concern* (M = 2.27, SD = 2.27). Therefore, these findings indicate that breast cancer patients are communicating with their spouse about distinct stressors in different ways.

Discussion

The goal of this study was to examine how emotional and cognitive reactions to stressors associated with breast cancer might contribute to communication patterns between relational partners about those stressors. In reviewing the literature on interventions that have been used to facilitate adjustment to a breast cancer diagnosis for breast cancer patients and their families and the scholarly work that identifies stressors associated with a breast cancer diagnosis, we highlighted the need to tailor interventions to specific types of stressors. In particular, we took a phenomenological approach to understanding how stressors associated with a diagnosis of breast cancer vary by the reactions they produce. Moreover, following from the logic of appraisal theories of emotion and the reasoning of attribution theories, we advanced two research questions about the nature of emotions and cognitions and communication in association with breast cancer stressors. In the following section, we review the results of this investigation and discuss their implications.

Emotional Reactivity, Communication, and Stressors Associated with Breast Cancer

Previous research on stressors associated with a breast cancer diagnosis indicates that women experience distress and concern throughout the trajectory of their disease. Using cluster analysis techniques we observed that breast cancer stressors fell into four categories: (a) *finding out,* (b) *fitting the cancer into one's life,* (c) *intrapersonal and identity concerns,* and (d) *life's other nuisances*. These findings suggest that certain types of stressors do produce similar profiles in terms of emotional and cognitive reactions, which is distinct from other types of stressors.

Following, we used the four clusters to predict communication behavior. We observed that encouraging communication, supportive communication, direct communication, and distressing communication varied by cluster. Moreover, conversations about *intrapersonal and identity concerns* were more encouraging, more supportive, and less distressing than discussions about *fitting the cancer into one's life,* and they were more direct than couples' discussions about *life's other nuisances.* These results suggest that couples are pulling from a broader repertoire of communicative techniques when discussing *interpersonal and identity concerns* than other types of stressors.

These findings suggest that interventions aimed at facilitating adjustment to breast cancer may need to consider how emotional and cognitive reactions to particular stressors shape communication between relational partners. Clearly, these findings indicate that people are talking relatively openly about *intrapersonal and identity concerns,* and in somewhat supportive and encouraging ways. On the flip side, however, other types of stressors appear to be more difficult for breast cancer patients and their partners to talk about. Perhaps interventions aimed at aiding families to cope with a breast cancer diagnosis should hone in on the difficulties that arise because of stressors not related to *interpersonal and identity concerns.* For example, *fitting the cancer into one's life* is a stressor that fosters particularly distressing communication.

In light of this book's aim to examine how health transitions shape day-to-day communication within families, our results suggest that for families touched by breast cancer, more nuanced interventions are needed. Specifically, interventions may need to spend extra time focusing on how to communicate about discussing circumstances that arise in association with concern about *fitting the cancer into one's life* in order to facilitate adjustment to this aspect of a breast cancer diagnosis, whereas less time may need to be spent unpacking *intrapersonal and identity concerns.* Ironically, much of the scholarly work currently aimed at identifying how to reduce stress associated with a breast cancer diagnosis focuses on elements of *intrapersonal and identity concerns* such as giving meaning to the diagnosis (Manne, Ostroff, Winkel, Goldstein, Fox, & Grana, 2004) or helping patients prepare for the changes that will occur to their body because of treatment (Scott, Halford, & Ward, 2004).

In addition to identifying specific stressors that may benefit from more developed interventions, our findings also provide insight into the mechanisms that underlie stressful experiences during transitional moments in relationships. In particular, the results from this study suggest that emotional reactions and cognitive reactions drive stressors associated with a breast cancer diagnosis. Future work should consider other intrapersonal and interpersonal factors that might exacerbate already stressful transitions that couples face. For example, Weber and Solomon (2007) suggest that experiencing relational uncertainty during a transition or having a partner interfere with one's daily goals during a breast cancer diagnosis can intensify communication exchanges between relational partners.

More broadly, the findings of this study provide insight into how couples or families cope together. Specifically, these findings indicate that the ways in which people react to different types of stressors shape the communication that couples are having about their experiences with breast cancer. To expand this understanding of communication about breast cancer stressors between dyads and within families, future work should consider the point of view of other family members including spouses and partners, children, siblings, parents, and grandparents. Additionally, documenting the ways in which family members are communicating with one another about the stressors that they face outside of discussions that are held with the breast cancer patient will allow for a more complete understanding of breast cancer as a family transition. Moreover, recognizing how a breast cancer diagnosis impacts all members of a family can assist in the daily management of the disease and facilitate family functioning.

Conclusion

Our research adds to the body of literature on adjustment to breast cancer by identifying distinct communication behaviors that characterize discussions of different stressors encountered during a breast cancer diagnosis. When considering the ways in which health transitions shape day-to-day communication within families, our findings suggest that different stressors associated with breast cancer evoke different emotional and cognitive reactions, and in turn, communication about stressors is not a uniform experience. This research has implications for couple interventions developed to assist breast cancer patients and their partners cope with a breast cancer diagnosis. Specifically, these interventions should note that not all stressors are being discussed by breast cancer patients and their partners in the same way, and the development of tailored interventions may be helpful to families who are going through breast cancer together.

References

American Cancer Society (2009). *How many women get breast cancer?* Retrieved from http://www.cancer.org/docroot/CRI/content/CRI_2_2_1X_How_many_people_get_breast_cancer_5.asp?sitearea=

Arnold, M. B. (1960). *Emotion and personality.* New York: Columbia University Press.

Ashing, K., Padilla, G., Tejero, J., & Kagawa-Singer, M. (2003). Understanding the breast cancer experience of Asian American women. *Psycho-Oncology, 12,* 38-58.

Avis, N., Crawford, S., & Manuel, J. (2004). Psychosocial problems among younger women with breast cancer. *Psycho-Oncology, 13,* 295-308.

Bloom, J., Stewart, S., Johnston, M., & Banks, P. (1998). Intrusiveness of illness and quality of life in young women with breast cancer. *Psycho-Oncology, 7,* 89-100.

Bradbury, A., Dignam, J., Ibe, C., Auh, S., Hlubocky, F., Cummings, S., White, M., Olopade, O., & Daugherty, C. (2007). How often do BRCA mutation carriers tell their young children of the family's risk for cancer? A study of parental disclosure of BRCA mutations to minors and young adults. *Journal of Clinical Oncology, 25,* 3705-3711.

Bultz, B., Speca, M., Brasher, P., Geggie, P., & Page, S. (2000). A randomized controlled trial of a brief psychoeducational support group for partners of early-stage breast cancer patients. *Psycho-Oncology, 9,* 303-313.

Carlson, L., Speca, M., Patel, K., & Goodey, E. (2003). Mindfulness-based stress reduction in relation to quality of life, mood, symptoms of stress, and immune parameters in breast and prostate cancer outpatients. *Psychosomatic Medicine, 65,* 571-581.

Chow, E., Tsao, M. & Harth, T. (2004). Does psychosocial intervention improve survival in cancer? A meta-analysis. *Palliative Medicine, 18,* 25-31.

Compas, B. E., Worsham, N. L., Epping-Jordan, J. E., Grant, K., Mireault, G., Howell, D. C., & Malcarne, V. L. (1994). When mom or dad has cancer: Markers of psychological distress in cancer patients, spouses, and children. *Health Psychology, 13,* 507-515.

Cowan, C., & Hoskins, R. (2007). Information preferences of women receiving chemotherapy for breast cancer. *European Journal of Cancer Care, 16,* 543-550.

Donnelly, J., Kornblith, A., Fleishman, S., Zuckerman, E., Raptis, G., Hudis, C., Hamilton, N., Payne, D., Massie, M., Norton, L., & Holland, J. (2000). A pilot study of interpersonal psychotherapy by telephone with cancer patients and their partners. *Psycho-Oncology, 9,* 44-56.

Edwards, B., & Clarke, V. (2004). The psychological impact of a cancer diagnosis on families: The influence of family functioning and patients' illness characteristics on depression and anxiety. *Psycho-Oncology, 13,* 562-576.

Feldman, G. (2007). Cognitive and behavioral therapies for depression: Overview, new directions, and practical recommendations for dissemination. *Psychiatric Clinic of North America, 30,* 39-50.

Fincham, F. D., Bradbury, T. N., & Grych, J. H. (1990). Conflict in close relationships: The role of intrapersonal phenomena. In V. Graham & S. Folkes (Eds.), *Attribution theory: Applications to achievement, mental health, and interpersonal conflict. Applied social psychology* (pp. 161-184). Hillsdale, NJ: Erlbaum.

Gil, K., Mishel, M., Belyea, M., Germino, B., Porter, L., LaNey, I., & Stewart, J. (2004). Triggers of uncertainty about recurrence and long-term treatment side effects in older African American and Caucasian breast cancer survivors. *Oncology Nursing Forum, 31,* 633-639.

Given, B., & Given, C. W. (1993). Patient and family caregiver reaction to new and recurrent breast cancer. *Journal of the American Medical Women's Association, 47,* 201-206.

Graham, S., & Folkes, V. S. (1990). *Attribution theory: Applications to achievement, mental health, and interpersonal conflict. Applied social psychology.* Hillsdale, NJ: Erlbaum.

Hair, J. F., Anderson, R. E, Tatham, R. L., & Black, W. C. (1998). *Multivariate data analyses* (5th ed., pp. 469–518). Upper Saddle River, NJ: Prentice Hall.

Helgeson, V., Cohen, S., Schulz, R., & Yasko, J. (2000). Group support interventions for women with breast cancer: Who benefits from what? *Health Psychology, 19,* 107-114.

Henry, D. B., Tolan, P. H., & Gorman-Smith, D. (2005). Cluster analysis in family psychology research. *Journal of Family Psychology, 19,* 121–132.

Hilton, B. A. (1988). The phenomenon of uncertainty in women with breast cancer. *Mental Health Nursing, 9,* 217-238.

Hodgkinson, K., Butow, P., Hunt, G., Wyse, R., Hobbs, F., & Wain, G. (2007). Life after cancer: Couples' and partners' psychological adjustment and supportive care needs. *Support Care Cancer, 15,* 405-415.

Kangas, M., Henry, J. L., & Bryant, R. A. (2002). Posttraumatic stress disorder following cancer: A conceptual and empirical review. *Clinical Psychology Review, 22,* 499–524.

Kash, K., Holland, J., Halper, M., Miller, D. (1992). Psychological distress and surveillance behaviors of women with a family history of breast cancer. *Journal of the National Cancer Institute, 84,* 24-30.

Keitel, M. A., Zevon, M. A., Rounds, J. B., Petrelli, N. J., & Karakousis, C. (1990). Spouse adjustment to cancer surgery: Distress and coping responses. *Journal of Surgical Oncology, 43,* 148-153.

Koopman, C., Hermanson, K., Diamond, S., Angell, K., & Spiegel, D. (1998). Social support, life stress, pain and emotional adjustment to advanced breast cancer. *Psycho-Oncology, 7,* 101-111.

Kuijer, R., Buunk, B., De Jong, G., Ybema, J., & Sanderman, R. (2004). Effects of a brief intervention program for patients with cancer and their partners on feelings of inequality, relationship quality and psychological distress. *Psycho-Oncology, 13,* 321-334.

La Raja, M., Virno, F., Mechella, M., D'Andrea, M., D'Alessio, A., Ranieri, E., & Pagni, P. (1997). Depression secondary to tumors in patients who underwent surgery for mammary carcinoma: Psycho-pharmaceutical and psychotherapeutic care. *Journal of Experimental and Clinical Cancer Research, 16,* 209-216.

Lauzier, S., Maunsell, E., Drolet, M., Coyle, D., Hébert-Croteau, J., Mâsse, B.,... Robert, J. (2008). Wage losses in the year after breast cancer: Extent and determinants among Canadian women. *Journal of the National Cancer Institute, 100,* 321-332.

Lazarus, R. S. (1968). Emotions and adaptation: Conceptual and empirical relations. In W. J. Arnold (Ed.), *Nebraska Symposium on Motivation* (pp. 175-266). Lincoln: University of Nebraska Press.

Lazarus, R. S., & Folkman, S. (1984) *Stress, appraisal, and coping*. New York: Springer.

Lazarus, R. S. (1991). *Emotion and Adaptation*. New York, NY: Oxford University Press.

Lebel, S., Rosberger, Z., Edgar, L., & Devins, G. (2007). Comparison of four common stressors across the breast cancer trajectory. *Journal of Psychosomatic Research, 63,* 225-232.

Leventhal, H., & Scherer, K. (1987). The relationship of emotion to cognition: A functional approach to a semantic controversy. *Communication and Emotion, 1,* 3-28.

Lewis, F., Cochrane, B., Fletcher, K., Zahlis, E., Shands, M., Gralow, J., Wu, S., & Schmitz, K. (2008). Helping her heal: A pilot study of an educational counseling intervention for spouses of women with breast cancer. *Psycho-Oncology, 17,* 131-137.

Ma, S., & Teasdale, J. (2004). Mindfulness-based cognitive therapy for depression: Replication and exploration of differential relapse prevention effects. *Journal of Consulting and Clinical Psychology, 72,* 31-40.

Mandelblatt, J., Handley, J., Kerner, J., Schulman, K., Gold, K., Dunmore-Griffith, J., Edge, S. Guadagnoll, E., Lynch, J., Meropol, N., Weeks, J., & Winn, R. (2000). Patterns of breast carcinoma treatment in older women: Patient preference and clinical and physician influences. *Cancer, 89,* 561-573.

Manne, S., Ostroff, J., Winkel, G., Fox, K., Grana, G., Miller, E., Ross, S., & Frazier, T. (2005). Couple-focused group intervention for women with early-stage breast cancer. *Journal of Consulting and Clinical Psychology, 73,* 634-646.

Manne, S., Ostroff, J., & Winkel, G. (2007). Social-cognitive processes as moderators of a couple focused group intervention for women with early-stage breast cancer. *Health Psychology, 26,* 735-744.

Manne, S., Ostroff, J., Winkel, G., Goldstein, L., Fox, K., & Grana, G. (2004). Posttraumatic growth after breast cancer: Patient, partner, and couple perspectives. *Psychosomatic Medicine, 66,* 442-454.

McGregor, B., Antoni, M., Boyers, A., Alferi, S., Blomberg, B., & Carver, C. (2004). Cognitive-behavioral stress management increases benefit finding and immune function among women with early-stage breast cancer. *Journal of Psychosomatic Research, 56,* 1-8.

Meijers-Heijboer, H., Brekelmans, C., Menke-Pluymers, M., Seynaeve, C., Baalbergen, A., Burger, C., …Klijn, J. (2003). Use of genetic testing prophylactic mastectomy and oophorectomy in women with breast or ovarian cancer from families with a BRCA1 or BRCA2 mutation. *Journal of Clinical Oncology, 21,* 1675-1681.

Northouse, L., & Swain, M. (1987). Adjustment of patients and husbands to the initial impact of breast cancer. *Nursing Research, 36,* 221-225.

Northouse, L., Dorris, G., & Charron-Moore, C. (1995). Factors affecting couples' adjustment to recurrent breast cancer. *Social Science and Medicine, 41,* 69-76.

Northouse, L., Kershaw, T., Mood, D., & Schafenacker, A. (2005). Effects of a family intervention on the question of life of women with recurrent breast cancer and their family caregivers. *Psycho-Oncology, 14,* 478-491.

Northouse, L., Laten, D., & Reddy, P. (1995). Adjustment of women and their husbands to recurrent breast cancer. *Research in Nursing & Health, 18,* 515-524.

Ohaeri, J. U., Campbell, O. B., Ilesanmil, A. O., & Ohaeri, B. M. (1998). Psychosocial concerns of Nigerian women with breast and cervical cancer. *Psycho-Oncology, 7,* 494-501.

Okamura, H., Fukui, S., Nagasaka, Y., Koike, M., & Uchitomi, Y. (2003). Psychoeducational intervention for patients with primary breast cancer and patient satisfaction with information: An exploratory analysis. *Breast Cancer Research and Treatment, 80,* 331-338.

Omne-Ponten, M., Holmberg, L., Bergstrom, R., Sjoden, P., & Burns, T. (1993). Psychosocial adjustment among husbands of women treated for breast cancer: Mastectomy vs. breast-conserving surgery. *European Journal of Cancer, 29A,* 1393-1397.

Partridge, A., Gelber, S., Peppercorn, J., Sampson, E., Knuden, K., Laufer, M., Rosenberg, R., Przypyszny, M., Rein, A., & Winer, E. (2004). Web-based survey of fertility issues in young women with breast cancer. *Journal of Clinical Oncology, 22,* 4174-4183.

Ravdin, P., Siminoff, I., & Harvey, J. (1998). Survey of breast cancer patients concerning their knowledge and expectations of adjuvant therapy. *Journal of Clinical Oncology, 16,* 515-521.

Scherer, K. R. (1982). Emotion as a process: Function, origin, and regulation. *Social Science Information, 21,* 555-570.

Scott, J., Halford, W., & Ward, B. (2004). United we stand? The effects of a couple-coping intervention on adjustment to early-stage breast or gynecological cancer. *Journal of Consulting and Clinical Psychology, 72,* 1122-1135.

Shands, M., Lewis, F., Sinsheimer, J., & Cochrane, B. (2006). Core concerns of couples living with early-stage breast cancer. *Psycho-Oncology, 15,* 1055-1064.

Smith, C. A., & Ellsworth, P. C. (1987). Patterns of appraisal and emotion related to taking an exam. *Journal of Personality and Social Psychology, 52,* 475–488.

Smith, C. A., & Lazarus, R. S. (1990). Emotion and adaptation. In L. A. Pervin (Ed.), *Handbook of personality: Theory and research* (pp. 609–637). New York: Guilford.

Stafford, D., Szczys, R., Becker, R., Anderson, J., & Bushfield, S. (1998). How breast cancer treatment decisions are made by women in North Dakota. *The American Journal of Surgery, 176,* 515-519.

Taylor, S., Fedoroff, I. C., Koch, W. J., Thordarson, D. S., Fecteau, G., & Nicki, R. M. (2001). Posttraumatic stress disorder arising after road traffic collisions: Patterns of response to cognitive behavior therapy. *Journal of Consulting and Clinical Psychology, 69,* 541–551.

Watson, M., St. James-Roberts, I., Ashley, S., Tilney, C., Brougham, B., Edwards, L., Baldus, C., & Romer, G. (2006). Factors associated with emotional and behavioral problems among school age children of breast cancer patients. *British Journal of Cancer, 94,* 43-50.

Weber, K. M., & Solomon, D. H. (2007, November). *A relational turbulence model of distress and communication associated with breast cancer.* Paper presented at the 93rd annual meeting of the National Communication Association, Interpersonal Communication Division, Chicago, IL.

Weber, K. M., & Solomon, D. H. (2008). Locating relationship and communication issues among stressors associated with breast cancer. *Health Communication,* 23, 548-559.

Weber, K. M., Solomon, D. H., & Goodwin, A. (2008, April). *Relational and communicative stressors among breast cancer patients.* Paper presented at the 10th biennial Kentucky Conference of Health Communication, Lexington, KY.

CHAPTER 4

The Role of Couple Communication in Managing Type 2 Diabetes

J. Lynne Brown

THE PENNSYLVANIA STATE UNIVERSITY

Type 2 diabetes is generally diagnosed in older adults and this is a time when family communication patterns are typically well established. This presents a problem for most adults diagnosed with type 2 diabetes because this disease requires tremendous skill adjustments to behavioral patterns if the diabetic is to meet medical treatment guidelines. As a result, the disease affects all household members. In this chapter I define diabetes and establish it as a public health problem, discuss current treatment guidelines, compliance, the role of family support in compliance, and the need for family-based interventions in managing type 2 diabetes. I then present the results of a qualitative study I conducted with couples where one partner had recently been diagnosed with type 2 diabetes. My goal is to illustrate how couple interaction and communication patterns impact disease management.

Occurrence, Treatment, and Compliance

Diabetes mellitus is diagnosed as an inability to reduce blood glucose to normal levels after an overnight fast although there are also physical warning symptoms associated with onset. These high levels of blood glucose damage body proteins and blood vessel walls and, over time, can lead to blindness, kidney function loss and poor wound healing with resultant extremity amputations. Two types are clinically distinguished: type 1 (5-10% of cases) resulting from complete loss of insulin production by the pancreas and type 2 (90-95% of cases) where the insulin that is produced is less effective in controlling blood glucose over time. Insulin is a hormone produced by the pancreas that is responsible for lowering blood glucose levels after a meal (AACE Diabetes Mellitus Clinical Practice Guidelines Taskforce, 2007).

An estimated 21% of the U.S. population is thought to have diabetes mellitus (7%) or be in preclinical mellitus (14%), a condition with a high probability of progression to full blown diabetes. Type 1 is typically a child's disease. Most cases diagnosed after age 40 are type 2 and the prevalence is highest in those age 65-74 years. Among ethnic and racial groups, non-Hispanic whites have the lowest risk and prevalence (AACE, 2007). In the last 20 years, the prevalence of overweight and obesity, risk factors for the development of diabetes, has risen in the US and now 32% of adults and 16% of children are overweight or obese (Hedley, Ogden, Johnson, Carroll, Curtin, & Flegal, 2004; Ogden, Carroll, Curtin, McDowell, Tabak, & Flegal, 2006). This rise in obesity is thought to be contributing to the increased prevalence of diabetes and especially the increase in diagnosis of type 2 in children (AACE, 2007).

Treatment focuses on patient self-management with the support of a health care team (dietitian, endocrinologist, family doctor, etc.) and should include first medical nutrition therapy (MNT) (American Dietetic Association [ADA], 2003), and then drugs plus MNT, increased exercise and self-care instruction on monitoring blood glucose, eyes and feet (AACE, 2007). Instruction may involve several visits with a dietitian to establish dietary goals plus attending group classes that focus on patient skills, although family members may also attend (Franz et al., 1995). The number of skills, lifestyle changes, new terms and goals to reach (hemoglobin A1c (HbA1c), blood glucose, blood lipids, etc.) can be overwhelming (ADA, 2000).

Intensive lifestyle interventions that increase exercise and weight loss (e.g., Knowler et al., 2002; Tuomilehto et al., 2001) or that tightly control blood glucose levels (Diabetes Control and Complications Trial Research Group [DCCTRG], 1993; Writing Team for the DCCT, 2002) do reduce disease progression or long-term complications but require large investments of clinical staff and patient time. In the UK Prospective Diabetes Study (UKPDS) trial, patients receiving just quarterly diet instruction did more poorly than those receiving one of several common drugs in addition to diet instruction suggesting that dietary control was difficult (UKPDS, 1998). Interventions conducted to improve self-management of type 2 diabetes have limited effects on blood glucose control (called glycemic control) after 6 months (Norris, Engelgau, & Narayan, 2001). Indeed, 24 hours of contact time by clinicians or dietitians were needed to reduce HbA1c by 1%, much more than most patients would receive in a year (Norris, Lau, Smith, Schmid, & Engelgau, 2002). Overall, reviews suggest that successful self-management requires much more professional support than is normally provided to insure long-term compliance (Norris et al., 2001). It is not surprising that in the U.S. in 2002, only 40% of adults with type 2 diabetes achieve a HbA1c of less than 7%, as recommended by the American Diabetes Association (Saaddine, Cadwell, Gregg, Engelgau, Vinicor, Imperatore, & Narayan, 2006). Even in academic, top of the line, health care settings, only 7% of patients achieved recommended goals for treatment of blood glucose, blood lipids and high blood pressure (Grant, Buse, & Meigs, 2005). The cost of noncompliance is high and is associated with greater cardiovascular problems, more hospitalizations and higher mortality rates than those in treatment compliance (Muszbek, Brixner, Benedict, Keskinaslan, & Khan, 2008). Better compliance decreases hospital costs, and the indirect costs of loss of workdays or lower productivity.

Why Is Compliance a Problem?

Patient adherence to lifestyle treatment recommendations is low. NHANES III data indicated nearly 70% of people with type 2 diabetes were overweight and not meeting exercise or dietary recommendations (Nelson, Reiber, & Boyko, 2002). Adherence to other treatment recommendations is also low and current efforts to improve this are not effective (Vermeire, Wens, Van Royen, Biot, Hearnshaw, & Lindemeyer, 2005). Although many barriers to treatment compliance have been identified, social support from family and friends is a consistent need reported by patients with type 2 diabetes of various ethnic backgrounds (Albarran, Ballesteros, Morales, & Ortega, 2006; Anderson, Wiggins, Rajawani, Holbrook, Blue, & Ng, 1995; Ary, Toobert, Wilson, & Glasgow, 1986; Kieffer, Willis, Odoms-Young, Guzman, Two Feathers, & Loveluck, 2004; Nagelkerk, Reick, & Meengs, 2006; Vincent, Clark, Zimmer, & Sanchez, 2006; Vijan et al., 2004).

Social support is the exchange of resources or aid between two persons such that the recipient has an increase in well–being. Support can be emotional, appraisal, informational or tangible (Taylor, 1999). Emotional or appraisal support may indirectly foster coping strategies that relieve stress while informational or tangible support may have direct effects on health (Cohen & Hoberman, 1983; Taylor, 1999). Friends, others with the same disease, members of social organizations and of family can all provide social support of various types. Only a half dozen randomized clinical trials have been conducted to examine the effect of social support on treatment adherence in patients with type 2 diabetes (van Dam, van der Horst, Knoops, Ryckman, Crebolder, & van den Borne, 2005). Among the various forms of social support tested, peer groups were most promising. One study found that spousal support (as spouse program attendance) was more effective for women's weight loss than men's, suggesting that women and men with diabetes may approach social support differently (Wing, Marcus, Epstein, & Jawad, 1991). Men may function better as an individual among peers, based on social expectations.

Marriage can affect health. Although the number of older adults who live alone has increased in the past 30 years, nearly 70% of adults, age 40-74, still live in households with a married partner (US Census, 2007). Non-Hispanic adults, age 50 or older, who live with only a spouse have better diet quality than those living alone or with other household arrangements (Davis, Murphy, Neuhaus, Gee, & Quiroga, 2000), indicating that marriage partners influence each other's dietary intake. Indeed, marriage has an impact on health, with positive and negative marital interactions playing a role (Kiecolt-Glaser & Newton, 2001). Higher positive marital adjustment has been associated with greater compliance with blood pressure medication, less weight gain after gastric bypass, better immune function, and fewer risky health habits.

Generally, married people have better health profiles than unmarried people and epidemiological studies indicate that marriage is more beneficial to men's health than women's. Although female personality traits, work/family stress and physiological responses to conflict have all been suggested as reasons why benefits accrue to men rather than women, the factors that explain this difference are still not clear (Kiecolt-Glaser & Newton, 2001). In long-married patients with type 2 diabetes, cross-sectional surveys indicated that degree of marital quality and family function was related to attitudes toward adjustment to diabetes (called psychosocial adaptation) (Fisher et al., 1998; Trief, Grant, Elbert, & Weinstock, 1998; Trief, Orendorff, Himes, & Weinstock, 2001). However, in a two-year study, although marital quality was related to some aspects of self-care at initial assessment and did predict satisfaction with some aspects of the treatment regimen, it did not predict blood glucose testing or control at year year (Trief, Ploutz-Snyder, Britton, & Weinstock, 2004; Trief, Wade, Dee Britton, & Weinstock, 2002). Pieper, Kushion and Gaida (1990) found a married partner's diagnosis of type 2 diabetes after age 40 was associated with more conflict around diet and medications. In particular, the higher the benefit of the dietary treatment to the non-diabetic spouse, the more likely difficulty working with the partner with diabetes was reported. Others have reported that marital conflict was often acted out through the medium of diabetes (Katz, 1969) and the importance of wives in insuring their husband's compliance (Shenkel, Rogers, Perfetto, & Levin, 1985).

Glasgow and Toobert (1988) reported that family support was the strongest predictor of treatment adherence in patients with diabetes. In other studies, patients indicate that, of the skills to master, dietary is the most difficult, exceeding the difficulty of exercise and blood glucose monitoring or insulin injection (Glasgow, Hampson, Strycker, & Ruggiero, 1997; Vijan et al., 2004). Patients with type 2 diabetes report that families could have positive or negative effects on dietary compliance (Albright et al., 2001; Gerstle, Varenne, & Contento, 2001) but lack of family support was a key barrier to maintaining the diet regardless if African American, White or Hispanic (Carter-Edwards, Skelly, Cagle, & Appel, 2004; Vijan et al., 2004; Wen, Parchman, & Shepherd, 2004). African American women reported their family and friends did not really understand "what a diabetic is." They felt pressured to eat inappropriate foods due to family member food preferences and unwillingness to adopt a healthful diet, and family member communication tactics (giving orders, treating them like children) also created conflict (Carter-Edwards et al., 2004). Cultural expectations about foods served at family meals limited some patients' ability to control their own eating patterns (Lawton, Ahmad, Hanna, Douglas, Bains, & Hallowell, 2008). Family members purchasing tempting foods or eating foods the patient should not eat were key problems as were social events, all indicating that families generally did not adopt the healthful diet plan prescribed for the patient (Schlundt, Rea, Kline, & Pichert, 1994; Vijan et al., 2004; Vincent et al., 2006; Wen, Shepherd, & Parchman, 2004). In contrast, family care givers of elderly diabetics reported two important hurdles to diabetes care management were dealing with patient moods and *non-compliance,* and decision making and communication with other family members (Hennessy, John, & Anderson, 1999). Thus reports from both patients and those providing care indicate the need to expand family member involvement in treatment and for effective communication.

Family-Centered Diabetes Management

The self-care focus of current diabetes management produces poor compliance, necessitating the examination of alternative approaches. Family centered, rather than patient centered, treatment of type 2 diabetes has been discussed for nearly 20 years (Patterson, & Garwick, 1994).

A chronic disease like diabetes affects the entire family system, as a change in one part of the system inadvertently changes other parts (Patterson & Garwick, 1994). The family system includes structures (e.g., boundaries that define who is or is not a member) and functional components (patterns of relationships among the members) described as cohesion, flexibility, problem solving style, etc. Chronic illness can impact family boundaries, alter relationships and create stress. Family adaptation requires resources. Among important family resources are clarity of rules and expectations, effective communication skills, flexibility and supportive relationships, most of which must be employed to cope with the chronic illness. Patterson and Garwick (1994) argued that treatment of chronic disease should be family focused and protocols should be developed and tested with various types of families. The working group on family–based interventions in chronic disease sponsored by the National Academy of Sciences (Fisher & Weihs, 2000) agreed and recommended a family-based approach to disease treatment in contrast to current self-care treatment aimed at the patient. With the diagnosis, families can reorganize to "own the disease" and support treatment or families can undermine disease management, isolating the patient and making compliance and positive outcomes more problematic. They identified three approaches for disease management: 1) family education about the disease, 2) work on family relationships and 3) psychotherapy, for especially dysfunctional families. However, the majority of family interventions focused on chronic disease have addressed diseases of childhood or adolescence. Although fewer family interventions to address adult chronic disease are available as models, these indicate that low family cohesion, high family conflict, extremes of family boundary permeability, poor communication and low spouse involvement contribute to poor disease outcomes (Fisher et al., 1998; Fisher & Weihs, 2000).

Similar factors have been found for type 2 diabetes. Cross-sectional surveys of samples of European American, Hispanic, Chinese American and African American families in which one adult partner had diabetes, revealed that conflict resolution was important for the patient's morale, satisfaction with diabetes management, quality of life and for reducing depression (Chesla et al., 2004; Fisher, Chesla, Chun, Skaff, Mullan, & Kanter, 2004; Fisher, Gudmundsdottir, Gilliss et al., 2000). Conflict resolution and the needed communication skills appear important for emotional management. Family organization (cohesion and sex-defined roles) was also related to positive disease outcomes in European American and Hispanic families (Fisher, Chesla, Skaff et al., 2000) suggesting that clear family roles help mediate conflict resolution and less conflict contributes to better health outcomes. Despite the consistent identification of conflict resolution as an important factor, how conflict is resolved is likely to differ among ethnic groups. Further work using videotaped discussions revealed that in Latino couples (Fisher, Gudmundsdotir, Gillis et al.), where traditional household roles dominate, discussion of problems and their resolution occurred more often for male than for female patients while for European American couples there was an opposite trend. This suggests that adjustment to diabetes may differ by gender.

Most actual family-based treatment interventions for diabetes mellitus have focused on type 1 diabetes. A majority of thirteen clinical trials targeting a parent (usually the mother) and the children with type 1 reduced HbA1c significantly, and some reduced conflict in families, while in three different intervention trials targeting disease management in adults with type 1, including the spouse appeared to increase diabetic compliance (Armour, Norris, Jack., Zhang, & Fisher, 2005). Despite the lack of family-based intervention data for type 2 diabetes, Fisher et al. (1998) proposed a family-based context for treatment of type 2 diabetes that would involve evaluation of family functioning, couple beliefs and allocation of disease management behaviors to guide clinical input into disease management. However, no data is available to support this approach.

Gender Differences in Diabetes Experience

The observation that men tend to die earlier than women but women tend to have higher rates of morbidity (chronic health problems) has been accepted as truth for many years (Verbrugge, 1982; Macintyre, Hunt, & Sweeting, 1996). Verbrugge suggested that this could be due to sex differences in genetic factors, environmental and lifestyle exposure, and socially defined health behaviors. Some think the morbidity observation is a simplification. Careful examination of British health survey data (Macintyre et al.) revealed that women were more likely to report certain malaise and physical symptoms significantly more often than men, but there were no sex differences in many other symptoms examined. Additionally only a few chronic diseases were more common in women than in men and the direction and magnitude of sex differences in health varied according to the symptom or disease and the lifecycle stage. Still, similar disease prevalence across the sexes does not mean the disease ramifications are the same for each sex.

As for diabetes, overall diabetes mellitus prevalence is nearly equal for men and women although prevalence varies greatly by race and ethnic group (Correa-de-Araujo et al., 2006). However, its prevalence is growing fastest among older minority women. Once diagnosed, compared to men, women have twice the risk for developing coronary artery disease, a higher risk of hypertension and a greater risk of death from cardiovascular disease. These outcomes plus other risk factors more prevalent in women than men suggest that the disease experience is different for men and women, and that management programs should be tailored to these differences (Legato et al., 2006). Yet household survey data indicates that women received some diabetes services significantly less frequently than men (Legato et al.), perhaps because most treatment regimens, developed using male subjects, are tied to men's treatment (Correa-de-Araujo et al.) or women ignore their own symptoms more than men.

Gendered role expectations affect response to a disease. Ballantyne (1999) argues that economic and social factors influence health outcomes in men and women because these are mediated through gender identities that define expected roles both in the workplace and in the home. Women often have jobs of lower quality (less power and control) than men, and the positive effect of paid employment on health is weaker for women than men. In particular, women face gender and economic inequities within households, where women often balance outside jobs with internal household labor in gender-defined roles of food production and family care giving. Women are more likely to experience role strain and stress overload due to unsuccessful balance of work and family responsibilities while occupational status and job-related stress are more likely to affect men's health. Household structure, access to resources, power differentials and cultural norms all play out in the family, where health is created and maintained through day-to-day decisions (Moss, 2002). Denton and Walters (1999) found that women living alone reported better perceived health than those living with a partner and children, while men living in a nuclear family reported better health than those living alone. In each case the relationship did not hold for the other sex. Although social support was important to the health of both sexes, it was significantly more important for women than men. Thus, the family situation and social support play different roles in men, and women's health and are likely to affect how they would respond to emergence of a chronic illness in a family member. While marriage is health enhancing for men, its gender-based inequities can produce gender-based stressors that could negatively affect women's health.

Focusing again on diabetes, married or cohabiting women face challenges regardless of who receives the diagnosis of diabetes because of their household and caretaking roles (Hepworth, 1999; Sarkadi & Rosenqvist, 2002; Wong, Gucciardi, Li, & Grace, 2005). More men than women generally comply with the treatment recommendation to exercise (Nelson et al., 2002; Whittemore, Melkus, & Grey, 2005). In qualitative interviews, women with type 2 diabetes indicated that household role expectations (preparing meals, caregiving of others) coupled with employment eliminated or reduced time for exercise (Sarkadi & Rosenqvist, 2002). While men might also face time restrictions from their jobs, their non-involvement in these household chores could leave more time for exercise. Dietary compliance, the most difficult of the lifestyle modifications that patients with diabetes face (Wong et al.), usually become the wife's job as women still do most of the food chores (Harnack, Story, Martinson, Neumark-Sztainer, & Stang, 1998; Wansink, 2006), even in families where one adult has type 2 diabetes (Miller & Brown, 2005; Wong et al.). Qualitative studies consistently indicate that men with diabetes are more likely to receive tangible dietary support from their wives, while women with diabetes face one of two situations: receiving passive support from her husband as she makes some meal modifications or retaining other family member favored meal patterns and making her personal dietary adjustments on the side (Hepworth, 1999; Miller & Brown; Wong et al.). Many women seem to put their dietary adjustment secondary to family food preferences both in shopping (Miller, Warland, & Achterberg, 1997) and cooking (Hepworth, 1999; Miller & Brown; Sarkadi & Rosenqvist; Wong et al.).

Hepworth (1999) outlined how married women with diabetes construct the positions they take in their own diet management. Generally, catering to the husband's preferences was based on beliefs that the husband had no cooking skills, that diabetes is the patient's (her) problem and that the partner's resistance to change makes the wife's efforts futile. In this situation, the wife would eat smaller portions of the same food or only certain of the dishes presented to avoid cooking herself a separate meal. If the husband was also subsequently diagnosed with diabetes, these wives with diabetes addressed his dietary requirements over their own although this allowed them to address their own needs secondarily. Deference to male food preferences could extend to sons whose meal preferences were satisfied to the determent of the diabetic mother's needs. Thus, women appear to construct their diabetes management within the framework of their gendered roles making it difficult for many to enact the behavioral changes necessary to control their own diabetic symptoms.

In contrast, both men and women with diabetes indicate that friends (and family) are often unsupportive and insensitive to their needs in social situations where food is served. Friends criticize what they choose to eat (Wong et al., 2005), or see the disease as a result of their faulty lifestyle habits (Sarkadi & Rosenqvist, 2002). Not surprisingly, diabetics were sensitive about identifying their condition at work or social gatherings (Miller & Brown, 2005; Sarkadi & Rosenqvist). Coping with these expectations and demands from family and friends can be stressful. Both problem- and emotion-oriented methods of coping with stressful situations have been identified and more effective stress reduction is based on use of a broader repertoire of strategies (Taylor, 1999). Early studies indicated that men with diabetes used more problem-solving strategies while women with diabetes relied on more emotional and social coping skills (Diehl, Coyle, & Labouvie-Vief, 1996; Kvam & Lyons, 1991). Recently, Gafvels and Wandell (2006) found that men and women with diabetes did not differ in use of problem solving but that women, of whom 70% were married, were significantly more likely to use resignation, protest and isolation as coping strategies than men. Overall women were more likely to use negative coping strategies than men although both were equally likely to use a repertoire of positive coping strategies as well. Unfortunately, use of the three negative strategies identified was positively correlated with HbA1c levels. Use of negative coping may be a result of women's restricted ability to manage their own diabetes because of traditional family role expectations.

The Study: Couple Adjustment to Type 2 Diabetes

In order to examine couples' adjustment to diabetes, semi-structured interviews were conducted with 20 married couples in which one had been recently diagnosed with diabetes. This study was conceptually guided by Olson's Circumplex Model of Family Functioning (Olson, McCubbin, Barnes, Larsen, Muxen, & Wilson, 1989), which proposes that the emotional closeness (*cohesion*) and *adaptability* of families are key to coping with a stressful event like the diagnosis of diabetes (Lavee & Olson, 1991). The interviews focused on adaptability (i.e., flexibility) in managing the stressor of diabetes, which could require altering family rules, roles and power structures (Gorell & Olson, 1995). Gorell and Olson point out that how the couple adapts to stressors is facilitated by and managed through communication. Given this theoretical framework, I posed the following research questions to guide the inquiry: Since diagnosis, how have couples adapted to the patient's diabetes? How does communication affect their adaptation?

Participants

Couples were recruited from several hospital diabetes education classes. Criteria were that 1) type 2 diabetes was diagnosed within one year of recruitment; 2) the person with diabetes was age 45 or older; 3) the couple was married or cohabiting; 4) both partners agreed to be interviewed; and 5) at least the patient had completed hospital-sponsored sessions on diabetes management. Sampling was purposeful to secure equal numbers of each sex with diabetes and a mix of those reporting success or difficulty adjusting to management. Interviews were conducted at two time points, initially (T1) and again a year later (T2), to understand more about adaptation as a process over time. Couples were interviewed together to investigate joint perceptions and then separately to investigate personal perceptions. The interview schedule was semi-structured employing open-ended questions to assess adjustment to the diagnosis and the new dietary regimen. A qualitative grounded thematic analysis using constant comparison was conducted (Glaser & Strauss, 1967) to identify ways in which the couple adapted to diabetes initially and over time. Determinations of each couple's types of interaction around the dietary regimen at both time 1 and time 2 were made to see if there were consistent patterns of adaptation. Then, within each pattern, qualitative content analysis was conducted (see Mayring, 2000) to identify communication patterns.

Findings

Time One (T1)

In this sample, men's mean age was 65 while women were generally ten years younger. Couples had been married a mean of 30 years and the majority had only a high school education. In the T1 interviews, many couples described an initial period of denial and mourning when the couple, but most importantly the diabetic, came to accept that the diagnosis was real. The length of this period varied but was still evident in some couples at T2, a year later. The findings did not suggest clear patterns of gender difference, but three distinct management styles of adjustment to the diabetic regimen emerged. Those three management styles were called "cohesive," "enmeshed," and "disengaged," borrowing terms from the Circumplex Model, and represent varying degrees of couple flexibility.[1] A description and discussion of distinct *management styles* are presented below, providing excerpts from the interviews to illustrate how communication patterns influenced couple adjustment to type 2 diabetes.

Couples with cohesive management style. Couples labeled as *"cohesive"* (n = 5 couples, 3 females and 2 males with diabetes) generally worked as a team to adjust to the dietary recommendations, although the degree of teamwork varied. Both partners in each of these five couples made many dietary changes in meals and snacks so that, in essence, both adopted the "diabetic diet" to some degree for themselves, especially at the main dinner or supper meal. For some, this meant both partners learned to like new food choices and new methods of cooking. The following exchange illustrates this change:

ND[2]: Well, when I found out that he had to start counting carbs I figured that it would be best if I went on it with him, to help him and we would count carbs together and we could keep track of each other and he could tell me and I could tell him and be a support for one another cause he knows I have been trying to lose weight and it is hard for me to lose weight. And that was one reason I wanted to go on it but basically to help him, to help motivate him to stay on it.

1 Editor's note: The management styles of "cohesive," "enmeshed," and "disengaged" refer to couple flexibility here in this chapter. This is in contrast to the original Circumplex model that would refer to these as levels of emotional bonding.

2 ND = non-diabetic partner; DB = diabetic partner; IN = interviewer.

IN: What was his reaction?

ND: Well, I think he appreciated that because he knows we both like to eat and he knows what a sacrifice that would be to cut down on things I really like, like baking. (Couple 5, male diabetic)

Among these couples, roles were adjusted so meal planning was shared and the couple worked together to understand the need for and to make cooperative decisions about food choices for daily meals. Some gave up cherished roles like baking, such as in the excerpt above. Yet others take on the new role of counting and monitoring carbohydrates for the diabetic patient. In the excerpt below a non-diabetic wife assumes the role of the monitor while the husband continues his role as cook.

ND: Well we usually talk it over. [DB agrees] About what we want to have and discuss how we are going to do it and I figure out how many carbs are in everything that we are gonna have and the fat and the protein and that is how we figure it out.

IN: How about shopping?

ND: We do that together and like I said, check the labels for the carbs now instead of the salt or whatever we are doing.

DB: Well I always did watch the salt. (Couple 5, male diabetic)

New rules were negotiated for snacks allowed in the house, what foods were served during family visits, meal schedules, meal preparation methods, and restaurant selection. Rules were also established about discussion of the diagnosis in social settings. No one particular set of rules fit all couples, especially around snacks, since what was tempting varied with the person. The following illustrates accommodation for non-tempting and tempting snacks:

IN: What about food he eats that is different than yours?

DB: It is mostly his candies. Since he can eat that kind of food, like I will get cupcakes and different things, which I will put in the side of the freezer door. If he wants something, he will go get it. It does not bother me. If we go to the store, he will get what he wants and he knows I will not

> get into it. There were [these] things in the house before I was diagnosed that did not bother me. Nuts and ice cream on the other hand they are tempting [and kept out of the house], but nothing else bothers me. (Couple 9, female diabetic)

Communication in these couples was considered to be conversational in quality and characterized by openness. Eating behaviors and food choices were discussed freely and in detail. Non-diabetic spouses learned and practiced softer monitoring messages so that these comments were seen as suggestions or gentle reminders of what the partner with diabetes should be doing. This is illustrated in the following exchange where a non-diabetic partner talked about the importance of "not harping" on the issue.

IN: Anything you might say that would make it more difficult for her?

ND: I don't know how to put it. Um, how can I say it? I am compassionate towards her feelings. I know what she likes and what she dislikes. I know what upsets her. I know what makes her happy. And I don't ask the wrong questions. [Like] I would say something dealing with her weight or with her sugar, her feet. The best thing would be "don't harp on the issue." You have to have an understanding that they're going through a hard time too, harder than what I am going through. (Couple 3, female diabetic)

Overall, both spouses in "cohesive" couples were attempting to master new dietary management skills, altering their roles to enable this mastery, and were practicing the communication principles of attentive and empathic listening, discussing options and feelings, and negotiating a set of agreeable rules.

Couples with enmeshed management style. In couples identified as *"enmeshed"* (*n* = 7 couples, 2 females and 5 males with diabetes), the spouse without diabetes (i.e., non-diabetic) was responsible for most of the management chores and day-to-day monitoring. In "enmeshed" couples, the non-diabetic partner typically demanded the compliance of the diabetic partner, and the diabetic partner was highly dependent on the non-diabetic partner. Most non-diabetic partners took over diet management because they were already the cooks in the family. Often the diabetic partner did not agree to the dietary changes made by the non-diabetic partner and these changes appeared to be imposed rather than discussed by the couple, as admitted in the following excerpt:

IN: She changed your diet pretty radically.

DB: I think I had to put a check on that too, you know the diet. She will say "well you are not supposed to do this." And I will say "hey wait a minute, that was not want was said at the meeting," you know what I mean. With the diet she would want to do more, I think, you follow me.

IN: Did you have disagreements about that?

DB: I guess you could call it disagreements. Like she said to me the other night, maybe your reading is high because you had a beer today. I say "when I talked to Jenny out here [at the hospital meeting], they did not want you to cut out everything completely," in other words you are permitted to. In fact I was surprised that they let you have as much to eat as they do. They are talking about three meals and snacks in between. (Couple 6, male diabetic)

While both spouses might benefit from following the more healthful diet needed to manage diabetes, frequent disagreement about its necessity was a challenge for the non-diabetic spouse who often perceived him- or herself as doing most of the work. The following non-diabetic partner stated:

ND: Well I know he gets resentful when I tell him you shouldn't eat something. It's been hard on me, you know. Of course we both need to be on diets, so it's been good for me. But mainly controlling what he eats falls, you know pretty much on me. He gets upset when I tell him he should not eat something or he is allowed to eat anything he wants to eat but you have to keep it within proportions. And if you want to eat one thing, you have to give up something else. Am I right that this is hard to do? (Couple 12, male diabetic)

For the "enmeshed" couples, food preparation roles were not shared and did not appear to change with the diagnosis. Years of experience and the cook's greater skills were often the diabetic's reasons for not taking on diet management responsibility. Sometimes the non-diabetic spouse continued in the well-worn role because the diabetic was easy to cook for and had no interest in either shopping or cooking. The non-diabetic spouse in one "enmeshed" couple did adopt new roles, but then he reconsidered the wisdom of that adaptation strategy in the following remarks.

ND: When it comes time for her to take her blood sugar, I get the stuff out, lay it out for her. I even put the needles in and take them out and get them ready. All she has to do is come over and take it. So I told her, "I think I do too much for you. I think that is the problem here."

DB: No you don't.

ND: I think I do overdo a bit too much in helping her. [Helping her with] things she should be doing herself. (Couple 8, female diabetic)

Many of the "enmeshed" non-diabetic spouses were dealing with a diabetic partner who resisted compliance with dietary restriction. Managing other's intake was frustrating and difficult, especially when taking on the task of managing portion size. One participant explained:

ND: Trying to keep her on her own limit of what she is allowed to have. Every once in a while she wants to cheat a bit on me… "Everything is measured out for you, right there." I said, "Look at the measuring cups." I got about four sets of [measuring cups] and I use two or three of them in a meal. She says, "I can have a little more." I say, "No, no you had enough. You don't need no more." (Couple 8, female diabetic)

For "enmeshed" couples, rules did not appear to be discussed but were often based on personal beliefs or assumptions of the non-diabetic spouse about how things should be managed. These included determining who should and should not be told about the partner's diabetes and the management of snacks and treats. Some couples reported that public comments about the diabetes triggered arguments. A non-diabetic wife recalled:

ND: He would prefer that I not mention it [his diabetes]. In fact, he gets very upset with me if I do talk about it. But, we have friends that also have that problem and I think that is probably why we should talk about it. But he gets upset if I do. He say, "I wish you wouldn't say anything!" So, I gotta learn to keep my mouth shut. (Couple 12, male diabetic)

Methods of handling sweets and treats were based on several assumptions, with no discussion of rules that might satisfy both partners' needs. One assumption of non-diabetics in "enmeshed" couples was that the diabetic could just ignore or learn to ignore tempting foods brought into the house. After all, the non-diabetic spouse could eat these foods. Another assumption was that if treats were hidden, there would be no temptation for the diabetic partner. Some non-diabetic spouses hid tempting foods in special spots (the bedroom, the back of the freezer, or a particular drawer) and would go out of the diabetic's sight (i.e., into another room) to indulge in the tempting food. Partners with diabetes, however, were usually aware of the location of the "secret" supply. While some diabetics felt keeping treats in the house was necessary to harden them against temptation, most reported they would have preferred tempting treats not be brought into the home.

IN: What if he stopped eating candy altogether?

DB: Oh I would love that. But he won't. (Couple 8, female diabetic)

Generally, in the "enmeshed" couples, non-diabetic spouses assumed they could continue eating, buying, or making tempting foods and that it was up to the diabetic to deal with the temptation.

For these couples, communication tended to be one sided, with one partner dominating the interview conversation. Closed channels of communication characterized these couples. One non-diabetic wife remembers:

ND: The last weekend I said, "Hey you are on your own and I will just set food on the table and just see." But that is the roughest times, letting him on his own.

IN: Are there other times when you get a better reaction from him?

ND: No. I can't say that he does not appreciate my cooking for him. He just does not like me telling him he is not allowed to eat something. I think he resents it. And he is definitely embarrassed by that fact that he has diabetes, it can't be happening to him, and it is an embarrassment to him. But, hey, this happens. You live with it. It is not something to be hidden. We all have problems. (Couple 12, male diabetic)

Many of the wives in this sample noted that changing their interaction style is difficult to do at this stage in their marriage. One wife said:

> ND: I am sometimes blunt to the point and sometimes to my own disadvantage. Or maybe I just treat him too much like I would a child. I don't know. Because you know with kids, you tell them, hey, this is the way it is gonna be. Maybe that is the mothering instinct in me. That is what we women are supposed to be doing. (Couple 12, male diabetic)

Another explained:

> ND: Oh he sort of gives a dirty look and does not like it but he is okay after that. I feel he knows I am working for his lifestyle, his diet and we have been married 54 years so after a while you get to know, he knows I am working for him and he appreciates it in his own way. But it is hard. (Couple 6, male diabetic)

Generally communication was considered closed because spouses were unwilling to openly discuss the prescribed diet or negotiate rules agreeable to both. Monitoring was also a contentious area and non-diabetic spouses did not seem overly willing to renegotiate ingrained patterns of eating, cooking, or interacting. This pattern of closed communication hindered effective rule-making and may have increased their diabetic partner's dependency. This pattern of communicating could also erode the non-diabetic partner's willingness to master the diet regimen skills needed to self-manage the diabetes.

Couples with disengaged management style. In *"disengaged" couples* (N = 8 couples; 3 male and 5 females with diabetes) the diabetic spouses were entirely responsible for their own disease management. Disengagement involved high levels of independence and separateness. For "disengaged" couples, if the diabetic spouse was the food preparer, their partner either passively accepted changes made in meals or refused to accept changes in the usual food pattern, forcing the diabetic to adjust on his or her own. The non-diabetic partners who cooked showed little interest in altering food preparation methods or menus to accommodate the diabetic diet plan. Some non-diabetic partners continued purchasing and eating tempting snacks or sweets or baking tempting desserts, which made it difficult for the diabetic spouse to manage their food choices. Since personal motivation is critical to addressing disease management, most diabetic spouses in "disengaged" couples were doing little or nothing to address their treatment regimen.

Personal independence and the need for personal agency in controlling the diabetes were the most prominent traits of "disengaged" partners with diabetes. Many personalized the disease and believed it was their problem alone and that they should manage it with no help or supervision. In some cases both partners endorsed independence and separateness from each other, such as in the following exchange:

IN: Does he ask your opinion on this?

ND: Not really that I can think of. Like do you think I should have this or do you think this would—No, because he is pretty independent. Like he sat here and said, and I didn't even realize, he has got it down pat how many carbohydrates and how many fats he is suppose to have. He knows what he has to do and what he is supposed to do and he will do it eventually.

IN: [Directed to the spouse] Would you change her level of involvement?

DB: I don't think I would probably change it at all because I would not want her to be more domineering as far as telling me what to do. I know what I have to do. And if it comes down to it, I will do it. On the other hand, I don't want her to have the attitude I don't care. So she is in between and it is just the way we do it. (Couple 7, male diabetic)

This independence also meant some diabetic spouses did nothing to address diet management and their partners would make no effort to try to help them. The following exchange illustrates how a non-diabetic partner can assume the attitude of "it's his/her problem, not mine:"

IN: What were your feelings about the diagnosis?

ND: Me? I don't know. I didn't really think about it I guess. I know she has been having problems, but she is usually in denial about all her problems. It did not matter what. Getting her to the doctor is a job. She never did go to the doctor. In fact, she does not follow plans very well, whether it is for weight problems or whether it is for diabetes.

DB: I am not a program person.

ND: She starts out meaning well, but it sort of fades off. In fact, I think this program has too. She is not really following it like she should be. (Couple 17, female diabetic)

Roles were generally not shared in these "disengaged" couples, although a few highly motivated diabetic men took on new shopping or meal planning roles to influence their wives. Sometimes, the non-diabetic spouse did not appreciate the efforts made by the diabetic partner, such as in the following example where the diabetic spouse now helps with the shopping.

ND: Shopping is taking more time and I don't have patience. I can't stand around a bunch of people or in close spaces so I want to get my shopping done and get out. And it is taking too much time [to read labels etc]. Cause he pokes around looking at stuff we don't even…we are not going to buy, and he is wasting more of my time. So I actually prefer to do it alone but I don't have the nerve to tell him because he likes to do it. (Couple 2, male diabetic)

In these "disengaged" couples, often the non-diabetic cook was making little or no accommodation for the meal plan needs of the diabetic. In this couple, the partner continued to cook as she had before the diagnosis and the male diabetic had to make his adjustments around the edges.

ND: We eat the same thing [at dinner]. I don't cook two different meals. This is why I would never go on any diets that the doctor gave me because I would have to had cook two different ways, one for him and one for me and I would not do that. So I did not go on the diet, now I will go with him.

DB: Last night we had rigatonis with sauce and this did not come out with enough carbohydrate so I ate a slice of bread with peanut butter on it to get the protein and we had cantaloupe and watermelon chunks for dessert.

ND: I did not eat the peanut butter and the stuff he does, but we eat the same thing. I just make sure he gets the fruit now where I was never sure of before, I did not bother putting fruit on before, but he is supposed to have that, so now I put that on and that is about it. (Couple 2, male diabetic)

Wives with diabetes who were cooks generally made meals that matched the husbands' expectations and then adjusting ingredients and portion sizes for themselves. One participant admitted this approach in the following exchange:

IN: So how did the diet work out—eating according to the diet plan?

DB: I just cook and he eats it.

IN: What about portioning?

ND: I eat as much as I want.

DB: He does [eat as much as he wants] and I measure...He probably does not notice a big difference because I am the one that does the cooking and I make sure the recipes taste right...It is a pain to make two meals. So we are just gonna eat the way he needs to eat and I kind of manipulate mine. (Couple 16, female diabetic)

For "disengaged" couples, rules that might help the diabetic adjust were not discussed or established. The most troublesome arena for these couples was establishing rules for sweets and snacks. Some non-diabetic partners recognized that foods they brought home were tempting, but they were not willing to give these up. In the excerpt below, the non-diabetic wife explains why she continues to have her snacks, the diabetic husband indicates why he does not push this issue, and the wife outlines an unsatisfactory strategy to deal with the snack problem.

IN: How do you expect to work this out in the future?" (This is in reference to her stash of snacks in her bedroom that he finds tempting.)

DB: Well, we will probably get better, either I will quit eating it or she will quit buying it.

ND: I will probably quit buying it, that is the only way he will quit eating it. I am getting used to not having this or that gradually. I am like a little kid; you got to wean me off this stuff. I have to have something to munch on.

The husband acknowledges he knows she leaves tempting items like zucchini bread and potato chips sitting on the counter, but he is not likely to say anything because...

DB: I don't want to get an argument started. Then she will say, "If you want some of it you will find it no matter where I put it," which I probably would. But if I say anything to her about nibbling all the time, then she gets upset and then she might not speak to me the rest of the day, you know, and I don't like that.

IN: What strategy would help with the snack problem?

ND: The only thing I can think of is to absolutely hide the darn things. And I don't purposely eat them in front of him because I feel guilty. So, I get them past him and into the bedroom quick enough and it is not really too bad. (Couple 2, male diabetic)

In other cases, the diabetic cannot face setting rules about the snack problem. In this example, both partners, but especially the non-diabetic husband, bring sweets and treats into the house although they both claim that they don't buy "that much" of the tempting food items.

IN: What would be a good solution to this [problem of sweets in the house]?

ND: Don't buy it, although he does this anyway.

DB: Yeah but I think if it was not there and I could not get a bite here and there it would be worse. Then I would really feel like I was deprived. I am never gonna just...

ND: Quit. (Couple 19, female diabetic)

For "disengaged" couples, communication about the diabetes regimen was generally closed. Sometimes the diabetic spouse fought with the non-diabetic spouse to establish their superior knowledge of diabetic treatment information and to maintain control of their disease management. Most often, though, there was no discussion of the meal plan at all. The diabetic partners in these couples tended to "own" the disease and preferred to take control of its management. One couple shared the following:

IN: You have an idea of how many [food] exchanges you are to have?

DB: I know what I am supposed to have. [He lists these off for each meal.]

IN: Do you talk about exchanges much?

ND: You mean between us? No, we don't discuss it.

DB: No, it isn't like you sit down and discuss, whether I should have a potato tonight or something else in its place, no.

IN: Do you comment much on each other's eating?

DB: Not really. (Couple 7, male diabetic)

In other cases, the non-diabetic partner had little or no interest in such a discussion, even if the diabetic partner would participate.

IN: How is communication about the diet?

DB: Not good. We are very different. He is a very structured person, very neat, extremely neat, very organized and very disciplined. I am those things in my own way. But I am not like him. We often have a hard time in crises, being able to talk to each other. We tend to handle things privately…We have been married 28 years. But it has been hard for both of us. But we talk better now than we used to, but probably not as well as we should, and as well as I would like us to talk. He tends to be real critical and he always thinks I am undisciplined, that I am messy. When I first came home [after the diagnosis], he said it was my problem and I had to take care of it, and he was not involved with it. This really floored me that he had that kind of attitude this time [because he previously helped me with my broken leg]. But, he has done better since that first day. (Couple 16, female diabetic)

Monitoring intake tended to be a difficult process and could lead to angry outbursts. In the following example, the diabetic makes a clear distinction between receiving messages of support and messages that are interpreted as directives or nagging.

DB: I don't need you *telling* me. Supporting me is one thing and telling me something else. You are very supportive. But that is why you are so out in left field there .....Mainly you hammer me about the exercise thing. It is not the eating. It is like, "Go out and walk," which I know, if you would quit telling me to. Like, even my smoking. I know I should not smoke. I get real defensive on that. That is me. Defiant. Cut off my nose to spite my own face. I am doing the harm to me but at the same time, it's like, "Don't tell me!" (Couple 10, female diabetic)

The issue of nagging in the monitoring process was reported as a constant source of tension. Nagging could result in demand-withdraw patterns, belligerence, and spiteful reactions. One participant explained this process,

IN: How often do you make suggestions to try and keep her on track?

ND: Probably as much as I can. I hate to nag her all the time. I know at times you hate to be bugging her all the time about what she eats. Sometimes I just back off and figure, let her do it and I guess now and then I will start making a comment and sometimes it feels I am nagging her too much. But I try to keep after her as much as I can.

IN: How does she respond?

ND: Sometimes negative, sometimes positive. Once in a while she will say, I know I should not be doing this and you know let me do what I want. I think if you push too hard sometimes it is worse than not pushing at all. I think she gets a little more belligerent, more in denial of what she should be doing. (Couple 17, female diabetic)

Another shared...

IN: What are not good things to say?

ND: You shouldn't eat that [in a disapproving voice]. Just to come right out and say you know, well you should not eat another portion or you should not eat that.

IN: Why?

ND: Well he would probably just eat it to spite me. It is more of a reason to eat it probably. (Couple 7, male diabetic)

While the "disengaged" diabetic spouse generally appreciated praise for some accomplishment around their treatment regimen, there were cases in which no support was expected from the spouse. Surprisingly, there were also instances where the diabetic spouse interpreted support as enabling behavior and was grateful to receive no support. One participant shared,

> DB: I never look for compliments or anything. It is just if I have to do it, I do it. I just got used to doing it on my own instead of depending on somebody for support. I don't really look for support. It would be a lot easier to support somebody who was looking for support. It is not that she does not want to be supportive. I just don't look for her to be supportive. (Couple 14, male diabetic)

Another explained,

> DB: I will come in and I will say, "Well, I don't feel good today" and she will say, "You are not getting any sympathy off me." And I think she did that just so I would help myself more. She did not want me to get dependent on somebody and I thank her for that. (Couple 2, male diabetic)

Overall, in these "disengaged" couples, the diabetic spouse faced numerous challenges for their disease management. Only if the diabetic was highly skilled, motivated and possessed strong willpower was he or she able to follow diabetes regimen recommendations. Moreover, if dialogue occurred about the diabetes, it was not about expressing expectations, setting rules, dealing with problematic behavior, or enabling a smooth adjustment to the diet regimen.

From the analysis of the interview data at Time 1, it appears that there are patterned ways that couples adapt to the onset of diabetes for one of its partners. The management practices were distinctive across the three management styles of couple adaptation: "cohesive," "enmeshed," and "disengaged."

Follow-up Interviews (T2)

Of the 20 couples who participated in T1 interviews, 19 were interviewed again a year later to learn progress in adjustment to the treatment regimen (T2). The interview analysis revealed that the couples originally categorized as *"disengaged"* couples remained disengaged in their management of diabetes at T2. Interestingly, seven additional couples (4 originally "cohesive" couples and 3 originally "enmeshed" couples) reported a disengaged approach to diabetes management. So, at T2, the disengaged pattern of diabetes management was the most prominent pattern, followed by "enmeshed" (n = 4), and "cohesive" (n = 1). Only one couple retained open communication about diabetes and had established rules acceptable to both partners. In this couple, the diabetic wife had taken more individual control of her regimen management in the 12-month period.

In this sample, the shift to a *disengaged style* of disease management was facilitated by a breakdown of rules, an unwillingness to set more acceptable rules, and a low level of interest in participating in discussions or working together to maintain the meal plan. For couples who previously reported an enmeshed style of disease management at T1 but shifted to a disengaged style at T2, blaming and disagreements were more common than for other couples at T2. For couples who previously reported a cohesive style of disease management at T1 but shifted to a disengaged style at T2, family health problems and financial problems increased more than for other couples. In most of these couples, the diet reverted or was reverting to pre-diabetic patterns. Even among the remaining "enmeshed" couples (n = 4) at T2, the caregiver was less careful about meal planning and the diabetic was less willing to abide by their rules. For all, the initial attention to the diabetic diet had lessened and communication about disease management had stopped altogether or was greatly diminished.

Although there was less communication about and attention paid to disease management at T2, diabetic partners in some couples managed to achieve some degree of dietary compliance across the 12-month period. There was no particular pattern related to this compliance, as one couple with a cohesive style, one with an enmeshed style, and five with a disengaged style of disease management achieved this. The couple with an enmeshed style to disease management attributed their success to the male diabetic's high adherence to his wife's rules and diet management methods. For those employing a disengaged style, the five successful diabetics (2 men and 3 women) were solely responsible for handling their diabetes (including food shopping and preparation) so there was no need to adjust roles and rules and partner food choices were not altered. By assuming the entire disease management burden, these diabetic partners reported that couple discussion of disease management was minimal. Regimen compliance in the other 12 couples remained low or deteriorated.

Summary

In this chapter, I illustrate how couple interaction and communication patterns impact disease management. Clearly, diabetes management research needs to move beyond the focus on just the partner with diabetes to include their adult partners. The findings from the study presented in this chapter reveal that, for adults, the ability to solve problems through discussion, negotiation, and rule setting may be major communication hurdles for successful diabetes disease management. Some of the problems identified by the couples in the study include managing tempting foods, portion control, monitoring intake, nagging or offering directives about food choices, and adjustments to cooking methods. Major disagreements about responsibility for disease management were identified in two styles of couple disease management. For these couples, there was an inability to discuss feelings, discuss food choice options, negotiate equitable rules and agreements about roles and social situations, and positively support changes. In all but six of these cases, these challenges were associated with low levels of regime compliance at T2. Lack of problem-solving skills and respectful communication in disease management styles should be addressed in future research and treatment plans for type 2 diabetes.

This chapter presents an exploratory, descriptive study that is heuristic in nature. The description outlines three management styles spouses can use to adjust to diabetes as a couple soon after the diagnosis in one partner. These three patterns of adaptation are reported when managing diabetes within the first year after diagnosis. The steep decline in the cohesive style and enrichment of the enmeshed and disengaged style after one year suggest that couple communication and problem solving skills found in the cohesive style may be critical to successful regimen adherence. Further research is needed to verify these management styles and explore their effect on regimen compliance.

References

AACE Diabetes Mellitus Clinical Practice Guidelines Taskforce. (2007). American Association of Clinical Endocrinologists medical guidelines for clinical practice for the management of diabetes mellitus. *Endocrine Practice, 13* (Suppl. 1), 3-68.

Albarran, N. B., Ballesteros, M. N., Morales, G. G., & Ortega, M. I. (2006). Dietary behavior and type 2 diabetes care. *Patient Education and Counseling, 61,* 191-199.

Albright ,T. L., Parchman, M., Burge, S. K., et al. (2001). Predictors of self-care behavior in adults with type 2 diabetes: An RRNeST Study. *Family Medicine, 33* (5), 354-360.

American Dietetic Association. (2000). Nutrition recommendations and principles for people with diabetes mellitus. *Diabetes Care, 23,* (Suppl.1), S43-46.

American Dietetic Association. (2003). Position of the American Dietetic Association: Integration of medical nutrition therapy and pharmacotherapy. *Journal of the American Dietetic Association, 103* (10), 1363-1370.

Anderson, J. M., Wiggins, W., Rajawani, R., Holbrook, A., Blue, G., & Ng, M. (1995). Living with a chronic illness: Chinese Canadian and Euro-Canadian women with diabetes-exploring factors that influence management. *Social Science Medicine, 41* (2), 181-195.

Armour, T. A., Norris, S. L., Jack, L., Zhang, X., & Fisher, L. (2005). The effectiveness of family interventions in people with diabetes mellitus: A systematic review. *Diabetic Medicine, 22,* 1295-1305.

Ary, D. V., Toobert, D., Wilson, W., & Glasgow, R. E. (1986). Patient perspective on factors contributing to non-adherence to diabetes regimen. *Diabetes Care, 9* (2), 168-172.

Ballantyne, P. J. (1999). The social determinants of health: A contribution to the analysis of gender differences in health and illness. *Scandinavian Journal of Public Health, 27,* 290-295.

Carter-Edwards, L., Skelly, A. H., Cagle, C. S., & Appel, S. J. (2004). "They care but don't understand": Family support of African American women with type 2 diabetes. *The Diabetes Educator, 30,* 493-501.

Chesla, C. A., Fisher, L., Mullan, J. T., Skaff, M. M., Gardiner, P., Chun, K., & Kanter, R. (2004). Family and disease management in African-American patients with type 2 diabetes. *Diabetes Care, 27* (12), 2850-2855.

Cohen, S., & Hoberman, H. M. (1983). Positive events and social supports as buffers of life change stress. *Journal of Applied Social Psychology, 13,* 99-125.

Correa-de-Araujo, R., McDermott, K., & Moy, E. (2006). Gender differences across racial and ethnic groups in the quality of care for diabetes. *Women's Health Issues, 16,* 56-65.

Davis, M. A., Murphy, S. P., Neuhaus, J. M., Gee, L., & Quiroga, S. S. (2000). Living arrangements and diet quality for US adults aged 50 years or older: NHANES III 1988-1994. *Journal of Nutrition, 130,* 2256-2264.

Denton, M., & Walters, V. (1999). Gender differences in structural and behavioral determinants of health: An analysis of the social production of health. *Social Science Medicine, 48,* 1221-1235.

Diabetes Control and Complications Trial Research Group. (1993). The effect of intensive treatment of diabetes on the development and progression of long-term complications in insulin-dependent diabetes mellitus. *New England Journal of Medicine, 329,* 977-986.

Diehl, M., Coyle, N., & Labouvie-Vief, G. (1996). Age and sex differences in strategies of coping and defense across the life span. *Psychological Aging, 11,* 127-139.

Fisher, L, Chesla, C. A., Bartz, R. J., Gilliss, C., Skaff, M. A., Sabogal, F., Kanter, R. A., & Lutz, C. P. (1998). The family and type 2 diabetes: A framework for intervention. *Diabetes Educator, 24* (5), 599-607.

Fisher, L., Chesla, C. A., Chun, K. M., Skaff, M. M., Mullan, J. T., & Kanter, R. A. (2004). Patient appraised couple emotional management and disease management among Chinese American patients with type 2 diabetes. *Journal of Family Psychology, 18* (2), 302-310.

Fisher, L., Chesla, C. A., Skaff, M. M., Gilliss, C., Mullan, J. T., Bartz, R. J., Kanter, R. A., & Lutz, C. P. (2000). The family and disease management in Hispanic and European-American patients with type 2 diabetes. *Diabetes Care, 23* (3), 267-272.

Fisher, L., Gudmundsdottir, M., Gilliss, C., Skaff, M., Mullan, J., Kanter, R., & Chesla, C. (2000). Resolving disease management problems in European-American and Latino couples with type 2 diabetes: The effects of ethnicity and patient gender. *Family Process, 39* (4), 403-416.

Fisher, L., & Weihs, K. L. (2000). Can addressing family relationships improve outcomes in chronic disease? *Journal of Family Practice, 49* (6), 561-566.

Franz, M. J., Monk, A., Barry, B., McClain, K., Weaver, T., Cooper, N., Upham, P., Bergenstal, R., & Mazze, R. S. (1995). Effectiveness of medical nutrition therapy provided by dietitians in the management of non-insulin-dependent diabetes mellitus: A randomized, controlled clinical trial. *Journal of the American Dietetic Association, 95* (9), 1009-1017.

Gafvels, C., & Wandell, P. E. (2006). Coping strategies in men and women with type 2 diabetes in Swedish primary care. *Diabetes Research Clinical Practice, 71,* 280-289.

Gerstle, J. G., Varenne, H., & Contento, I. (2001). Post-diagnosis family adaptation influences glycemic control in women with type 2 diabetes mellitus. *Journal of the American Dietetic Association, 101,* 918-922.

Glasgow, R. E., Hampson, S. E., Strycker, L. A., & Ruggiero, L. (1997). Personal-model beliefs and social environmental barriers to diabetes self-management. *Diabetes Care, 20* (4), 556-561.

Glasgow, R. E., & Toobert, D. J. (1988). Social environment and regimen adherence among type II diabetic patients. *Diabetes Care, 11*, 377-386.

Glaser B. G., & Strauss A. L. (1967) The Discovery of Grounded Theory: Strategies for qualitative research. Chicago, IL: Aldine de Gruyter.

Gorell, D. M., & Olson, D. H. (1995). Circumplex Model of Family Systems: Integrating ethnic diversity and other social systems. In R. H. Mikesell, D. Lusterman & S. H. McDaniel (Eds.), *Integrating family therapy: Handbook of family psychology and systems theory* (p. 217). Washington DC: American Psychological Association.

Grant, R. W., Buse, J. B., & Meigs, J. B. (2005). Quality of diabetes care in the US academic medical centers: Low rates of medical regimen change. *Diabetes Care, 28*, 337-442.

Harnack, L., Story, M., Martinson, B., Neumark-Sztainer, D., & Stang, J. (1998). Guess who's cooking? The role of men in meal planning, shopping and preparation in US families. *Journal of the American Dietetic Association, 98*, 995-1000.

Hedley, A. A., Ogden, C. L., Johnson, C. L., Carroll, M. D., Curtin, L. R., & Flegal, K. M. (2004). Prevalence of overweight and obesity among US children, adolescents and adults, 1999-2002. *Journal of the American Medical Association, 291*, 2847-2850.

Hennessy, C. H., John, R., & Anderson, L. A. (1999). Diabetes education needs of family members caring for American Indian elders. *The Diabetes Educator, 25*, 747-754.

Hepworth, J. (1999). Gender and capacity of women with NIDDM to implement dietary advice. *Scandinavian Journal of Public Health, 27* (4), 260-266.

Katz, A. M. (1969). Wives of diabetic men. *Bulletin Menninger Clinic, 33*, 279-294.

Kiecolt-Glaser, J. K., & Newton, T. L. (2001). Marriage and health: His and hers. *Psychological Bulletin, 127*, 472-503.

Kieffer, E. C., Willis, S. K., Odoms-Young, A. M., Guzman, J. R., Two Feathers, J., & Loveluck, J. (2004). Reducing disparities in diabetes among African American and Latino residents of Detroit: The essential role of community planning focus groups. *Ethnicity & Disease, 14* (3 Suppl. 1), S27-37.

Knowler, W. C., Barrett-Connor, E., Fowler, S. E., Hamman, R. F., Lachin, J. M., Walker, E. A., & Nathan D. M. (2002). Reduction in the incidence of type 2 diabetes with lifestyle intervention or metformin. *New England Journal of Medicine*, 346, 393-403.

Kvam, S. H., & Lyons, J. H. (1991). Assessment of coping strategies, social support and general health status in individuals with diabetes mellitus. *Psychological Reports, 68*, 623-632.

Lavee, Y., & Olson, D. H. (1991). Family types and response to stress. *Journal of Marriage and the Family, 53*, 786-798.

Lawton, J., Ahmad, N., Hanna, L., Douglas, M., Bains, H., & Hallowell, N. (2008). "We could change ourselves, but we can't": Accounts of food and eating practices amongst British Pakistanis and Indians with type 2 diabetes. *Ethnicity & Health, 13* (4), 305-319.

Legato, M. J., Gelzer, A., Goland, R., Ebner, S. A., Rajan, S., Villagra, V., & Kosowski, M. (2006). Gender-specific care of the patient with diabetes: Review and recommendations. *Gender Medicine, 3* (2), 131-158.

Macintyre, S., Hunt, K., & Sweeting, H. (1996). Gender differences in health: Are things really as simple as they seem? *Social Science Medicine, 42* (4), 617-624.

Mayring, P. (2000). Qualitative Content Analysis [28 paragraphs]. *Forum Qualitative Sozialforschung / Forum: Qualitative Social Research, 1*(2), Art. 20.

Miller, C., Warland, R., & Achterberg, C. (1997). Food purchase decision-making typologies of women with non-insulin-dependent diabetes mellitus. *Patient Education and Counseling, 30,* 271-281.

Miller, D., & Brown, J. L. (2005). Marital interactions in the process of dietary change for type 2 diabetes. *Journal of Nutrition Education and Behavior, 37*(5), 226-234.

Moss, N. E. (2002). Gender equity and socioeconomic inequality: A framework for the patterning of women's health. *Social Science Medicine, 54,* 649-661.

Muszbek, N., Brixner, D., Benedict, A., Keskinaslan, A., & Khan, Z. M. (2008). The economic consequences of noncompliance in cardiovascular disease and related conditions: A literature review. *International Journal of Clinical Practice, 62* (2), 338-351

Nagelkerk, J., Reick, K., & Meengs, L. (2006). Perceived barriers and effective strategies to diabetes self-management. *Journal of Advanced Nursing, 54* (2), 151-158.

Nelson, K. M., Reiber, G., & Boyko, E. J. (2002). Diet and exercise among adults with type 2 diabetes: Findings from the third national health and examination survey (NHANES III). *Diabetes Care, 25* (10), 1722-1728.

Norris, S. L., Engelgau, M. M., & Narayan, K. M. (2001). Effectiveness of self-management training in type 2 diabetes: A systematic review of randomized controlled trials. *Diabetes Care, 24* (3), 561-587.

Norris, S. L., Lau, J., Smith, S. J., Schmid, C. H., & Engelgau, M. M. (2002). Self-management education for adults with type 2 diabetes. *Diabetes Care, 25* (7), 1159-1171.

Ogden, C. L., Carroll, M. D., Curtin, L. R., Mcdowell, M. A., Tabak, C. J., & Flegal, K. M. (2006). Prevalence of overweight and obesity in the US, 1999-2004. *Journal of the American Medical Association, 295* (13), 1549-1555.

Olson, D. H., McCubbin, H. I., Barnes, H. L., Larsen, A. S., Muxen, M. J., & Wilson, M. A. (1989). *Families: What makes them work.* Newbury Park, Ca: Sage Publications.

Patterson, J. M., & Garwick, A. W. (1994). The impact of chronic illness on families: A family systems perspective. *Annals of Behavioral Medicine, 16,* 131-142.

Pieper, B. A., Kushion, W., & Gaida, S. (1990). The relationship between a couple's marital adjustment and beliefs about diabetes mellitus. *Diabetes Educator, 16* (2), 108-112.

Saaddine, J. B., Cadwell, B., Gregg, E. W., Engelgau, M. M., Vinicor, F., Imperatore, G., & Narayan, K. M. (2006). Improvements in diabetes processes of care and immediate outcomes: United States, 1988-2002. *Annals of Internal Medicine, 144,* 465-474.

Sarkadi, A., & Rosenqvist, U. (2002). Social network and role demands in women's type 2 diabetes: A model. *Health Care for Women International, 23,* 600-611.

Schlundt, D. G., Rea, M. R., Kline, S. S., & Pichert, J. W. (1994). Situational obstacles to dietary adherence for adults with diabetes. *Journal of the American Dietetic Association, 94,* 874-879.

Shenkel, R. J., Rogers, J. P., Perfetto, G. M., & Levin, R. A. (1985). Importance of "significant others" in predicting cooperation with the diabetic regimen. *International Journal of Psychiatry Medicine,* 15, 149-155.

Taylor, S. E. (1999). *Health Psychology,* 4th edition. Boston: McGraw-Hill.

Trief, P. M., Grant, W., Elbert, K., & Weinstock, R. S. (1998). Family environment, glycemic control and the psychosocial adaptation of adults with diabetes. *Diabetes Care, 21* (2), 241-245.

Trief, P. M., Orendorff, R., Himes, C. L., & Weinstock, R. S. (2001). The marital relationship and psychosocial adaptation and glycemic control of individuals with diabetes. *Diabetes Care, 24* (8), 1384-1389.

Trief, P. M., Ploutz-Snyder, R., Britton, K. D., & Weinstock, R. S. (2004). The relationship between marital quality and adherence to the diabetes care regimen. *Annals of Behavioral Medicine, 17* (3), 148-154.

Trief, P. M., Wade, M. J., Dee Britton, K., & Weinstock, R. S. (2002). A prospective analysis of marital relationship factors and quality of life in diabetes. *Diabetes Care, 25,* 1154-1158.

Tuomilehto, J., Lindstrom, J., Eriksson, J. G., Valle T. T., Hamalainen, H., Ilanne-Parikka, P.,... Uusitupa, M. (2001). Prevention of type 2 diabetes mellitus by changes in lifestyle among subjects with impaired glucose tolerance. *New England Journal of Medicine, 344,* 1343-1350.

UK Prospective Diabetes Study (UKPDS) Group (1998). Intensive blood-glucose control with sulphonylureas or insulin compared with conventional treatment and risk of complications in patients with type 2 diabetes (UIPDS 33). *Lancet, 352,* 837-853.

US Census. (2007). *American families and living arrangements.* Table A-1. Accessed at www.census.gov/population/www/socdemo/hh-fam/cps2007.html

van Dam, H. A., van der Horst, F. G., Knoops, L., Ryckman, R. M., Crebolder, H. F., & van den Borne, B. H. (2005). Social support in diabetes: A systematic review of controlled intervention studies. *Patient Education and Counseling, 59,* 1-12.

Verbrugge, L. M. (1982). Sex differentials in health. *Public Health Reports, 97*(5), 417-437.

Vermeire, E., Wens, J., Van Royen, P., Biot, Y., Hearnshaw, H., & Lindemeyer, A. (2005). Interventions for improving adherence to treatment recommendations in people with type 2 diabetes mellitus. *Cochrane Database System Reviews, 18* (2), CD003638.

Vijan, S., Stuart, N. S., Fitzgerald, J. T., Ronis, D. L., Hayward, R. A., Slater, S., & Hofer, T. P. (2004). Barriers to following dietary recommendations in type 2 diabetes. *Diabetic Medicine, 22*, 32-38.

Vincent, D., Clark, L., Zimmer, L. M., & Sanchez, J. (2006). Using focus groups to develop a culturally competent diabetes self-management program for Mexican Americans. *Diabetes Educator, 32*, 89-97.

Wansink, B. (2006). Nutritional gatekeepers and the 72% solution. *Journal of the American Dietetic Association, 106*, 1324-1327.

Wen, L. K., Parchman, M. L., & Shepherd, M. D. (2004). Family support and diet barriers among older Hispanic adults with type 2 diabetes. *Family Medicine, 36* (6), 423-430.

Wen, L. K., Shepherd, M. D., & Parchman, M. L. (2004). Family support, diet and exercise among older Mexican Americans with type 2 diabetes. *Diabetes Educator, 30* (6), 980-993.

Whittemore, R., Melkus, G. E., & Grey, M. (2005). Metabolic control, self-management and psychosocial adjustment in women with type 2 diabetes. *Journal of Clinical Nursing, 14*,195-203.

Wing, R. R., Marcus, M. D., Epstein, L. H., & Jawad, A. (1991). A family-based approach to treatment of obese type II diabetic patients. *Journal of Consulting Clinical Psychology, 59*, 156-62.

Wong, M., Gucciardi, E., Li, L., & Grace, S. L. (2005). Gender and nutrition management in type 2 diabetes. *Canadian Journal of Dietetic Practice and Research, 66* (4), 215-220.

Writing Team for the Diabetes Control and Complications Trial/Epidemiology of Diabetes Interventions and Complications Research Group. (2002). Effect of intensive therapy on the micro-vascular complications of type 1 diabetes mellitus. *Journal of the American Medical Association, 287*, 2563-2569.

CHAPTER 5

Working It Out Together: The Role of Family Support in the Management of Postpartum Depression

LaKesha Anderson Dearmen

GEROGE MASON UNIVERSITY

Postpartum depression (PPD) is a deeply personal experience. Mental health disorders carry stigma (Hinshaw & Cicchetti, 2000), and women's emotional disorders may be even more stigmatized simply because women are expected to behave in a socially accepted way that involves shouldering an inordinate work-life balance (The Boston Women's Health Book Collective, 1998). Until recently, female conditions traditionally received less attention than male conditions, partially because of the omission of women from medical studies ("How Far We've Come," 1999; Sargent & Brettell, 1996) that has also contributed to substandard medical care for women (Schur & Nicolette, 1997). In particular, less may be known about the gynecological and other related disorders that affect women because more emphasis has been placed on the development of the fetus than the woman carrying the fetus (Kinser, 1997). For example, premenstrual syndrome (PMS) and its more severe form premenstrual dysphoric disorder (PMDD) went unrecognized for many decades, despite evidence that these were very real problems (Ussher, 2003). As another example, endometriosis is often misdiagnosed or undiagnosed and women are told their pain is merely a symptom of being female, exaggerated, or "all in their heads" (Taylor, 2003). PPD carries a particular stigma; often minimized, the sufferer is often blamed when she cannot "snap out of it" and enjoy her baby. PPD is very real and is very personal. Women with PPD feel guilt, shame, and self-loathing, and are often afraid to seek help (Venis & McCloskey, 2007). No scholarly treatment of PPD should be undertaken without a firm grounding in this emotional site. PPD cannot be understood if it is sanitized; it must be grasped with full comprehension of its pain and desolation.

My Standpoint

I always wanted to be a mother. Like so many young women, I had this rosy image of how motherhood was supposed to be: peaceful no-fuss baby sleeping in the arms of her perfect multi-tasking mother. So imagine my dismay when the endometriosis I had been struggling with since my early teens made it difficult to get pregnant. Imagine again the shock, confusion, and horror I felt when I finally did give birth to a beautiful baby girl only to discover that not only was I not perfect, neither was she. Things were actually very different from perfect.

The grim reality of motherhood began setting in only hours after we brought her home from the hospital. My daughter had a horrible case of colic and neither one of us could stop crying. Motherhood was nothing like I had anticipated: rather than the peaceful baby I looked forward to rocking to sleep at night, I had a screaming infant who slept for 45 minutes at a time. Instead of being the perfect multi-tasking mother, I found myself immobilized by fear and sheer exhaustion. Some days, I even wanted to die.

Thankfully, my rational side won the battle, and I sit here writing a very personal chapter on how families manage PPD. Still, I find it difficult to verbalize my emotions during the years following the birth of my first child. Like many women, I found it reprehensible to say that I had visions of harming my daughter. I feared that if I said aloud what I felt inside that I would lose my baby, whom I loved very much. I had constant thoughts of my daughter's head shattering like a melon being dropped on concrete. Paradoxically, I did not want anyone else holding her, for fear they may harm her. Frighteningly, I did not think I was capable of caring for her. I was scared to be alone with her; her constant crying was like nails on a chalkboard. I despised the sound and wanted it to go away. I lived life as a prisoner to my thoughts. I felt scared, irrational, guilty, incompetent, and confused all at once.

I knew I was supposed to feel a little down for a couple of weeks postpartum. However, my postpartum baby blues were getting worse each day. The longer the feelings lasted, the more upset I became: with myself, with the baby, with my husband, and with anyone else who acknowledged that I might not be acting "normal." Despite feeling anything but, I certainly did not want anyone else to see that I was not at my best. At work, with extended family, and with friends, I became good at smiling through the pain. My husband, however, bore the brunt of my unstable condition. I was enraged with him because I knew he did not understand. How could he? I was not going to tell the father of this precious child that I had visions of harming her. After months of crying and fruitless attempts to explain my condition without truly explaining every thought, I sunk into a very deep depression and some days I honestly felt that the only way out was to leave, no matter what that meant.

It was not until I was pregnant with my second child nine months after giving birth that I knew with certainty that I needed help. I tried explaining to my husband exactly how I felt. I told him I knew I needed help but I was too scared to tell anyone how I felt. I met with my church pastor, a safe choice I felt. I thought that maybe everything that I was experiencing was some form of punishment. Of course, he assured me that was not the case, but I left thinking I simply needed to go to church more often. I felt if I were a better Christian, this agony would cease. I tried that. It did not stop. It got worse.

In April 2006, a little piece of me was better. My daughter was well past her colicky days, I had taken a new job that I really enjoyed, and my new son was a joy. But, something still was not fully right. Rather than simply feeling depressed all the time, I was also feeling overwhelmingly nervous as well. I felt a little more comfortable telling people about my feelings because I could blame it on anxiety, which sounds much better than "I have suicidal thoughts and visions of hurting my baby." I began to slowly confide in a close colleague. To my surprise, she disclosed that she had been battling general depression and suggested I visit her doctor. She actually made the appointment for me and one week later, I was on my way to getting the help I knew I needed.

As if a divine force knew I needed reassurance that I was doing the right thing, I had my first actual panic attack on my way to the doctor's office. Stopped at a traffic light I became frozen. I could not move the steering wheel because I just knew that the oncoming vehicles were not going to stop. I could see them crashing full speed into my car, killing me instantly. This thought led to the idea that I should just stop driving because if I lived through this traffic light, the accident would surely happen at a different one, and what if my children were in the car at the time? I made it to the doctor's office and cried; expressions of guilt, pain, anger, confusion, and despair came pouring out of me. I left the office with a plan, which included an antidepressant. She informed me that I was not only suffering with PPD but postpartum anxiety as well. "Wow," I thought, "someone finally understands me."

I was lucky. My physician had experienced something similar and could empathize with me. Many women never say anything about their feelings, and not all doctors understand how to screen or diagnose PPD. In addition, I had a very supportive family. My husband was my biggest advocate when I decided to seek help from a physician. I knew he wanted me to be happy and find peace, but he simply could not provide that to me. He knew I needed more support than he could offer. It took me a little longer to come to the same conclusion, but I am so thankful that I did.

When I agreed to write this piece, I had no idea how difficult it would be to write about my personal experience. I talked through how I felt with my husband and mother, telling them things I had never told either of them about what I went through and the things I thought about my sweet girl. Talking it out with my family, however, made me want to tell my story. Through the extraordinarily difficult process of expressing my feelings, I began to see even more clearly the purpose for scholarly works such as this one. As someone who has experienced PPD, I have a responsibility to tell my story, to use my scholarly endeavors to provide a foundation for mandatory PPD screening, reduce the stigma of the condition, and prevent the physical and emotional harm that both women with PPD and their babies suffer. I have a mission. Self-discovery is hard, but it is my hope that my pain will help other women experiencing PPD to get the medical attention they need and deserve.

What Is PPD?

PPD is a very real, very severe mood disorder affecting as many as one in every eight new mothers each year (Wisner, Parry, & Piontek, 2002). This figure is likely an understatement, however, because as many as 50 percent of cases of PPD may go undetected (Ramsay, 1993). PPD is marked by sadness, lack of energy, lack of concentration, tiredness, inability to sleep, nightmares, change in appetite, difficulty caring for the baby, feelings of worthlessness or inadequacy, thoughts of harming the baby or oneself, and excessive fear or anxiety for the baby (Curtis & Schuler, 2004; Pryke, 2002; Reisser, 1997; Stone & Eddleman, 2003; Williamson & McCutcheon, 2004; Young, 2005). Because many of those feelings can also be attributed to the demands of caring for an infant 24 hours a day, PPD often goes unrecognized.

Most new mothers experience a brief period of "baby blues." This occurs as hormone levels diminish and the new mother's body adjusts to no longer being pregnant. PPD, though often confused with "baby blues," is a more serious condition that continues on after the "blues" have passed. In fact, PPD can manifest as late as one year after childbirth. The condition significantly impacts the mother, her infant, and her relationships with the child's father and other family, co-workers, and friends. These effects can be both physical and mental, leading to suicide, infanticide, other mental disorders, social and emotional withdrawal, and lack of involvement in interpersonal relationships. Not surprisingly, these interpersonal relationships are essential for both preventing and treating postpartum depression.

Just as PPD should not be confused with "baby blues," it should not be confused with postpartum psychosis (PPP) either, a more rare and serious disorder affecting one in 500 to 1,000 women each year (Silberner, 2002). Unfortunately, much of the information people receive about postpartum illnesses is related to PPP, the condition from which Andrea Yates suffered. The Texas mother was convicted in 2002 of drowning her five children. Since Yates' trial, PPP has often been mislabeled in the media and in the vernacular as PPD (Venis & McCloskey, 2007), likely due to a lack of knowledge by people discussing the conditions. Misinterpretations of these distinctions can hinder medical treatment, as women experiencing PPD may be misled to believe that their symptoms are normal or less severe than what they may have seen reported in the media about PPD cases.

Like me, there are scores of women with PPD who rarely speak to others in their social support network about their feelings. Bennett and Indman (2003) reported that one woman contrasted her cancer treatment to PPD: when undergoing cancer treatment she verbalized her concerns and fears, sought the support of friends and family, and spoke about treatment options. When experiencing PPD, however, she did not tell anyone about her emotional symptoms and did not seek help from friends or family because she felt guilty and ashamed. As a result, she did not have treatment options. This happens to many women each year whose PPD is apparent only to them. Like many mental illnesses, PPD is often thought of as a problem that is easily overcome simply by "thinking happier thoughts" or as one that is not "real" (Venis & McCloskey, 2007). The postpartum period is one in which many women feel isolated and alone. One reason for this, according to Beck (2001), a seasoned PPD researcher, is that women lack social support during the postpartum period. In fact, many studies have listed a lack of social support as a risk factor for PPD (Beck, 1993; Beck, 2001; Robertson, Grace, Wallington, & Stewart, 2004; Scrandis, 2005; Stice, Ragan, & Randall, 2004).

It Takes a Village: Social Support and PPD

Many scholars have studied the impact of social support on health outcomes, generally finding that social support benefits individuals both physically and mentally (Achat, et al., 1998; Cornman, Goldman, Glei, Weinstein, & Change, 2003; Wright & Bell, 2003; VanderVoort & Skorikov, 2002). Studies have linked perceived social support to decreases in depression following heart attacks (Frasure-Smith, et al., 2000), the depression levels of parents of disabled children (Mickelson, 2001), and even immunity from diseases (Cohen & Williamson, 1991). Research on PPD, however, is limited in scope, focusing mostly on how one would identify symptoms of the condition. PPD clearly deserves examination in nonmedical research that considers the importance of effective communication strategies, including the role of interpersonal communication and family support, on improved PPD care and prevention efforts.

Women suffering with PPD represent an understudied group. Studies of the relationship between postpartum health and social support are nearly absent from social science literature, which is unfortunate given the vast amount of social science research on the benefits of social support and the growing body of work on social support and health care outcomes. Studies that do examine social support during the postpartum period tend to focus on the quantity of a woman's social support network, rather than the quality of social support received. In addition, literature on the impact that PPD has on the sufferer's family is virtually nonexistent. These gaps in the literature present a number of barriers to diagnosing, treating, and communicating about the condition, not just for patients and their physicians, but for partners, children, and friends of afflicted mothers, as well.

Mother-Partner Relations

As any partner in a committed relationship knows, maintaining a relationship takes work. The many obstacles that couples face have been well documented in social science literature, and it is no surprise that adding a newborn to the family can also add stress (Fincham, 2003; Hackel & Ruble, 1992; Lavee, Sharlin, & Katz, 1996; Majewski, 1986). Couples spend months and even years planning for the day their child is born, but spend little, if any, time addressing the changes that come with moving from lovers to parents, a couple to a family. This is unfortunate given the significant impact that the couples' interpersonal relationship has on the new mother's health. Research shows that marital dissatisfaction and lack of social support are risk factors for depression both during pregnancy and in the postpartum period (Beck, 2001; Buultjens & Liamputtong, 2007; Henshaw, 2006).

One can flip through the pages of any parenting magazine and find tips for new mothers on how to manage new-baby stressors: make time for yourself, spend time with your partner away from the baby, and get sleep when the baby does. However, much less information exists on how partners adapt to the stressors of having a new baby. In fact, the emotional lives of fathers has been overlooked and are typically discussed only as a small part of a larger discussion about the mother's postpartum lives (Goodman, 2004).

For the partners of new mothers, stressors may be somewhat different than those experienced by the mother. Despite the fact that partners want to take an active role and participate equally in parenting duties, much of what an infant requires is typically provided by the mother. This can cause partners to feel angry, ignored, rejected, or emotionally disconnected from the mother (Venis & McCloskey, 2007). Further, partners may worry over finances, as the introduction of a new child means there is another mouth to feed and an education to finance. The father, who typically returns to work before the new mother, may also find it difficult to work because of sleep interruptions at home. In families where the mother is experiencing PPD, partners can also suffer from frustration and an overall sense of powerlessness (Ross, Dennis, Blackmore, & Stewart, 2005), as well as feel resentment from taking on childcare duties while the mother manages her depression (Meighan, Davis, Thomas, & Droppleman, 1999). Studies have found that partners of women with PPD are likely to report being depressed as well (Bennett, 2007; Goodman, 2004; Venis & McCloskey).

Many women (like me) are unaware that their partners are experiencing these feelings. After my daughter was born, I was completely unaware of my husband's feelings, and I honestly did not care about them. I was too overwhelmed by my inability to manage my own feelings and care for my baby to be concerned with what I perceived as "his" problems. After months of watching me cry and yell about my feelings, he finally exploded with his own. For months, he had worried silently about the high cost of daycare and the rising price of rent in our too-small apartment; he had watched me cry without being able to help despite his best efforts to assist with household chores, listen and provide emotional support; and he had spent days at work nearly asleep at his desk because our colicky new daughter slept only 45 minutes at a time (on a good day). I was shocked and saddened by his disclosure, but for the wrong reasons. I listened to him, but what I heard was him blaming me for his problems. I felt like such a failure as a mother that I just assumed it was also my fault that he felt the way he did.

Milgrom, Martin, and Negri (1999) explained that women delineate between *practical* and *emotional* support. Practical support includes helping with physical activities: changing and feeding the baby, shopping, and taking care of finances. Conversely, women are emotionally supported when they are given opportunities to express their concerns and feelings and believe that those issues are understood. Despite their need for both physical and emotional support, women with PPD are less likely to receive emotional support because they do not disclose their feelings. This was certainly true in my experience. My husband was helping, as best he knew how. Of course, I felt like he should simply try harder to help me around the house. But, what I wanted more than anything was for him to stop asking, "What is wrong?" I explained that if I knew the answer, I would tell him. But that was not true. How was I supposed to tell him that I wanted to leave, without him, without our beautiful, helpless daughter? How do you tell your husband that you want to die, or that you are afraid to be left alone with his child? I was angry that he could not provide me emotional support, but how could he? I kept him in the dark about my true feelings.

Research has also shown that marital satisfaction decreases after the birth of the first child (Belsky & Rovine, 1990). Kendall-Tackett (2005) referenced several studies that demonstrate the critical role that partners play in helping women overcome PPD. In particular, Cutrona (1996) explained that support from one's spouse can prevent the onset of significant depression as well as the negative behaviors that may lead to depression, such as self-pity and irritability. Though largely overlooked by PPD researchers, partners can also experience depression during the postpartum period. Goodman (2004) claimed that as many as 24 to 50 percent of men whose partners experience PPD also experience PPD. Meighan, Davis, Thomas, and Droppleman (1999) explained that fathers experience both a loss and a gain upon the birth of a child. Specifically, fathers lose the relationship they once shared with the new mother. In their study, they found that new fathers described a number of other losses including those of control and intimacy. Figure 5.1 identifies eight themes, and quotes, that describe the father's experiences of PPD reported in this study.

Table 5.1 Summary

Theme	Quote
She Becomes An Alien	She…within one afternoon became a completely different person.
He Attempts to Fix the Problem	I was trying to find something wrong, you know, I wanted a wrong we could fix.
He Makes Sacrifices	You think 'oh God, I could just sit down, I'm so mentally exhausted,' but that's when you suck it up and go on.
His World Collapses	I thought her suicide would be an answer, then I felt guilty for [having] those feelings.
Loss of Control	There wasn't any time for me to do what I wanted to do or needed to do…I felt trapped.
Loss of Intimacy	I understand that there is a medical reason or a hormonal reason, it's not because she doesn't love you, but for the heart and those natural desires that a man should have for his wife—to be rejected continually—that's a tough one.
Altered Relationship	I'm learning now that I cannot make her happy.
A Real Crisis	I felt like I was out there all on my own, without anybody to guide me, or anybody to talk to. There was no where I could go.

Note: Based on findings from "Living with postpartum depression: The father's experience." By M. Meighan, M. W. Davis, S. P. Thomas, and P. G. Droppleman, 1999, *The American Journal of Maternal/Child Nursing, 24*, pp. 202-208.

Kendall-Tackett (2005) suggested that including partners in interventions can help open lines of communication between mothers and their partners, thereby helping both partners overcome their depression. Additionally, Cutrona (1996) reported that couples who continue to provide support during times of great stress are likely to prevent emotional withdrawal by either partner. She emphasized the importance of managing stress as a "whole" rather than as individuals. Indeed, research shows that couples sensitive to and supportive of one another's needs for emotional support are less likely to experience both significant marital discord and depression.

Ross, Dennis, Blackmore, and Stewart (2005) also explained that health care providers should spend time with partners reassuring them. Specifically, they state that service providers should help partners realize that:

1. They cannot take the mother's illness personally.

2. They are not responsible for the mother's depression.

3. They cannot cure the mother of her depression; instead they need to encourage the mother to seek professional treatment.

4. They can best help the mother by listening, offering support, and organizing help from others.

5. They need to take occasional breaks.

In summary, both marital satisfaction and social support are significant factors in predicting a woman's chances of having PPD as well as overcoming PPD. This need for support presents an interesting paradox. Indeed, having higher marital satisfaction and social support are critical in helping a woman move past her PPD. However, having a strong support network before childbirth can help prevent a woman from ever developing PPD. This paradox is all the more reason for practitioners to sensitively take a family-based approach, recognizing that the occurrence of PPD may very well be an indication that the relational skills needed to manage and overcome PPD are likely underdeveloped to begin with.

In committed relationships, it is often expected that partners are one another's primary source of social support. Therefore, ensuring that partners have the tools necessary to provide adequate social support is vital to helping women overcome PPD. Lacking this support network can lead to a downward spiral where a woman is not only more likely to suffer PPD, but less likely to seek and receive help for PPD. While understanding the role partners play in both prevention and recovery of PPD is important, it is equally important to understand how partners are affected by PPD and the steps they can take to protect themselves against depression, keep their partnership strong, and reduce the impacts that a mother's depression can have on their child(ren), which is the subject of the next section.

Mother-Child Relations

It has been five years since my daughter was born and nearly four since I began treatment for PPD. While I no longer worry that someone will drop her and I no longer want to die, I often wonder what impact my condition had on her development. My daughter and I have butted heads since she was born and I often blame myself for that. I listen intently to other mothers talk about their daughters and feel a sense of relief each time I hear that they, too, struggle. I often wonder if she knows what I went through, if she knows what she went through, and how those experiences shape both my parenting of her and her interactions with me. While only time will tell how my experience shapes my relationship with my daughter, research shows that having PPD has significant impacts for both new mothers and their infants.

A mother serves a distinct and important role in the life of her newborn. She acts as a mediator between her new child and his/her outside world, she determines who will comprise his/her social network, and serves as the primary source for both emotional and physical stimulation (Grace, Evindar, & Stewart, 2003). Children depend on their mothers to meet their every need, especially in the first weeks and months of the child's life. However, PPD can seriously impair what are considered normal interactions between a new mother and her child (Dennis, 2003; Milgrom, Erickson, McCarthy, & Gemmill, 2006). Women suffering with PPD may lack energy and concentration, be irritable, eat poorly, and be unable to meet their child's emotional needs, or form a bond with their baby (Moline, Kahn, Ross, Altschuler, & Cohen, 2001). This, in turn, can cause women to lose confidence in their ability to parent, thereby deepening their depression.

Cheryl Tatano Beck, a pioneer in research on PPD, has written extensively on the experiences of women with PPD. In a 1996 study, she examined the experiences of women with PPD interacting with their children. In the study, Beck found that women with this condition were overcome daily with thoughts of guilt, irrational ideas and images, and anger. She found that those emotions negatively impacted how these mothers interacted with their children, explaining that mothers acted "like robots" when providing care for their infants and failed to always respond to their infant child. Beck found that women with PPD experienced more negative interactions with their older children as well.

In addition to impairing the maternal-child relationship, there are a number of other ways that PPD can affect infants. Among those are delays in language development, diminished cognitive ability, inability to emotionally bond to others, behavioral problems, sleep problems, and distress. One study found that infants may be able to detect their mother's depressed behavior, and respond in a similar manner by demonstrating depressed affect and lower activity levels (Field, 2002). There is conflicting research about infant sex and effects of PPD. PPD more negatively impacts infant boys than infant girls (Cohn, Campbell, Matias, & Hopkins, 1990; Murray, Kempton, Woolgar, & Hooper, 1993) and may affect women giving birth to males at a greater rate than those giving birth to females (de Tychey, et al., 2008). In addition to myriad emotional and behavioral problems, infants may experience physical effects stemming from their mothers' PPD. Research has shown that infants whose mothers suffer with PPD are also more likely to die from Sudden Infant Death Syndrome (SIDS) (Mitchell, 2008). Studies have long indicated that children of depressed individuals are more likely to experience physical abuse. Unfortunately, for children of postpartum depressed mothers, infanticide, or infant death, is a possibility.

Perhaps the most well known case of infanticide (and filicide, the murder of a child over the age of one) in America is the previously mentioned case of Andrea Yates. Yates suffered from PPP when she killed her children, but she had previously been diagnosed with PPD. Left untreated, PPD can lead to PPP (Wynszynsky & Lusskin, 2005); therefore, it is important to examine her case as a chilling reminder of the importance of treating PPD. Yates is a former nurse who, in June 2001, drowned her five young children. The news received instant media coverage and Yates was quickly judged in the court of public opinion. People of all ages, parents and non-parents, responded in outrage, asking *How could a mother kill her children?* Yates was deemed a "murderer" by society long before her trial concluded. One individual close to the case was Margaret Spinelli, who has written extensively about both infanticide and the Yates case. Spinelli (2005a) says it is natural that people debate infanticide, stating that the topic is both "compelling and repulsive…It demands retribution. That is the law. Yet the perpetrator of the act is a victim too, and that makes for a more paradoxical response" (p. 18). Spinelli's view of the perpetrator as a victim developed in part from the lack of a formal definition for either PPD or PPP and the fact that the U.S. legal system does not recognize psychosis as being "insane."

Spinelli has argued for the benefit of a formal diagnosis for PPD. The *Diagnostic and Statistical Manual of Mental Disorders* (DSM), also used by the legal community to determine one's ability to provide testimony, does not provide diagnostic standards for PPD or PPP, making these conditions difficult, and at times impossible, to diagnose and treat. Yates herself had been treated for depression and psychosis and hospitalized multiple times for psychiatric care and repeated suicide attempts. Despite her continuing decline in health, her psychiatrist discontinued some of her medication and drastically reduced other medications (O'Malley, 2004), and Yates continued to care for five young children with limited family intervention and medical assistance. Spinelli thus argued that the American society shares responsibility for death of Yates' children. Specifically, Spinelli (2005b) stated:

> We as a society share responsibility for this tragedy. Friends, neighbors, and family failed to see or report as Mrs. Yates continued to decompensate. The medical community failed to provide appropriate protection, social work assistance and child services to a severely psychotic mother of five children. When the legal community and her state failed to appreciate the severity of her illness, they eliminated her last opportunity for appropriate treatment." (p. 22)

While Spinelli frequently discusses a flaw in society and government handling of the Yates case, Moore (2008), a consultant to the Yates trial, has argued that Yates' husband, Rusty, is also at fault for the deaths of their children. While she does not dispute that Ms. Yates murdered her children, she posits that she did so in order to escape physical, emotional, and sexual abuse by her husband. She explains that Mr. Yates controlled every aspect of his wife's life: her religious convictions, her employment status, and her friendships and visitors. In addition, she claims his oppressive behavior included uprooting the family to advance his career and selling their home, without consulting his wife, to move the seven-member family to a small trailer, and eventually a bus. Explaining the vast difference between the image Mr. Yates presented to the public and the one Ms. Yates described, Moore wrote "… while Russell Yates presented an image of himself as someone who emotionally supported and assisted Andrea in caring for their children, the image was not consistent with the reality of their daily lives (p. 27)" in which she claims Mr. Yates really thought that "all people with depression need is a swift kick in the pants" (p. 28). Further, regarding Ms. Yates' participation in a group therapy, Moore stated:

> The group encouraged Andrea to assert herself with Rusty. Her response was illuminating. She told the group that although she wanted to communicate with Rusty, when he was home he turned on the television… More importantly, when being discharged from out-patient care, Andrea told her therapy group that she was sorry she had to leave them because they supported her. There was an unmistakable implication: Rusty did not and had not been supporting her. She realized what it meant to receive emotional support, yet until she attended group therapy, she had not verbalized its conspicuous absence from her marriage to Rusty. Arguably, this was one of the first times during her marriage Andrea experienced a genuine ethic of care and support. She felt "safe." (p. 27)

Just as Andrea Yates should be held in our consciousness as a constant reminder of where PPD can lead, Russell Yates should remain there as an exemplar of the centrality of partner support to successful PPD treatment, the necessity of educating family members on both the need for appropriate support and the skills to provide it, and the importance of external intervention into the lives of PPD sufferers whose family lives are detrimental to their treatment. The lives of children of PPD literally depend on these things.

Children of depressed women are at greater risk of experiencing physical abuse. In 2001, Mahar-Sylvestre, a Canadian doula, childbirth educator, and social worker, wrote about her experience with

PPD. She explained that during the early months of her son's life, she was not only emotionally unable to care for him, but that she also fantasized about killing herself and her child, as well as finding her child dead from SIDS. When I first read her article, a year after my daughter was born, I felt that my own thoughts of harming my child had finally been recognized; someone finally understood. I could especially relate to her description of PPD fantasies as "like having a VCR in your head, repeating the same images again and again." Yet, merely knowing others shared my experiences did not eliminate them. By that point, I had also become so depressed that I actually thought my family would be happier if I were dead.

Identifying and treating PPD is vital to the health of a new mother as well as to the health of the infant. Suicide is a leading cause of maternal death. Also, as Oates (2003a, 2003b) explains, perinatal psychiatric disorders, including PPD, are known to cause poor maternal health outcomes, including death. As mentioned earlier, untreated PPD can lead to PPP. Psychosis sufferers experience an altered reality and often report hearing voices telling them to hurt their children or themselves, as in the case of Yates, who reported that Satan told her to kill her children in order to save them from eternal damnation (Roche, 2002). In Yates' altered reality she believed that to protect her children, the ultimate maternal good, she had to commit the ultimate maternal evil.

The Yates case is commonly cited as evidence of the importance of illuminating the plight of women with perinatal mental disorders. After Yates was found guilty and sentenced to life in prison, the American Psychiatric Association, despite their exclusion of formal diagnostic standards for PPD and PPP in the DSM, issued a public statement about mental illness and insanity pleas. The announcement explained that mentally impaired people who commit crimes should be treated in a hospital rather than placed in a prison or on death row (Spinelli, 2004). Since then, the Yates ruling was overturned. In 2006, Yates was found not guilty by reason of insanity and now spends her days in a low-security mental hospital.

Cases like that of Andrea Yates, as well as the many mothers who have appeared recently in the news for similar crimes (for instance, Dr. Suzanne Killinger-Johnson, Susan Smith, and Dena Schlosser all murdered their children while suffering with PPD), highlight the need for a standard definitions of PPD and PPP. These women have become "poster children" for what can happen when suffering with untreated depression and psychosis. Their cases draw attention to a potentially fatal, but treatable condition that can severely harm both mothers and their children, emotionally, mentally, and physically.

Relations with Other Family Members

In addition to my husband, I received heavy support from my father, my mother-in-law, and especially my mother after the birth of my first child. However, I received the most support in the first postpartum week. After that week, I was on my own. I started demonstrating symptoms of PPD within that first week but assumed those symptoms were "normal." In the weeks that followed, I sank deeper into my depression; however, I never mentioned it to anyone. My mother sensed that something was not quite right, but I assured her things were fine. By the time my second child was born, my husband, parents, and mother-in-law knew about my condition and we were better able to plan. Also, in the time since my daughter was born, my husband and I had become better educated about my condition and we knew the importance of a strong social support network. I definitely benefited from my family's willingness to learn about the condition and to work with me to ensure I had support in the weeks after my son was born. Unfortunately, not all women have the understanding and supportive family I do.

After my son was born, my mother stayed for a week, my husband the next, and my mother-in-law the third week. Having support for an extended period of time, as opposed to that one week, helped jumpstart my recovery from PPD. The structured support-system we created ensured I had not just instrumental help but emotional help for a greater period of time. Research has shown that many women turn to family for support during this time (Chan & Levy, 2004; Thome, 2003); therefore, it is important to recognize the contributions of family support, as well as the problems these support providers may experience.

Though research on PPD is growing, research on the effects of the condition on family members other than the woman's partner and children is practically non-existent. The impact of mental health disorders on partners and relationships is well documented, and the impact of maternal depression on infants is a hot topic for medical and psychology researchers. However, PPD can affect the woman's household members and radiate through the family and social network. In fact, research shows that depression can significantly affect other family members and caregivers (Beck, 2002; Ross, et al., 2005).

Despite having access to extended family, some women may not seek support from their family because they are embarrassed or feel vulnerable (Venis & McCloskey, 2007). This can create confusion and concern amongst family members who offer their support or question the woman about her well-being. As I previously mentioned, my mother frequently asked me how I was doing, but I refused to say much. She often tells me how she wishes I had confided in her earlier. It was not that I did not think she would try to help. Rather, I had the same concerns as many other mothers with PPD: I was afraid of disappointing the people who expected me to be a good at motherhood. Social norming and myths about motherhood have created strong ideas of what motherhood should look like (Bennett, 2007; Clay, 2001; Dobris & White-Mills, 2006; Venis & McCloskey, 2007), and it does not look like a crying, depressed mother unable, or unwilling, to care for her child.

It may be the case that family members, particularly mothers, hurt the new mother more than help by telling stories about "how things used to be," which perpetuate motherhood myths. For me, these stories were of days when women did not take time off work for childbirth, breastfed with ease for a full year, and took care of a home, a husband, and a baby without help. These stories, while often shared in an effort to bond to the new mother, may cause the new mother to question her own parenting behavior. Story-telling acts, according to Savage (2001), serve to provide expectant mothers with knowledge about childbirth and mothering and these stories, while serving as a means of "connecting" women and sharing concerns about the experience of becoming and being a mother (Callister, 2003), help shape how expectant mothers view their transition to motherhood.

Storytelling is often associated with collectivist societies (Harkins & Ray, 2004). While the U.S. does still have collectivist co-cultures,

America is largely individualistic. Parents in Western cultures encourage physical and emotional independence from an early age (Harkins & Ray) which may encourage women to stay silent about their depressive symptoms. While individualistic cultures do engage in storytelling, stories may be told for different reasons or with different outcomes. Many of the cultural norms and beliefs of collectivistic societies are reported to serve a protective role in helping women transition to motherhood (Sayil, Gure, & Ucanok, 2006). Women in collectivist societies may be at an advantage because women in these cultures are more likely to have larger support networks than those living in individualistic societies, thus making social support more accessible (VanderVoort & Skorikov, 2002). However, simply having social support available does not always mean the woman is comfortable receiving it, or even perceives it as being available. Dunkel-Schetter, Sagrestano, Feldman, and Killingsworth (1996) explain that collectivism and individualism can be as much a personality trait as a cultural variable. Kendall-Tackett (2005) provides the following quote from Christine, who felt uncomfortable having her mother-in-law help after the birth of her child:

> Everyone was really helping with the baby but me. They were *too* supportive. I know my husband wouldn't want to think that. I felt like they were taking over everything, that I had to be able to do it all. I kept trying to be the perfect wife. I'm a very private person. I felt like everything was exposed. (p. 119)

Given the cultural norms and the many myths that guide what women come to believe is the "ideal mother," it is no wonder women find it difficult to seek support, explain their weaknesses, or not compare themselves to the women who came before them.

Regardless of how women with PPD react to family members' attempts to provide social support, it is important that women have a strong social support network both during and after pregnancy. Milgrom, et al. (1999) highlighted the importance of continued social support outreach for mothers who experience PPD. They cite inadequate social support as a risk factor for relapses of PPD. However, providing social support to a depressed individual can be stressful and exhausting (Venis & McCloskey, 2007). While it is certainly important for women to have social support it is also imperative that caretakers also care for themselves and their own mental health. Families should work together to ensure each caretaker has opportunities to take breaks and tend to their own support needs.

Summary

The importance of providing positive support has been discussed in social science literature for over 30 years. The emphasis on providing social support to improve health outcomes, however, is a relatively new area of study. The impact of social support in health care has become increasingly evident, as researchers discover the many ways in which social support networks, consisting of both strong and weak ties, are positively linked to improvements in personal health care. Lakey and Lutz (1996) explain that one of the primary goals of social support is to ensure the provision of successful interventions. One such intervention might be for women with PPD, whose lives are dramatically altered during what they expected to be, and what could be, a joyous time in their lives. PPD, as explained here, can wreak havoc on very important interpersonal relationships. The accessibility of positive, supportive relationships is highlighted by many researchers as a remedy for PPD while the absence of these relationships serves as a risk factor for PPD. Women without these relationships are thus doubly at risk.

This chapter has highlighted the importance of three key relationships: the relationship between the mother and her partner, the mother and her new infant, and the mother and other family members. Each is fundamentally important to the mother: her ability to overcome PPD hinges, to some extent, on the accessibility of strong support networks. In addition, these relationships are important to the healthy development of the new infant, who may lack proper care from the depressed mother, and therefore rely on the support of his/her father and other family members.

When a couple becomes a family, the mother-partner relationship is drastically changed and each partner must redefine his/her role and negotiate new rules and norms for how to behave within the context of a new family. While mothers are the ones who experience PPD itself, partners do experience feelings of loss and can enter into a depressive state, as well. It is also speculated that mothers with PPD are more likely to have depressed infants. Researchers have identified a number of developmental and behavioral problems that often manifest in infants of postpartum depressed mothers (Grace, et al., 2006; Moline, et al., 2001). Many studies document the severe impacts that untreated PPD can have on the infant, including physical abuse and infanticide (Spinelli, 2005a). Other family members, including and especially grandparents and in-laws, are also affected by a mother's experience with PPD. Family members, and in particular, mothers and mothers-in-law, provide much-needed support during the postpartum period. However, this does not always equate to women disclosing their feelings to their family members. In fact, the fear of disappointing her family may lead the new mother to remain silent, suffering alone (Venis & McCloskey, 2007).

Despite what we know about PPD and the crucial role of family in both preventing and overcoming PPD, the question remains: how can families help women suffering with PPD? How can they provide the practical and emotional support needed to help lessen the new mothers' stress? Ross, et al. (2005, p. 80) provide the following list of suggestions for partners, and other family members, helping mothers suffering with PPD.

1. Help her work with her health care provider to make informed decisions about the treatment plan that is best for her.

2. Ask her which kind of support she prefers; ask her for a list that details how people can help her the most.

3. Help with household tasks without being asked, and, as Curtis and Schuler (2003) explain, without expecting much in return.

4. Provide her with reassurance: tell her you are there for her, emphasize that she is a good mother, tell her you love her, and that you will get through this together.

5. Encourage her to talk about her feelings and explain to her that you want to understand and are trying to do so.

6. Explain to her that her depression is not her fault and that she is not at fault.

Conclusion

Everyone has a "moving" story. These stories tell tales about how people moved away from their friends at a young age, or how they adjusted to their friends moving away, or how they left college and moved away with nary a friend or family member for support. Some of us can relate to all three situations, but most can relate to at least one. It is unlikely that one's social support network will remain the same across the lifespan; it is constantly changing as we change and grow as people, as we move to different locations and meet new people, as we move in and out of social and professional networks. However, despite change and adaptation characterizing our social support networks, it is likely that one means of social support is constant: family. While friends and colleagues come and go, families typically provide for a fairly consistent form of social support. Yet, families today are often geographically dispersed, making it even more difficult to provide the interpersonal face-to-face support family members may be accustomed to receiving. Thankfully, though, new technologies, such as the Internet, are making it easier to stay in touch with family and friends.

Interpersonal "talk" therapy has been shown effective in not only treating but potentially preventing PPD (Mazure & Keita, 2006). Therefore, it is important that scholars research all channels of interpersonal support rather than only the face-to-face interactions women have with their physicians, or other closer ties such as family members. Given the scores of women using the Internet for health information seeking, and the fact that PPD is a condition often undiagnosed in part due to women's decisions to remain silent about their symptoms, it is important to understand where women are receiving support during the postpartum period and from whom they are receiving such support. This information may lead to the development of preventative strategies that include arranging social support prior to the postpartum period, rather than merely during a brief postpartum period. Looking back at the differences in how we planned for support after my two deliveries, the outcomes are clear.

We arranged for extended familial support to be available in my home after the birth of my second child; this was much more effective than having a family member available for only one week postpartum, as was the case during my first delivery. I wish someone had explained to me the value of having support available in the immediate postpartum period. I also wish I had known that my symptoms were not "normal" and that I needed to ask for help. As a woman experienced in the art of saying "I can handle it," I wonder just how many women silently suffer with postpartum depression simply because they feel they will be seen as weak or as incapable of dealing with motherhood. Certainly, there is no justifiable reason for this lack of education about PPD. A simple conversation with a health care provider during a prenatal visit could lead women to further educate themselves about the condition, or at minimum, set the stage for any future conversations about PPD. In the same vein, childbirth educators could easily discuss PPD and its warning signs during one session of a childbirth class. It is important that a woman be educated about PPD during the prenatal period so that she is informed before her symptoms begin and is aware of resources available to her for diagnosing and treating the condition.

Many women are forced to raise their children alone without the built-in support that comes with a spouse or partner. Others lack supportive families, do not have access to adequate medical care, and do not know about myriad social support groups, both in-person and online, that exist for postpartum depression. I, however, have a supportive husband and family. I have insurance and can easily access medical care and mental health specialists. I am also well educated and have access to resources. Despite my life-changing experience with PPD, I consider myself lucky to have the support system I do.

In sum, it is important to understand the impact that PPD has on mothers, their infants, and their families. Women must rely heavily on their social support networks to successfully navigate treatment for PPD and prevent PPP. There is a growing body of research on women's health care, and women's mental health. In addition, the media are highlighting PPD more than in years past, and some are taking an active role to de-stigmatize the condition. Still, there is misinformation about PPD reaching new mothers each day, and each day another woman suffers in silence, her feelings invalidated by medical professionals or others who brush off her symptoms as "normal." Hopefully, the causes of PPD will soon be discovered. Until then, we can focus on how to increase the prevention behaviors we already know of and to study these behaviors inside a woman-centered framework. It is also important to understand the very deep scars this condition can leave on the relationships depressed women have with family members, particularly their partners who often suffer from depression as well. It is important to generate dialogue about this condition and give voice to the thousands of women, and their families, who lack the ability to express their symptoms and who are afraid to tell their stories, and to ensure no more women or babies lose their lives to this immobilizing, yet treatable, condition.

References

Achat, H., Kawachi, I., Levine, S., Berkey, C., Coakley, E., & Colditz, G. (1998). Social networks, stress, and health-related quality of life. *Quality of Life Research, 7*, 735-750.

Beck, C. T. (1993). Teetering on the edge: A substantive theory of postpartum depression. *Nursing Research, 42*, 42-48.

Beck, C. T. (1996). Postpartum depressed mothers' experiences interacting with their children. *Nursing Research, 45*, 98-104.

Beck, C. T. (2001). Predictors of postpartum depression: An update. *Nursing Research, 50*, 275-285.

Beck, C. T. (2002). Revision of the postpartum depression predictors inventory. *Journal of Obstetric, Gynecologic, and Neonatal Nursing, 31*, 394-402.

Belsky, J., & Rovine, M. (1990). Patterns of change across the transition to parenthood: Pregnancy to three years postpartum. *Journal of Marriage & Family, 52*, 5-19.

Bennett, S. S. (2007). *Postpartum depression for dummies.* Hoboken, NJ: Wiley.

Bennett, S. S., & Indman, P. (2003). *Beyond the blues—a guide to understanding and treating prenatal and postpartum depression.* San Jose, CA: Moodswings Press.

Buultjens, M., & Liamputtong, P. (2007). When giving life starts to take the life out of you: Women's experiences of depression after childbirth. *Midwifery, 23*, 77-91.

Callister, L. C. (2003). Making meaning: Women's birth narratives. *Journal of Obstetric, Gynecologic, & Neonatal Nursing, 33*, 508-518.

Chan, S., & Levy, V. (2004). Postnatal depression: A qualitative study of the experiences of a group of Hong Kong Chinese women. *Journal of Clinical Nursing, 13*, 120-123.

Clay, R. A. (2001). Fulfilling an unmet need. [Electronic version]. *Monitor on Psychology, 32*. Retrieved from http://www.apa.org/ monitor/feb01/postpartum.html.

Cohen, S., & Williamson, G. M. (1991). Stress and infectious disease in humans. *Psychological Bulletin, 109,* 5-24.

Cohn, J. F., Campbell, S. A., Matias, R., & Hopkins, J. (1990). Face to face interactions of postpartum depressed and nondepressed mother-infant pairs at 2 months. *Developmental Psychology, 26,* 15-23.

Cornman, J. C., Goldman, N., Glei, D. A., Weinstein, M., & Change, M. C. (2003). Social ties and perceived support: Two dimensions of social relationships and health among the elderly in Taiwan. *Journal of Aging and Health, 15,* 616-644.

Curtis, G. B., & Schuler, J. (2003). *Your pregnancy and the father to be*. New York, NY: Da Capo Press.

Curtis, G. B., & Schuler, J. (2004). *Your pregnancy week by week* (5th ed.). Cambridge, MA: Da Capo Press.

Cutrona, C. E. (1996). Social support as a determinant of marital quality: The interplay of negative and supportive behaviors. In G. R. Pierce, B. R. Sarason, & I. G. Sarason (Eds.), *Handbook of social support and the family* (pp. 173-194). New York, NY: Plenum.

Dennis, C-L. (2003). The effect of peer support on postpartum depression: A pilot randomized controlled trial. *Canadian Journal of Psychiatry, 48,* 115-124.

de Tychey, C., Briancon, S., Lighezzolo, J., Sptiz, E., Kabuth, B., de Luigi, V., ...Vincent, S. (2008). Quality of life, postnatal depression, and baby gender. *Journal of Clinical Nursing, 17,* 312-322.

Dobris, C. A., & White-Mills, K. (2006). Rhetorical visions of motherhood: A feminist analysis of the what to expect series. *Women and Language, 29,* 26-37.

Dunkel-Schetter, C., Sagrestano, L. M., Feldman, P., & Killingsworth, C. (1996). Social support and pregnancy: A comprehensive review focusing on ethnicity and culture. In G. R. Pierce, B. R. Sarason, & I. G. Sarason (Eds.), *Handbook of social support and the family* (pp. 375-412). New York, NY: Plenum.

Field, T. M. (2002). Early interactions between infants and their postpartum depressed mothers. *Infant Behavior & Development, 25,* 25-29.

Fincham, F. D. (2003). Marital conflict: Correlates, structure, and context. *Current Directions in Psychological Science, 12,* 23-27.

Frasure-Smith, N., Lesperance, F., Gravel, G., Masson, A., Juneau, M., Talajic, M., & Bourassa, M. G. (2000). Social support, depression, and mortality during the first year after myocardial infarction. *Circulation, 101,* 1919-1924.

Goodman, J. H. (2004). Paternal postpartum depression, its relationship to maternal postpartum depression, and implications for family health. *Journal of Advanced Nursing, 45,* 26-35.

Grace, S. L., Evindar, A., & Stewart, D. E. (2003). The effect of postpartum depression on child cognitive development and behavior: A review and critical analysis of the literature. *Archives of Women's Mental Health, 6,* 263-274.

Hackel, L. S., & Ruble, D. N. (1992). Changes in the marital relationship after the first baby is born: Predicting the impact of expectancy disconfirmation. *Journal of Personality and Social Psychology, 62,* 944-957.

Harkins, D. A., & Ray, S. (2004). An exploratory study of mother-child storytelling in east India and northeast United States. *Narrative Inquiry, 14,* 347-367.

Henshaw, C. (2006). Psychological and social approaches to treatment. *Psychiatry, 5,* 21-24.

Hinshaw, S. P., & Cicchetti, D. (2000). Stigma and mental disorder: Conceptions of illness, public attitudes, personal disclosure, and social policy. *Development and Psychopathology, 12,* 555-598.

How far we've come. (1999, December). *Harvard Women's Health Watch, 6,* 2.

Kendall-Tackett, K. A. (2005). *Depression in new mothers: Causes, consequences, and treatment alternatives.* Binghamton, NY: Haworth Press.

Kinser, A. E. (1997). *Pregnant with meaning: An interpretive analysis of women's pregnancy discourse.* Unpublished doctoral dissertation, Purdue University.

Lakey, B., & Lutz, C. J. (1996). Social support and preventative and therapeutic interventions. In G. R. Pierce, B. R. Sarason, & I. G. Sarason (Eds.), *Handbook of social support and the family* (pp. 435-466). New York, NY: Plenum.

Lavee, Y., Sharlin, S., & Katz, R. (1996). The effect of parenting stress on marital quality: An integrated mother-father model. *Journal of Family Issues, 17,* 114-135.

Mahar-Sylvestre, C. (2001, Winter). When sadness follows childbirth: Postpartum depression. [Electronic version]. *The Canadian Women's' Health Network Magazine, 4,* 3. Retrieved October 9, 2006 from http://www.cwhm.ca/network-reseau/4-1/4-1pg3.html.

Majewski, J. L. (1986). Conflicts, satisfactions, and attitudes during transition to the maternal role. *Nursing Research, 35,* 10-14.

Mazure, C. M., & Keita, G. P. (2006). *Understanding depression in women: Applying empirical research to practice and policy.* Washington, DC: American Psychological Association.

Meighan, M., Davis, M. W., Thomas, S. P., & Droppleman, P. G. (1999). Living with postpartum depression: The father's experience. *The American Journal of Maternal/Child Nursing, 24,* 202-208.

Mickelson, K. D. (2001). Perceived stigma, social support, and depression. *Personality and Social Psychology Bulletin, 27,* 1046-1056.

Milgrom, J., Ericksen, J., McCarthy, R., & Gemmill, A. W. (2006). Stressful impact of depression on early mother-infant relations. *Stress and Health, 22,* 229-238.

Milgrom, J., Martin, P. R., & Negri, L. M. (1999). *Treating postnatal depression: A psychological approach for health care practitioners.* West Sussex, England: John Wiley & Sons.

Mitchell, E. A., Thompson, J. M. D., Stewart, A. W., Webster, M. L., Taylor, B. J., Hassall, I. B., ... Becroft, D. M. O. (2008). Postnatal depression and SIDS: A prospective study. *Journal of Paediatrics and Child Health, 28,* S13-S16.

Moline, M. L., Kahn, D. A., Ross, R. W., Altshuler, L. L., & Cohen, L. S. (2001). *Postpartum depression: A guide for patients and families.* A Postgraduate Medicine Special Report: Treatment of Depression in Women, pp. 112-113. Retrieved from http://www.psychguides.com/DinW%20postpartum.pdf#search=%22definition%20for%20postpartum%20depression%22.

Moore, S. A. D. (2008). *An inconvenient truth: Recognizing Andrea Yates was a victim of spousal abuse: She killed her children to save her life.* Retrieved from website: http://works.bepress.com/shelby_moore/1.

Murray, L., Kempton, C., Woolgar, M., & Hooper, R. (1993). Depressed mothers' speech to their infants and its relation to infant gender and cognitive development. *Journal of Child Psychology and Psychiatry, 34,* 1083–1101.

Oates, M. (2003a). Perinatal psychiatric disorders: A leading cause of maternal morbidity and mortality. *British Medical Journal, 67,* 219-229.

Oates, M. (2003b). Suicide: the leading cause of maternal death. *British Medical Journal, 183,* 279-281.

O'Malley, S. (2004). *Are you there alone: The unspeakable crimes of Andrea Yates.* New York, NY: Simon & Schuster.

Pryke, R. (2002). A patient-centered approach to postnatal depression. *Pulse,* 37.

Ramsay, R. (1993). *Postnatal depression. Lancet, 341,* 1358.

Reisser, P. C. (1997). *Complete book for baby & child care.* Wheaton, IL: Tyndale House Publishers, Inc.

Robertson, E., Grace, S., Wallington, T., & Stewart, D. (2004). Antenatal risk factors for postpartum depression: A synthesis of recent literature. *General Hospital Psychiatry, 26,* 289-295.

Roche, T. (2002). *Andrea Yates: More to the story.* Retrieved October 29, 2008, from http://www.time.com.

Ross, L. E., Dennis, C-L., Blackmore, E. R., & Stewart, D. E. (2005). *Postpartum depression: A guide for front-line health and social service providers.* Toronto, Canada: Centre for Addiction and Mental Health.

Sargent, C. F., & Brettell, C. B. (1996). *Gender and health: An international perspective.* Upper Saddle River, NJ: Prentice Hall.

Savage, J. S. (2001). Birth stories: A way of knowing in childbirth education. *Journal of Perinatal Education, 10,* 3-7.

Sayil, M., Gure, A., & Ucanok, Z. (2006). First time mothers' anxiety and depressive symptoms across the transition to motherhood: Associations with maternal and environmental characteristics. *Women & Health, 44,* 61-77.

Schur, E., & Nicolette, J. (1997). Medical students and the future of women's health. *The Journal of the American Medical Association, 277,* 1406-1408.

Scrandis, D. A. (2005). Normalizing postpartum depressive symptoms with social support. *American Psychiatric Nurses Association Journal, 11,* 223.

Silberner, J. (2002). *One mother's story. Postpartum psychosis: Rare, frightening, and treatable.* Retrieved October 9, 2006 from http://www.npr.org/programs/morning/features/2002/feb/postpartum/020218.postpartum.html

Spinelli, M. (2004). Maternal infanticide associated with mental illness: Prevention and the promise of saved lives. *American Journal of Psychiatry, 161,* 1548-1157.

Spinelli, M. (2005a). Infanticide: Contrasting views. *Archives of Women's Mental Health, 8,* 15-24.

Spinelli, M. (2005b). Perinatal infanticide and suicide. In A. Riecher-Rossler & M. Steiner (Eds), *Perinatal stress, mood, and anxiety disorders: From bench to bedside* (pp. 85-99). Basel, Switzerland: Karger.

Stice, E., Ragan, J., & Randall, P. (2004). Prospective relations between social support and depression: Differential direction of effects for parents and peer support? *Journal of Abnormal Psychology, 113,* 155-159.

Stone, J., & Eddleman, K. (2003). *The pregnancy bible: Your complete guide to pregnancy and early parenthood.* Buffalo, NY: Firefly Books.

Taylor, M. M. (2003). Endometriosis—a missed malady. *AORN Journal, 77,* 297-311.

The Boston Women's Health Book Collective. (1998). *Our bodies, ourselves for the new century.* New York, NY: Simon & Schuster, Inc.

Thome, M. (2003). Severe postpartum distress in Icelandic mothers with difficult infants: A follow-up study on their health care. *Scandinavian Journal of Caring, 17,* 104-112.

Ussher, J. M. (2003). The role of premenstrual dysphoric disorder in the subjectification of women. *Journal of Medical Humanities, 24,* 131-146.

VanderVoort, D. J., & Skorikov, V. B. (2002). Physical health and social network characteristics as determinants of mental health across cultures. *Current Psychology, 21,* 50-67.

Venis, J. A., & McCloskey, S. (2007). *Postpartum depression demystified: An essential guide for understanding and overcoming the most common complication after birth.* New York, NY: Marlowe & Company.

Williamson, V., & McCutcheon, H. (2004). Postnatal depression: A review of current literature. *Australian Midwifery Journal, 17,* 11-16.

Wisner, K. L., Parry, B. L., & Piontek, C. M. (2002). Postpartum depression. *The New England Journal of Medicine, 347,* 194-199.

Wright, K., & Bell, S. B. (2003). Health-related support groups on the internet: Linking empirical findings to social support and computer-mediated communication theory. *Journal of Health Psychology, 8,* 39-54.

Wynszynski, A. A., & Lusskin, S. I. (2005). *Manual of psychiatric care for the medically ill.* Arlington, CA: American Psychiatric Publishing.

Young, E. (2005). State takes arms against postpartum depression. *The Record.* Retrieved from http://www.lexisnexis.com

PART 2

Stigma

CHAPTER 6

Stigma and Politeness: Challenging Family Health Discussions

Kelly Rossetto

BOSTON COLLEGE

Rachel A. Smith

THE PENNSYLVANIA STATE UNIVERSITY

Barbara Jones

THE UNIVERSITY OF TEXAS AT AUSTIN

Learning that someone in your family has a serious health condition is a difficult situation to face. For professionals, providing this information to families can be emotionally challenging. These discussions can be especially tough when the topic is taboo or the person is at risk of stigmatization. This chapter highlights how politeness and co-ownership of health information can help us to understand the challenges facing families when they discuss taboo or stigmatized health conditions.

Stigma and Taboos

Stigma processes are considered significant barriers to health promotion, treatment, and support (e.g., World Health Organization, 2001) and are also the least understood (e.g., UNAIDS, 2004). What is a stigma? It is a "simplified, standardized image of the disgrace of certain people that is held in common by a community at large" (Smith, 2007, p. 464). The disgrace imbedded in a stigma relates to taboos, which are defined as a prohibited condition or act (Oxford English Dictionary). Goffman (1963) argued that stigmas generate an intense form of devaluation such that a member of a stigmatized group may be considered no longer human. Because of dehumanization, communities exercise a number of discrimination choices that ultimately limit stigmatized people's quality of life and possibly their lives (Goffman, 1963).

The most salient example of stigmatized health issues in the past few decades has been HIV/AIDS. People living with HIV/AIDS often experience uncertainty about others' reactions (Brashers, Neidig, & Goldsmith, 2004) and often choose not to disclose their status because of the stigma attached to the illness and concerns about others' reactions (e.g., Alonzo & Reynolds, 1995; Derlega et al., 2004) and rejection (Brashers, Neidig, & Goldsmith, 2004). HIV/AIDS is not the only illness in which such challenging conversations occur. Women battling cancer express reluctance about sharing their results because of family communication barriers (e.g., Green, Richards, Murton, Statham, & Hallowell, 1997) or family relationship problems (e.g., Hughes et al., 2002). Partners, other family members, friends, children, and co-workers may be eager to get past the disruptions created by discovery of cancer and its treatment so life can return to normal (Lewis & Deal, 1995). These significant others, therefore, may discourage discussion of cancer, leaving women to work through their unresolved questions and feelings in isolation (Lewis & Deal, 1995). Indeed, a family's social norms can discourage health practices (e.g., Ajzen & Fishbein, 1980). These barriers may be why the practice of initiating cancer conversations, such as disclosing that one carries genetic mutations for breast cancer, may be burdensome on the carrier (see Hallowell et al., 2005 for a review). For example, families may expect that providing for the family may take precedence over taking time to be screened for cancer. As such, stigma and uncertainty can act as barriers to important benefits of disclosure such as support and medical care.

People want to avoid being targets of stigmatization (Herek, 2007). People who find themselves in a situation in which they have conditions that can categorize them as members of a stigmatized group (i.e., labeled) anticipate these judgments of responsibility, the categorization and labeling, as well as the potential for devaluation-discrimination. Consequently, potential targets engage in coping strategies (e.g., compensation, avoidance, comparison, deception, denial, secrecy, withdrawal) aimed at preventing negative reactions (Herek, 1996; Link, 1987; Link, Cullen, Streuning, Shrout, & Dohrenwend, 1989; Markowitz, 1998; Miller & Major, 2000; Smith, 2007).

Individual and Familial Diagnosis Disclosure

With denial, secrecy, avoidance, and deception as possible coping strategies for individuals anticipating stigma, disclosure or non-disclosure becomes an important communication process for consideration. Recently, Smith and Hipper (in press) proposed a model that explains the advice unlabeled confidants give their labeled (e.g., members of a stigmatized group) loved ones about how to use withdrawal, secrecy, and education to cope with labeling and potential stigmatization. Label management (LM) presumes that when a person discloses his/her labeling condition to an unlabeled confidant, the two become co-owners of this information (Petronio, 2002, Petronio, Sargent, Andea, Reganis, & Cichocki, 2004). Co-owners share in the knowledge of the discloser's labeled status, regulation of this knowledge, as well as its consequences. In LM (Smith & Hipper, in press), it is argued that confidants consider the label, its stereotypes and potential consequences, in similar fashion to those bearing the label, because this is socialized among all members of a community (Link et al., 1989; Smith, 2007). As predicted by LM, empirically, unlabeled confidants reported greater intentions to advise their labeled loved ones to use secrecy to cope with stigmatization as they held more devaluation-discrimination beliefs about the labeling condition and they felt that the labeling condition was more personally relevant (Smith & Hipper, in press; Smith, Moore, Catona, & Priem, 2009). In a different setting, respondents in Namibia, South Africa, in two studies, two years apart, reported greater desires to keep a family member's HIV-positive status a secret as they perceived their own risk of contracting HIV as higher and anticipated great HIV stigmatization (Smith & Niedermyer, 2009).

Similarly, Tasker (1992) created a phase-model of the process parents go through when they consider disclosing the parent's, child's, and/or another family member's HIV+ diagnosis. The phases, including secrecy, exploration, readiness, and final disclosure, imply a sequential stage model (from secrecy to final disclosure), but disclosers do not have to travel through each phase. The secrecy phase involves nondisclosure, or keeping the diagnosis a secret from the child. In this phase, there is also a resistance to attending outside support groups. In the exploration phase, parents maintain secrecy but with less intensity. Parents become more ambivalent about the secrecy but still affirm that it is best for the child not to know. They begin to discuss the illness with children using euphemisms and descriptions, but not using the words HIV/AIDS. During the readiness phase parents come closer to the disclosure and begin preparing for the disclosure interaction. They create plans for disclosing the diagnosis and sometimes enlist professional help in preparing for the disclosure. In the final disclosure phase, parents disclose the diagnosis to the child. The disclosure may involve structured plans and collaboration with a professional or it may stem from the child's direct questions (Tasker, 1992). Tasker's (1992) model illustrates the complex nature of disclosing illness diagnoses, explaining the process leading to and following diagnosis disclosure. However, it does not demonstrate how people enact disclosure communicatively and how the disclosures are interpreted.

Such family dynamics appear with other health conditions such as cancer. For example, family members and survivors make decisions about whether or not and with whom to disclose a cancer diagnosis. Often coupled/married pairs may decide not to tell their children until they have to (Bloom, Stewart, Chang, & Banks, 2004; Hallowell et al., 2005; Mellon, Berry-Bobovski, Gold, Levin, & Tainsky, 2006).

Doctor-Patient Diagnosis Disclosures

Many patients report preferences for open and full disclosure of a cancer diagnosis from their physician (Miyata et al., 2005; Schofield et al., 2001). In one study, adult patients rated the following items as highly important in the disclosure process: being told the diagnosis face-to-face, feeling confident about treatment options, being allowed to ask questions, and being given the information without delay (Schofield et al., 2001). Some disclosure characteristics, such as unhurried, honest, balanced, and empathic, may even improve patients' experiences with learning their diagnosis (Ellis & Tattersall, 1999). These characteristics facilitate the ability of the doctor and patient to explore expectations and concerns and increase patients' satisfaction with the disclosure interaction (Ellis & Tattersall, 1999).

There is some evidence that open and full disclosure may also be an optimal strategy with child patients (Clarke, Davies, Jenney, Glaser, & Eiser, 2005). In one study (Hooker, 1997), teenagers reported that having information about their diagnosis, prognosis, and treatment were top priorities for them. These priorities about disclosure processes were rated higher than other criteria, such as impact on lifestyle and appearance (Hooker, 1997). Another study (Dunsmore & Quine, 1995) found that childhood cancer survivors (aged 12-24) wanted to know whether or not treatments were effective and whether or not they were dying. This information may help reduce negative feelings and uncertainty (Claflin & Barbarin, 1991). It may also help child patients feel more involved in the treatment and decision-making process (Dunsmore & Quine, 1995; Ishibashi, 2001). Early cancer disclosure has been associated with improved emotional health, better parent-child relationships, and increased self-esteem (Chesler, Paris, & Barbarin, 1986).

When children are not old enough to consent to treatment, parents serve as proxy decision makers and also control the level of disclosure of information to the child. Despite the benefits of initially and fully disclosing cancer diagnoses, Clarke and her colleagues (2005) found that mothers differed in the communication styles they employed to inform their children (aged 3 to 18) about the child's leukemia. Older children (approximately 10 years old) were given a clearer time frame for their treatment and more detailed information. In addition, mothers' perceptions of cancer influenced which diagnosis strategy they used. For example, mothers who believed the cancer was not curable were less likely to fully disclose the child's disease to him/her. Consequently, children who do not receive full disclosures may believe the illness is taboo and cannot be talked about (Claflin & Barbarin, 1991). Child patients may also learn of their illness in other ways, including overhearing, sensing distress, and/or drawing their own conclusions (Kendrick, Culling, Oakhill, & Mott, 1986), which can lead to stress and suspicion (Atesci et al., 2004). These information-gaining strategies undermine the reason for nondisclosure, which is often protection from fear or worry (Clarke et al., 2005).

Based on the multiple considerations that caregivers and practitioners have regarding disclosure of cancer diagnoses, it is not surprising that there are multiple fears and anxieties (Clarke et al., 2005) about disclosure. Although most doctors in the U.S., Australia, and Europe endorse disclosing cancer diagnoses, many doctors still report difficulties with the interaction (Ellis & Tattersall, 1999). Because doctors want to protect children from pain, and avoid problems with compliance, avoid worsening children's symptoms, they may fear disclosing the diagnosis (Manos & Christakis, 1980). Disclosing illnesses to children produces a variety of concerns for both parents and doctors who hold the information. Parents and doctors worry about disclosing HIV diagnosis to children because they are afraid that children will not understand, will react poorly, and will be adversely affected by the disclosure (Lester et al., 2002).

Disclosers' strategies impact more than patients' satisfaction with the diagnosis disclosure; they also influence patients' mental health (Schofield et al., 2003) and psychological adjustment (Slavin et al., 1982). Strategies that have been shown to reduce anxiety in adult patients include: preparing the patient for potential diagnosis, providing a desired amount of information, giving written information, clearly stating the information, answering questions as they arise, talking about feelings, and providing reassurance (Schofield et al., 2003). Other skills such as using the word "cancer," honestly discussing the diagnosis and prognosis, and encouraging patient involvement are communication practices associated with lower levels of depression in adults (Schofield et al., 2003) and children (Ishibashi, 2001). Perhaps most importantly, studies have shown that improved understanding of the illness, which can come from diagnosis disclosures, increases compliance to treatment regimens and health care outcomes in adults (Marelich & Murphy, 2003; Miura et al., 2000) and hope in children (Ishibashi, 2001; Last & vanVeldhuisen, 1996). As such, disclosure becomes the access point for information, support, and treatment; yet it also opens the door to potential labeling and stigma.

The communication adolescent patients receive is especially important because they face the diagnosis during a fundamental developmental stage associated with developing trust and autonomy. Cancer diagnosis during adolescence poses particular challenges because coping with the diagnosis and treatment is complicated by developmental tasks completed at the same time (Hooker, 1997). Cancer diagnosis in adolescents can also lead to problematic psychological and psychosocial outcomes, such as depression, anxiety, post-traumatic stress disorder (PTSD), distorted self-image, lower self-esteem, isolation from peers, and reduced social skills (Hewitt, Weiner, & Simone, 2003; Zebrack & Chesler, 2001). Further, communicative factors, such as coping, meaning making, and social support, can facilitate or inhibit resilience in adolescents faced with cancer (Woodgate, 1999).

Creating Polite Disclosures

Due to doctors' and parents' concerns and the complex nature of disclosing diagnosis information to children, they are likely to provide diagnosis information in a way that attends to the feelings and needs of the child resulting from the imposing act of cancer diagnosis (Spiers, 1998). Politeness theory (Brown & Levinson, 1978, 1987) provides a framework for understanding the diagnosis disclosure process and provides a means through which to understand patients' recall of the communicative actions of practitioners and caregivers. Although politeness theory is not often used in health literature (Spiers, 1998), diagnosis disclosure fits this theory because, most importantly, the disclosure can be considered a face-threatening act. In other words, the diagnosis disclosure involves unwanted and potentially damaging or imposing news. Face-threatening acts "by their very nature run contrary to the face wants of the addressee and/or the speaker" (Brown & Levinson, 1978, p. 70).

A person's face wants are twofold: the need to maintain positive face and the need to maintain negative face. Face-threatening acts can be performed against one's positive face or negative face. *Positive face* involves the desire to be liked and respected (Brown & Levinson, 1978, 1987; Goffman, 1967; Lim & Bowers, 1991). For example, children may want their parents to show concern and love during doctor's visits and treatments. As they anticipate treatments, children may also be concerned with not being liked as they go through physical changes. Children experience disruptions in their social lives that can lead to decreases in confidence and sociability (Clarke et al.,

2005). To reduce these threats, adults may provide support, love, and compliments to children as they face their cancer diagnosis and treatment.

Negative face entails the desire to be autonomous and independent (Brown & Levinson, 1978, 1987; Goffman, 1967; Lim & Bowers, 1991). The diagnosis itself is an imposing realization for children. Children will likely experience an inability to do tasks that were once easy for them and require extra help (Clarke et al., 2005), so disclosers may address prognoses in more optimistic ways to highlight future autonomy. Honesty and realism may also help the child feel "grown up" in that they are capable of hearing the truth. Honest, full disclosures also allow the patient to feel more involved in the treatment and decision-making process (Dunsmore & Quine, 1995; Ishibashi, 2001). These strategies are all aimed at mitigating negative face threats.

Politeness theory (Brown & Levinson, 1978, 1987) posits that messages vary in politeness based on a scale of directness. Direct messages, also known as bald-on-record, are messages that do not attempt to reduce the face-threatening act (Brown & Levinson, 1978). Rather, they issue the news, requests, or demands bluntly, with no attention to hearer's needs (Brown & Levinson, 1978). Thus, direct strategies are considered least polite and indirect strategies are more polite when delivering face-threatening messages. When face-threats are intense, people may not deliver the message at all. In these cases, the message deliverer avoids the interaction or delivers the message indirectly. Indirect, or off-the-record, messages involve hinting and vagueness so the message can be denied if it is acknowledged (Brown & Levinson, 1978). Between direct and indirect messages are positive and negative politeness strategies.

When communication acts involve threats to positive face, people respond with positive politeness. Strategies for positive politeness include indirect forms of communication, such as seeking agreement, avoiding disagreement, displaying interest, and showing approval. These strategies appeal to the other's desire to be liked and enhance feelings of rapport and connection. On the other hand, when communication acts involve negative face threats, people respond with negative politeness. Negative politeness includes indirect strategies, such as hedging, deferring to authority, apologizing, giving options, and minimizing assumptions (Brown & Levinson, 1978, 1987).

Caregivers and practitioners may exhibit strategies consistent with positive or negative politeness. However, with the push toward truthful, full disclosures (Atesci et al., 2004; Lester et al., 2002), disclosers may also produce more direct messages in an attempt to portray the full diagnosis disclosure to increase patient understanding and improve compliance (Gambosi & Berlin Ray, 1990; Lester et al., 2002; Manos & Christakis, 1980). Unfortunately, direct disclosure can "appear to the receiver to be a cold and distant response to a very traumatic and emotional situation" (Clark & LaBeff, 1982, p. 371). Direct disclosure is similar to "direct telling" in the breaking bad news literature, where "the deliverer is not looking for any outs or giving any; the fact of a death is simply stated" (Clark & LaBeff, 1982, p. 371). Thus, the disclosure of diagnoses presents a double bind for disclosers. With indirect strategies they risk appearing dishonest, and with direct strategies they risk being insensitive and cold.

This double bind likely contributes to the challenge associated with choices caregivers and providers must make when disclosing cancer diagnoses. Thus, it is logical to assess the cancer diagnoses adolescents are receiving through a lens of politeness theory. Brown and Levinson's (1978) original theory posits that face-threatening acts are either threatening to positive face or to negative face. However, disclosing cancer diagnosis involves a threat to both positive and negative face. According to Erbert and Floyd (2003), a single act can threaten both positive and negative face, or threaten one type of face (e.g., positive) in multiple ways. For example, child patients may want to be part of the treatment and decision-making process while simultaneously seeking support and love.

Using politeness theory, we assessed the diagnosis messages that adolescent patients recalled receiving and evaluated how the adolescents recalled different strategies affecting them at the time of the disclosure. The extant literature on disclosures of cancer diagnosis in children and adults suggests multiple ways for patients to experience this communication event.

Example from Cancer Diagnosis Disclosures to Latino/a Adolescents

Two of the authors conducted a study of Latino/a adolescent cancer survivors to understand the meaning of the experience for this population. Data from this study provides useful examples of the issues of diagnosis and disclosure. For this exploratory study, nine adolescent cancer survivors who were treated at two children's hospitals in the south/southwest provided in-depth interviews about their experiences with cancer diagnosis, treatment and survival. Of the participants, seven were female and two were male. All identified themselves as Latino/a. Participants ranged in age between 14 and 21 years old, and years since diagnosis ranged between two and six years. For the purposes of this chapter, data were analyzed from responses to the questions: "How did you first hear that you had cancer," "What helped you get through it and what didn't," and "What meaning do you make out of facing an illness?"

In-depth interviews were transcribed and data were analyzed qualitatively using both inductive and deductive approaches. The data were analyzed inductively through constant-comparative analysis (Lindlof & Taylor, 2002). Open and axial coding techniques were applied in order to discover themes that emerged from the data and then categorize those themes (Strauss & Corbin, 1998). The first stage of constant-comparative analysis involved the creation of multiple categories extrapolated from the data using open coding (Strauss, 1987). During this process, categories were discovered, named, and explained (Lindlof & Taylor, 2002). Then, responses were compared across other responses in order to place them within their appropriate categories, based on thematic properties. Finally, data were revisited using axial coding, which included the integration or collapsing of multiple categories into a more inclusive and manageable list of themes (Strauss & Corbin, 1990). The data were also examined deductively, looking for specific disclosure strategies within the adolescents' diagnosis disclosure descriptions. These disclosure strategies were then labeled according to their directness, or literality. For example, "You have cancer" is a direct strategy, while not sharing the diagnosis information is an indirect strategy. Although the data were analyzed deductively in terms of disclosure strategy directness, sub-themes emerged from the data. In other words, adolescents did not term diagnosis disclosures "indirect" or "direct," so within each categorization a variety of disclosure strategies emerged. Four themes, along with sub-themes, are discussed: 1) source and time, 2) direct/indirect disclosure strategies, 3) reactions, and 4) self-disclosure as patients and survivors.

Case Study Disclosure Themes

Source and time. Adolescents reported that cancer diagnoses occurred over time, between different people, and in different ways. Cancer diagnoses were not simply communicated within one interaction; the information was received over time and often through different channels. In other words, discussing "when you first found out about your cancer diagnosis" was a complicated task. Parents and doctors were the primary sources of diagnosis disclosures, but other health care workers and family members were also involved in the diagnosis process. Participants' reports indicate that parents were co-owners of the diagnosis information from the point of knowing. According to the adolescents, parents were often informed before the child, and parents were then given the assumed ability to choose the disclosure source and strategy. These findings support the assumption in label management (Smith & Hipper, in press) and communication privacy management (Petronio, 2002) that health information is co-owned and managed. The source and time of the disclosures can be noted in the quotes provided below. As expected based on politeness theory (Brown & Levenson, 1978, 1987), disclosure types could be categorized as both direct and indirect; sub-themes within each category are discussed.

Direct and indirect strategies. Direct disclosure strategies involve the communication of information about the cancer diagnosis, explanation of the disease and procedures, and use of the word "cancer." Doctors were recalled as using direct communication strategies when disclosing cancer diagnoses (1) to the participants, and (2) to their parents. Diagnoses were often disclosed directly to the parent(s) first, followed by disclosure to the adolescent. Then, in some cases with parents as the disclosers, participants recalled their parents using direct communication strategies when discussing the cancer diagnosis with them. First, one participant (CS7) illustrated direct disclosure from his doctor:

> He was like, "Well, we diagnosed you with Hodgkin's lymphoma"...And he was like, "It's the most treatable—it's really treatable," and then he said chemotherapy. And right when he said that I was like—that like hit me. And I asked him, I said, "It's cancer?" He said, "It's a type of cancer."

Another participant (CS4) also noted direct disclosure: "I mean there was always somebody explaining, you know a lot of explanation that went on there. They tell you...They would tell me exactly what was going on, why, and how it works, or how this medication works to fight for this."

Noting how parents were the initial receivers of the diagnosis, one participant (CS2) said, "My parents were called into a meeting. They let them know exactly what needed to be done. How long of time needed to be taken, you know, specific." And illustrating the parents "control" over the disclosure, another participant (CS1) stated, "They [parents] told the doctors, 'Don't tell her.' We want to break it to her." Although this plan was not altogether successful (the adolescent learned her diagnosis from a medical student), the family had intentions to tell this participant about her diagnosis. After this participant learned about her diagnosis elsewhere (i.e., indirectly from a medical student, as noted below), her mother came in and said, "We need to tell you something. You have cancer" (CS1).

In addition to direct diagnosis disclosures, participants reported learning about their cancer diagnosis indirectly. Two sub-themes within indirect communication strategies emerged from the data: 1) late or secondhand diagnoses and 2) hopeful information and prognoses. One participant (CS6) noted that she did not hear about her diagnosis until years after she had been through treatment, perhaps because she was too young to understand what it meant to have cancer. She said, "I remember going to the doctors. Nobody ever told me I had cancer until about two years ago." Two participants first heard about their diagnosis by overhearing conversations between doctors and family members. These adolescents witnessed both nonverbal and verbal communication that revealed the intensity of their diagnosis before they knew it was cancer. For example, one participant (CS3) recalled,

> I was waiting there and then I hear...I can hear my mom crying. And the nurse is like, "Can I have some nurses in this?" And I was like, "What's going on?" I thought it was something wrong with them because I had no idea what was going on with me because I didn't feel sick.

Another adolescent (CS1) stated,

> And when I was waking up from my surgery, before they had told me, I knew it was something really bad because I could hear my brother crying, and he was outside my door...They would just go in and they would hug me, tell me they loved me, and you know, just—they wouldn't tell me anything.

Adolescents also overheard verbal communication regarding diagnoses. Before the actual diagnosis, one participant overheard a doctor talking to a nurse about her illness. This participant (CS1) recalled,

> I was around 19, and when you go into a 20 or 21, that is complete liver failure. So, he looked at that, and he told the nurse, "Oh, she's in liver failure; I don't think she is going to make it." I was on the bed, and he was at the door, and I was like, "Ahhhh!"...I'm not sure if he realized I was awake.

This adolescent also later received the cancer diagnosis accidentally from a medical student. She (CS1) said,

> Who finally did end up telling me was, I want to say, what happened was one of the doctors, one of the med students, came in and he was talking to me, and he was like, "Yeah, so chemo, you scared?" And I'm like, "Huh?"

These indirect accidental and overheard disclosures relate to politeness theory in a few ways. Although the primary disclosers are attempting to avoid a face-threatening act by using an off-the-record strategy, the disclosure occurs. These disclosures are in line with both positive and negative politeness strategies. Positive politeness strategies attempt to accommodate the receiver's need to be liked and admired. Hearing they are loved, receiving affection, and being engaged in conversation about the diagnosis helps reduce threats to positive face. On the other hand, these indirect strategies also enact communicative strategies such as hedging and avoidance that are more indicative of negative politeness in that they attempt to reduce infringing on the patient's needs for independence.

Hopeful communication. Second, adolescents recalled learning about their diagnoses indirectly through hopeful communication, information, and prognoses. This form of disclosure was most often directed from parents to child. For example, one participant (CS1) stated,

> It never occurred to me, "Oh, I am going to die," because they never let me think like that. It's always, "You're going to be fine. Don't worry about it. You're going to be fine." Every time I went into the hospital, "Don't worry, it's just a setback. You're going to be fine."

Another adolescent (CS5) explained, "[My family] always supported me, kept telling me I'll be okay, and I'll get through it, and I'll be alright. [They said], 'It'll be fine. It'll be over.'"

These hopeful disclosures from parents exhibit both positive and negative politeness strategies. Positive politeness can be seen in the support and encouragement participants recalled. Negative politeness is also demonstrated in parents' attempts to make the participants feel like they would "be alright." This strategy enables participants to maintain a positive outlook on their abilities to function as normal.

It is tempting to assume that parents are more likely to employ hopeful communication strategies and prognoses because they are more interested in protecting the child's face. However, participants also recalled hopeful disclosures and prognoses from doctors, nurses, and caregivers. One participant (CS2) recalled,

> They were always so positive. Always. I'm very positive, too, but they always talked to me very comfortably. Even if it was a bad situation and they thought it was going to be something that was going to freak me out, they still put it in a very good way. They gave me different alternatives to where they were like, "Well, it's a bad thing, but it's not that bad because you can do this to make it better."

Another (CS7) said,

> He goes, "If you want to have cancer, which you don't, this is the one you want to get, the most treatable"...So I don't know from the very beginning I've had like a strong mentality, I mean like this isn't going to kill me. So I never really had to face my mortality I guess.

Again, both positive and negative politeness strategies are at work. Rapport building and positivity contribute to positive face, and giving alternatives and control to the patient help maintain negative face.

Reactions. In addition to describing the diagnosis process, adolescents also discussed the consequences of different types of cancer disclosures. Specifically, they recalled learning more and understanding their diagnoses better after receiving direct disclosures, and they described increased fear and awareness of being sick after receiving indirect disclosure strategies.

Direct disclosure strategies led the adolescents to feel more complete understanding of their diagnoses because they learned from the disclosures. One participant (CS4) stated, "You learn everything. You learn about different medications, you learn about different types of tests, blood tests, echos, stuff that people don't really know about." Another participant (CS4) stated that hearing clear information was helpful when learning about the cancer diagnosis. She said, "I guess not keeping secrets from me helped a lot...So, I guess being happy that you have people explaining it to you instead of trying to keep it a secret from you."

In response to indirect disclosures, adolescents' responses were varied. Following overhearing or accidentally receiving the diagnosis without getting direct information, participants reported a heightened awareness of and fear about being sick. In response to indirect strategies that involved hopeful communication, however, adolescents noted a sense of reassurance and comfort. In terms of receiving limited to no information, one adolescent (CS1) said, "I knew something was wrong. And for no one to tell me, it scared me. That scared me because I mean...they told me [later] I was probably going to die, and I never knew." Another participant (CS3) stated, "I didn't know what was going on at all. I had no idea. The thing that was kind of scary was that they put me in a separate room, and they asked my parents to go in another room." Separating this adolescent from his family, and consequently from the diagnosis information, produced fear within him. As a result of not receiving the information, these adolescents felt more afraid, which is likely the outcome that parents are trying to avoid. These findings support the idea in label management that it is not just those living with the challenging condition, but their close confidants that decide to use withdrawal/isolation or secrecy (Smith & Hipper, in press).

These reactions also highlight the actual impact indirect strategies had on the participants' positive and negative face, rather than the idealized consequences of politeness strategies. Although indirectness is thought to help maintain face, it also appears to have negative effects. Participants felt separated and alone (positive face threats), as well as afraid of the potential outcomes (negative face threats) because they did not receive the information they needed.

In response to indirect strategies using hopeful communication, however, adolescents felt a sense of reassurance and comfort. One participant (CS1) stated,

> My mom actually took me to church, and we just prayed, and she's like, "It's going to be okay, you know, it's just a setback; you're going to be fine. Nothing to worry about, you know. It's in God's hands. You're going to be fine, I can feel it. You're going to be okay." And it's just reassuring, you know, because you have your own thoughts, but to be able to just go, "Yeah, it's going to be okay."

Another participant (CS5) stated that she felt supported by her family because "they kept telling [her] that [she'd] be okay." And lastly, one participant (CS2) stated,

> ...They gave me different alternatives to where they were like, "Well, it's a bad thing, but it's not that bad because you can do this to make it better." They always were there to comfort me and there was always a bunch of doctors around, so if one doctor was gone, I could always just go grab another doctor and be like, "Hey, there's a problem." ...They were very helpful...They were my second family.

According to these adolescents, hearing positive and hopeful communication provided reassurance and comfort, which corresponds to positive face. They also received information and options, which helped maintain negative face.

Self-disclosure of patients and survivors. Participants often said they did not disclose their own diagnosis to others when they were patients and do not disclose now that they are out of treatment and living as "survivors." Some said they wanted to be treated normally, as a person, not as a disease or victim or patient. They got sick of hearing, "How are you?" or "Are you ok?" because they want their own identity, separate from being a cancer patient or cancer survivor. While social rejection or stigmatization may not be the reason behind withholding this information, it is still the fear of a reaction that contradicted participants' own beliefs about themselves. So even though reactions may be, "Wow! You are a survivor!" (CS2) rather than "Ewww, you have a disease," these adolescents wanted to maintain an identity separate from their cancer rather than feel a sense of separation and standardization that associated them with social categories, stereotypes, and stigma. One participant (CS7) noted,

> So I didn't like the feeling like it was like I'm bald, people can tell, you know like poor him. I didn't like pity…I just really wanted to have as much of a normal life as I could. And I always wore a hat…I just couldn't stand the idea of me, people maybe not looking down on me negatively it was just you know that pity or "Oh, he's going through something right now." I just wanted to have some sort of normal life that I could have.

Other participants also illustrated these feelings and decisions about disclosure: "I really don't tell my friends because then they start to feel sorry for you and I'm like I'm a normal person, so they don't need to feel sorry for me" (CS5).

> I remember just sort of coming back to normal life and it wasn't; you don't really feel like you have a normal life being at the hospital every day or every other day…And then you have some people who will treat you different. You go, "Oh yeah, I just went through cancer treatment," and they're like, "Ohhh, are you OK?" I think I got really really tired of people saying, "How are you feeeeeling?" I'm feeling OK, you know, you get tired of people treating you different…I didn't choose to tell a lot of people when I went back to school. The only people that really knew were close friends that knew me before I got sick. But it wasn't—I didn't go back and want to be treated like I just had—I didn't really tell anybody.

Expanding on the idea of wanting to feel and be "normal," one participant (CS8) said, "But, and the people around you, too. You know, they have to know, like you're not—you're still a person. You're not the sickness, you know. I think that was a big deal. It's not like you're going to break or something." These reactions speak strongly to tensions and anguish associated with being labeled and identified as one's health condition.

Discussion

Almost no one goes through cancer diagnosis, treatment, and survivorship alone. Rather, members of the cancer survivor's social network are involved at every step. For example, three-person consultations (physician, patient, and relative) appear frequently in cancer care (Lienard et al., 2008). Moreover, cancer survivors often bear the central responsibility to share their diagnosis with other family members (e.g., Velicer & Taplin, 2001; Mellon et al., 2006), and even to spur their social networks to preventative action, such as cancer screening (e.g, Myers, Vernon, Tilley, Lu, & Watts, 1998). This is not to suggest that the medical team does not impact these discussions. As cancer survivors report more problems interacting with their medical teams, they reported more stress, less emotional support from family, friends, and spouse, more aversive reactions from their networks, and less informational support (e.g., Han et al., 2005).

The issues of disclosure play integral roles in how patients and their families manage the outcomes associated with taboo activities, labeled as members of stigmatized groups, or stigmatization. In a modified labeling theory (MLT), Link and colleagues (1987, 1989) explain that labeled people cope with the aversive outcomes of stigmatization through secrecy, withdrawal, and/or education.

Diagnosed women often want to understand their own risk before communicating it to their families (Forrest et al., 2003). This caution may be warranted. Caregivers' poor adjustment to cancer has been linked with patients' poor social rehabilitation, poor treatment adherence, and increased emotional distress (see Merckaert et al., 2008). In one study, if at least one family member or friend discouraged a woman from having a mammogram, she expressed less favorable views of mammography a year later (Pearlman et al., 1997). Aversive reactions, secrecy, stigma, and social isolation can increase stress, which has been linked to neuroendocrine and cardiovascular responses, suppression of immune functioning, and interference with the performance of health behaviors (Cohen, 1988; Uchino et al., 1996).

Positive Possibilities

Although this discussion has focused primarily on how discussions can generate problematic outcomes, it is possible for these discussions to have very positive ones. For example, the size and diversity of one's social support system has been implicated in men and women getting screened for cancer (Kang & Bloom, 1993; Kang, Bloom, & Romano, 1994; Leach & Schoenberg, 2007), disease development (Seeman & Syme, 1987), psychological and social adaptation to diagnosis and its treatment (e.g., Bloom et al., 1991; Neuling & Winefield, 1988), compliance with cancer prevention and treatments (e.g., Gravell, Zapka, & Mamon, 1985; Kang & Bloom, 1993; Zhu et al., 2002), quality of life (Bloom, 1986), and even mortality (e.g., Berkman & Syme, 1979; Ell, Mishimoto, Mediansky, Mantell, & Hamovitch, 1992; Maunsell, Brisson, & Deschenes, 1995; Spiegel, Bloom, Kraemer, & Gottheil, 1989). The literature provides three possible reasons for *positive* effects of social networks: resources, normative influences, and stress-buffering.

People who maintain larger, diverse social networks have an advantage in garnering social support. They can more easily gain *information,* or knowledge relevant to the situation (Granovetter, 1976; Schaeffer, Coyne, & Lazarus, 1981), such as where to get the name of a specialist. Theories of behavior, such as the theory of reasoned action (e.g., Ajzen & Fishbein, 1980), explain that one reason people may engage in behavior comes from their impression that other people want, expect, or require them to do so. For example, a woman's decision to have a mammogram is influenced, in part, by opinions of significant others and similar others' screening behaviors (Pearlman et al., 1997). Social connections may benefit one's health by providing psychological and material resources needed to cope with stress (Cohen, 2004). People's networks can provide *emotional* support: feeling loved, esteemed, valued, and cared for regardless of achievement (Bloom et al., 1991. This support can aid in emotional regulation by limiting the intensity and duration of negative affective states (Cohen et al., 1998). Positive cognitions and emotions can reduce psychological despair, result in greater motivation to care for oneself, and result in suppressed neuroendocrine response and enhanced immune function (e.g., Cohen, 1988).

As a relational phenomenon, it may be no surprise to see concordance in patient and caregiver responses to network support. For example, when family caregivers and survivors report more resources available in the family and bigger networks of support, they both report more positive meanings associated with cancer (Mellon et al., 2006). Not surprisingly, caregivers with smaller, homogenous social networks report more caregiver burden (e.g., Goldstein et al., 2004). The same process of stress described for patients can appear with caregivers. For example, parents of children with cancer, versus healthy children, showed compromised immune regulation (Miller, Cohen, & Ritchey, 2002).

Summary

The disclosure of a diagnosis such as cancer or HIV/AIDS is a life-altering event for the patient and family. This chapter offers preliminary discussion about how and why disclosure may be difficult and socially curtailed for patients, physicians, and families. It considers strategies for disclosure that may help family members (as co-owners of the information) and practitioners with their decisions regarding how to communicate diagnoses to adolescent patients, how adolescent patients may react to different diagnosis disclosures, and adolescents' perspectives on their own decisions about disclosing information about their (past) illnesses. Overall it is clear that disclosure matters, in terms of both positive and negative consequences, but there is not a one-size-fits-all approach to disclosure. For example, strategies that may be considered *polite* may also be misinterpreted and evoke fear and uncertainty, while more direct strategies may help encourage understanding. Recognizing that culture and religion may also play a large part in patient's desire for disclosure, it is important to conduct a full trans-disciplinary, culturally relevant, psychosocial assessment of each patient and family to understand their disclosure needs. Then, health care professionals can tailor their information delivery to support each patient and his/her family. The communication involved in the diagnosis process should be patient-driven; there is a need for healthcare providers to be fully present to their patients' needs, compassionate, and flexible as they deliver diagnoses of life-threatening conditions.

References

Ajzen, I., & Fishbein, M. (1980). *Understanding Attitudes and Predicting Social Behavior.* Upper Saddle River, NJ: Prentice-Hall.

Alonzo, A. A., & Reynolds, N. R. (1995). Stigma, HIV and AIDS: An exploration and elaboration of a stigma trajectory. *Social Science & Medicine, 41,* 303–315.

Atesci, F. C., Baltalarli, B., Oguzhanoglu, N. K., Karadag, N. K., Ozdel, O., & Karagoz, N. (2004). Psychiatric morbidity among cancer patients and awareness of illness. *Support Care Cancer, 12,* 161-167.

Berkman, L., & Syme, S. L. (1979). Social networks host resistance and mortality: A nine-year follow-up study of Alameda county residents. *American Journal of Epidemiology, 109,* 186–204.

Bloom, J. R. (1986). Social support and adjustment to breast cancer. In B. L. Andersen (Ed.), *Women with cancer psychological perspectives* (pp. 204–229). New York: Springer.

Bloom, J. R., Fobair, P., Spiegel, D., Cox, R. S., Varghese, A., & Hoppe, R. (1991). Social supports and the social wellbeing of cancer survivors. *Advances in Medical Sociology, 2,* 95–114.

Bloom, J. R, Stewart, S. L., Chang, S., & Banks, P. J. (2004). Then and now: Quality of life of young breast cancer survivors. *Psycho-Oncology, 13,* 147-60.

Brashers, D. E., Neidig, J. L., & Goldsmith, D. J. (2004). Social support and the management of uncertainty for people living with HIV or AIDS. *Health Communication, 16,* 305-331.

Brown, P., & Levinson, S. C. (1978). Universals in language use: Politeness phenomena. In E. N. Goody (Ed.), *Questions and politeness: Strategies in social interaction* (pp. 56-289). London: Cambridge University Press.

Brown, P., & Levinson, S. C. (1987). *Politeness: Some universals in language.* Cambridge, UK: Cambridge University Press.

Chesler, M., Paris, J., & Barbarin, O. (1986). Telling the child with cancer: Parental choices to share information with ill children. *Journal of Pediatric Psychology, 11,* 497-516.

Claflin, C. J., & Barbarin, O. A. (1991). Does "telling" less protect more? Relationships among age, information disclosure, and what children with cancer see and feel. *Journal of Pediatric Psychology, 16,* 169-191.

Clark, R. E., & LaBeff, E. E. (1982). Death telling: Managing the delivery of bad news. *Journal of Health and Social Behavior, 23,* 366-380.

Clarke, S. A., Davies, H., Jenney, M., Glaser, A., & Eiser, C. (2005). Parental communication and children's behaviour following diagnoses of childhood leukaemia. *Psycho-Oncology, 14,* 274-281.

Cohen, S. (1988). Psychosocial models of social support in the etiology of physical disease. *Health Psychology, 7,* 269–297.

Cohen, S. (2004). Social relationships and health. *American Psychologist, 59.* 676-684.

Cohen, S., Frank, E., Doyle, W. J., Skoner, D. P., Rabin, B. S., & Gwaltney, J. M., Jr. (1998). Types of stressors that increase susceptibility to the common cold in adults. *Health Psychology, 17,* 214–223.

Derlega, V. J., Winstead, B. A., Greene, K., Serovich, J., & Elwood, W. N. (2004). Reasons for HIV disclosure/nondisclosure in close relationships: Testing a model of HIV-disclosure decision making. *Journal of Social and Clinical Psychology, 23,* 747-767.

Dunsmore, J., & Quine, S. (1995). Information, support, and decision-making needs and preferences of adolescents with cancer: Implications for health professionals. *Journal of Psychosocial Oncology, 13,* 39-56.

Ell, K., Mishimoto, R., Mediansky, L., Mantell, J., & Hamovitch, M. (1992). Social relations, social support and survival among patients with cancer. *Journal of Psychosomatic Research, 36,* 531–541.

Ellis, P. M., & Tattersall, M. H. N. (1999). How should doctors communicate the diagnosis of cancer to patients? *Annals of Medicine, 31,* 336-341.

Erbert, L. A., & Floyd, K. (2003). Affectionate expressions as face-threatening acts: Receiver assessments. *Communication Studies, 55,* 254-270.

Forrest, K., Simpson, S. A., Wilson B. J., Van Teijlingen, E. R., McKee, L., Haites, N., Matthews, E. (2003). To tell or not to tell: Barriers and facilitators in family communication about genetic risk. *Clinical Genetics, 64,* 317–326.

Gambosi, J. R., & Berlin Ray, E. (1990). Professional ideology and physicians' perceived disclosure patterns toward cancer patients. *Communication Research Reports, 7,* 132-138.

Goffman, E. (1963). *Stigma: Notes on the management of spoiled identity.* New York: Simon & Schuster.

Goffman, E. (1967). *Interaction ritual: Essays in face-to-face behavior.* Garden City, NY: Anchor.

Goldstein, N. E., Concato, J., Fried, T. R., Kasl, S. V., Johnson-Hurzeler, R., Bradley, E. H. (2004). Factors associated with caregiver burden among caregivers of terminally ill patients with cancer. *Journal of Palliative Care, 20,* 38-43.

Granovetter, M. S. (1976). The strength of weak ties. *American Journal of Sociology, 78,* 1360–1380.

Gravell, J., Zapka, J. G., & Mamon, J. A. (1985). Impact of breast self-examination planned educational messages on social network communications: An exploratory study. *Health Education Quarterly*, 12, 51—64.

Green, J., Richards, M., Murton, F., Statham, H., & Hallowell, N. (1997). Family communication and genetic counseling: The case of hereditary breast and ovarian cancer. *Journal of Genetic Counseling, 6*, 45–60.

Hallowell, N., Ardern-Jones, A., Eeles, R., Foster, C., Lucassen, A., Moynihan, C., & Watson, M. (2005). Communication about genetic testing in families of male BRCA1/2 carriers and non-carriers: Patterns, priorities and problems. *Clinical Genetics, 67*, 492-502.

Han, W. T., Collie, K., Koopman, C., Azarow, J., Classen, C., Morrow, G. R., ... Spiegel, D. (2005). Breast cancer and problems with medical interactions: Relationships with traumatic stress, emotional self-efficacy, and social support. *Psycho-Oncology, 14*, 318-30.

Herek, G. M. (1996). Why tell if you're not asked? Self-disclosure, intergroup contact, and heterosexuals' attitudes toward lesbians and gay men. In G. M. Herek, J. Jobe, & R. Carney (Eds.), *Out in force: Sexual orientation and the military* (pp. 197-225). Chicago: University of Chicago Press.

Herek, G. M. (2007). Confronting sexual stigma and prejudice: Theory and practice. *Journal of Social Issues, 63*, 905-925.

Hewitt, M., Weiner, S., & Simone, J. V. (2003). *Childhood cancer survivorship: Improving care and quality of life.* Washington, DC: National Research Council of the National Academies.

Hooker, L. (1997). Information needs of teenagers with cancer: Developing a tool to explore the perceptions of patients and professionals. *Journal of Cancer Nursing, 1*, 160-168.

Hughes, C., Lerman, C., Schwartz, M., Peshkin, B. N., Wenzel, L., Narod, S., ... Main, D. (2002). All in the family: evaluation of the process and content of sisters' communication about BRCA1 and BRCA2 genetic test results. *American Journal of Medical Genetics, 107*, 143–150.

Ishibashi, A. (2001). The needs of children and adolescents with cancer for information and social support. *Cancer Nursing, 24*, 61-67.

Kang, S. H., & Bloom, J. R. (1993). Social support and cancer screening among older Black Americans. *Journal of the National Cancer Institute, 85*, 737–742.

Kang, S. H., Bloom, J. R., & Romano, P. S. (1994). Cancer screening among African American women: Their use of tests and social support. *American Journal of Public Health, 84*, 104–106.

Kendrick, C., Culling, J., Oakhill, T., & Mott, M. (1986). Children's understanding of their illness and its treatment within a pediatric oncology unit. *Association of Child Psychology and Psychiatry, Newsletter 8*, 16-20.

Last, B. F., & vanVeldhuisen, A. M. H. (1996). Information about diagnosis and prognosis related to anxiety and depression in children with cancer aged 16 years. *European Journal of Cancer, 32,* 290-294.

Leach, C. R, & Schoenberg, N. E. (2007). The vicious cycle of inadequate early detection: A complementary study on barriers to cervical cancer screening among middle-aged and older women. *Preventing Chronic Disease, 4,* A95.

Lester, P., Chesney, M., Cooke, M., Whalley, P., Perez, B., Petru, A., Dorenbaum, A., & Wara, D. (2002). Diagnostic disclosure to HIV-infected children: How parents decide when and what to tell. *Clinical Child Psychology and Psychiatry, 7,* 85-99.

Lewis, F. M., & Deal, L. W. (1995). Balancing our lives: A study of the married couple's experience with breast cancer recurrence. *Oncology Nursing Forum, 22,* 943–953.

Lienard, A., Merckaert, I., Libert, Y., Delvaux, N., Marchal, S., Boniver, J., ... Razavi, D. (2008). Factors that influence cancer patients' and relatives' anxiety following a three-person medical consultation: Impact of a communication skills training program for physicians. *Psycho-Oncology, 17,* 488-496.

Lim, T. S., & Bowers, J. W. (1991). Facework: Solidarity, approbation, and tact. *Human Communication Research, 17,* 415-450.

Lindlof, T. R., & Taylor, B. C. (2002). *Qualitative Communication Research Methods.* Thousand Oaks, CA: Sage.

Link, B. G. (1987). Understanding labeling effects in the area of mental disorders: An assessment of the effects of expectations of rejection. *American Sociological Review, 52,* 96-112.

Link, B. G., Cullen, F. T., Struening, E. L., Shrout, P. E., & Dohrenwend, B. P. (1989). A modified labeling theory approach to mental disorders: An empirical assessment. *American Sociological Review, 54,* 400-423.

Manos, N., & Christakis, J. (1980). Attitudes of cancer specialists toward their patients in Greece. *International Journal of Psychiatry in Medicine, 10,* 305-313.

Marelich, W. D., & Murphy, D. A. (2003). Effects of empowerment among HIV positive women on the patient provider relationship. *AIDS care, 15,* 475-481.

Markowitz, F. E. (1998). The effects of stigma on the psychological well-being and life satisfaction of persons with mental illness. Journal of Health and Social Behavior, 39, 335–348.

Maunsell, E., Brisson, J., & Deschenes, L. (1995). Social support and survival among women with breast cancer. *Cancer, 76,* 631–637.

Mellon, S., Berry-Bobovski, L., Gold, R., Levin, N., & Tainsky, M. A. (2006). Communication and decision-making about seeking inherited cancer risk information: Findings from female survivor-relative focus groups. *Psycho-Oncology, 15,* 193-208.

Merckaert, I., Libert, Y., Delvaux, N., Marchal, S., Boniver, J., Etienne, A. M., ...Razavi, D. (2008). Factors influencing physicians' detection of cancer patients' and relatives' distress: Can a communication skills training program improve physicians' detection? *Psycho-Oncology, 17,* 260-269.

Miller, G. E., Cohen, S., & Ritchey, A. K. (2002). Chronic psychological stress and the regulation of pro-inflammatory cytokines: A glucocorticoid-resistance model. *Health Psychology, 21,* 531-41.

Miller, C. T., & Major, B. (2000). Coping with stigma and prejudice. In T. F. Heatherton, R. E. Kleck, M. R. Hebl, & J. G. Hull (Ed.), *The social psychology of stigma* (pp. 243-272). New York: The Guilford Press.

Miura, T., Kojima, R., Sugiura, Y., Mizutani, M., Takatsu, F., & Suzuki, Y. (2000). Incidence of non-compliance and its influencing factors in patients receiving Digoxin. *Clinical Drug Investment, 19,* 123-130.

Miyata, H., Takahashi, M., Saito, T., Tachimori, H., & Kai, I. (2005). Disclosure preferences regarding cancer diagnosis and prognosis: To tell or not to tell? *Journal of Medical Ethics, 31,* 447-451.

Myers, R. E., Vernon, S. W., Tilley, B. C., Lu, M., & Watts, B. G. (1998). Intention to screen for colorectal cancer among white male employees. *Preventative Medicine, 27,* 279–287.

Neuling, S., & Winefield, H. (1988). Social support and recovery after surgery for breast cancer: Frequency and correlates of supportive behaviors by family, friends, and surgeons. *Social Science and Medicine, 27,* 385–392.

Pearlman, D. N., Rakowski, W., Clark, M. A., Ehrich, B., Rimer, B. K., Goldstein, M. G., Woolverton, H., & Dube, C. E. (1997). Why do women's attitudes toward mammography change over time? Implications for physician-patient communication. *Cancer Epidemiology, Biomarkers, & Prevention, 6,* 451-457.

Petronio, S. (2002). *Boundaries of privacy: Dialectics of disclosure.* New York: State University of New York Press.

Petronio, S., Sargent, J., Andea, L., Reganis, P., & Cichocki, D. (2004). Family and friends as healthcare advocates: Dilemmas of confidentiality and privacy. *Journal of Social and Personal Relationships, 21,* 33-52.

Schaeffer, C., Coyne, J., & Lazarus, R. (1981). The health related functions of social support. *Journal of Behavioural Medicine, 4,* 381–406.

Schofield, P. E., Beeney, L. J., Thompson, J. F., Butow, P. N., Tattersall, M. H. N., & Dunn, S. M. (2001). Hearing the bad news of a cancer diagnosis: The Australian melanoma patient's perspective. *Annals of Oncology, 12,* 365-371.

Schofield, P. E., Butow, P. N., Thompson, J. F., Tattersall, M. H. N., Beeney, L. J., & Dunn, S. M. (2003). Psychological responses of patients receiving a diagnosis of cancer. *Annals of Oncology, 14,* 48-56.

Seeman, T. E., & Syme, S. L. (1987). Social networks and coronary artery disease: A comparison of the structure and function of social relations as predictors of disease. *Psychosomatic Medicine, 49,* 341–354.

Slavin, L. A., O'Malley, J. E., Koocher, G. P., & Foster, D. J. (1982). Communication of the cancer diagnosis to pediatric patients: Impact on long-term adjustment. *American Journal of Psychiatry, 139,* 179-183.

Smith, R. A. (2007). Language of the lost: An explication of stigma communication. *Communication Theory, 17,* 462-485.

Smith, R. A., & Hipper, T. (in press). Label management: Investigating how confidants encourage the use of communication strategies to avoid stigmatization. *Health Communication.*

Smith, R. A., Moore, J., Catona, D., & Priem, J. (2009). *Advising label management: Understanding unlabeled confidants' encouragement of communication strategies to avoid stigmatization.* Paper presented at the annual meeting of the National Communication Association: Chicago, IL.

Smith, R. A., & Niedermyer, A. J. (2009). Keepers of the secret: Desire to conceal a family member's HIV+ status in Namibia, Africa. *Health Communication, 24,* 459-47.

Spiegel, D., Bloom, J. R., Kraemer, H. C., & Gottheil, E. (1989). Effect of psychosocial treatment on survival of patients with metastatic breast cancer. *Lancet, 2,* 888–891.

Spiers, J. A. (1998). The use of facework and politeness theory. *Qualitative Health Research, 8,* 25-47.

Strauss, A. (1987). *Qualitative Analysis for Social Scientists.* Cambridge, UK: Cambridge University Press.

Strauss, A., & Corbin, J. (1990). *Basics of Qualitative Research.* Newbury Park, CA: Sage.

Strauss, A., & Corbin, J. (1998). *Basics of Qualitative Research: Techniques and Procedures for Developing Grounded Theory.* Thousand Oaks, CA: Sage.

Tasker, M. (1992). *How Can I Tell You? Secrecy and Disclosure with Children When a Family Member has AIDS.* Bethesda, MD: Association for the Care of Children's Health.

Uchino, B. N., Cacioppo, J. T., & Kiecolt-Glaser, J. K. (1996). The relationship between social support and physiological processes: A review with emphasis on underlying mechanisms and implications for health. *Psychological Bulletin, 119,* 488-531.

UNAIDS (2004, September). *Epidemiological fact sheets on HIV/AIDS and sexually transmitted infections.* Geneva, Switzerland: Author.

Velicer, C. M., & Taplin, S. (2001). Genetic testing for breast cancer: where are health care providers in the decision process? *Genetic Medicine, 3,* 112-119.

Woodgate, R. L. (1999). A review of the literature on resilience in the adolescent with cancer: Part II. *Journal of Pediatric Oncology Nursing, 16,* 78-89.

World Health Organization (2001). *The world health report 2001—Mental health: New understanding, new hope.* Geneva, Switzerland: World Health Organization.

Zebrack, B. J., & Chesler, M. (2001). Health-related worries, self-image, and life outlooks of long-term survivors of childhood cancer. *Health and Social Work, 26*, 245-256.

Zhu, K., Hunter, S., Bernard, L. J., Payne-Wilks, K., Roland, C. L., Elam, L. C., Feng, Z., & Levine, R. S. (2002) An intervention study on screening for breast cancer among single African American women aged 65 and older. *Preventative Medicine, 34*, 536-545.

CHAPTER 7

Mental Illness, Stigma, and Disclosure

Erica Bauer

UNIVERSITY OF ILLINOIS AT CHAMPAIGN-URBANA

Historically, people who were diagnosed with a mental illness were separated from society. They were removed from their families and placed in mental institutions to receive treatment (Awad & Voruganit, 2008; Kohn-Wood & Wilson, 2005; Kreisman & Joy, 1974). This system has largely been replaced. Now, people with mental illnesses receive treatment in their communities through hospitals, clinics, and family members (Awad & Voruganit, 2008; Kreisman & Joy, 1974). Despite the fact that people with mental illnesses are no longer separated from society physically, they are separated in another way, through mental illness stigma (Rüsch, Angermeyer, & Corrigan, 2005).

Over 57 million adults currently are living with a mental illness in the United States according to the National Institute of Mental Health (NIMH, 2008). Corrigan and O'Shaughnessy (2007) pointed out that "despite [the statistics], the general population is largely unaware of the number of people with psychiatric disorders because it is a largely hidden stigma" (p. 93). These researchers also revealed that there are three categories to describe mental illness stigma—self (stigma against oneself), structural (systemic or institutionalized stigma), and public (discrimination or public reactions in response to stigma). In this chapter I will focus on public stigma and how it affects familial disclosure of mental illness, beginning with an overview of stigma and disclosure literature and ending with a study designed to examine the relationship between mental illness stigma and disclosure in families.

Stigma

One of the most widely used definitions of stigma is "an attribute that is deeply discrediting" (Goffman, 1990/1963, p. 3) and unacceptable by society (Weiss, Ramakrishna, & Somma, 2006). The stigmatized condition may be rejected or found to be objectionable based on some criterion to which others may or may not subscribe. According to Parker and Aggleton (2003), stigma is what one would find at the intersection of culture, power, and difference; reflecting societal disdain at such a level that it can remove any credibility an individual once had (Herek, 2002). Link and Phelan (2001) summarized the key elements of stigmatization, saying that it occurs when:

> (1) people distinguish and label human differences; (2) dominant cultural beliefs link labeled persons to undesirable characteristics…; (3) labeled persons are placed in distinct categories…; (4) labeled persons experience status loss and discrimination…and is (5) …entirely contingent on access to social, economic, and political power that allows the identification of differentness, the construction of stereotypes, the separation of labeled persons into distinct categories, and the full execution of disapproval, rejection, exclusion, and discrimination. (p. 367)

Communication is central to the process of stigmatization (Corrigan & Rüsch, 2002; Parker & Aggleton, 2003) because the manner in which health conditions are discussed by society are instrumental in shaping how society understands and views these conditions. For example, AIDS used to be referred to as the Gay Related Immune Deficiency Syndrome, which communicated that the disease only affected the gay community, stigmatizing the community as a whole (Elmore, 2006). In this case, the label was the stereotype, endorsing inaccurate beliefs not just about AIDS, but about an entire community of people. This example also illustrates how stigma often is perpetuated by the powerful (e.g., health care professionals, medical staff, social workers, or media) because these groups have credibility and access to the public. As Rüsch and colleagues (2005) stated, "Whether patterns of behavior, thinking and feeling are being noticed at all and if so, whether they are described in moral, psychosocial or medical terms is influenced by societal discourse and usually varies over time" (p. 530). Society can both endorse and reject negative stereotypes associated with a group of people through discourse (Corrigan & Rüsch; Gray, 2002; Rüsch et al., 2005), evidenced by the fact that AIDS is no longer referred to as the Gay Related Immune Deficiency Syndrome.

Another way in which stigma is communicative is related to disclosure. Many mental illnesses are not visible to the naked eye (Corrigan & O'Shaughnessy. 2007), meaning that before a person can stigmatize someone living with a mental illness, he or she first must be made aware that the illness exists. This typically occurs when people decide to disclose their condition to others. The next section will define disclosure, discuss how people disclose, and provide reasons for disclosing a stigmatized health condition.

Disclosure

The term *disclosure* generally refers to sharing or revealing information about one's self with someone who otherwise would not have access to that information or perspective (Derlega, Winstead, Wong, & Greenspan, 1987; Jourard, 1959; Petronio, 2002; Stiles, 1978). Communication scholars also understand it as a process, rather than an event (Baxter & Montgomery, 1996; Dindia, 2000; Miller, 1990; Petronio, 2002). For example, a person first may disclose that he or she is ill and later disclose the label of that illness.

Disclosure is required when making personal information, perspectives, or experiences known. It also is required when making a mental illness known, particularly since they are considered to be invisible. Thus, one's disclosure patterns are directly related to one's stigma experiences. How people living with stigmatized health conditions decide to disclose can depend on a number of factors such as timing, context, and the person to whom the disclosure is being made (Chaikin & Derlega, 1974). For example, a literature review of maternal disclosure of HIV to non-infected offspring found that once mothers decide to disclose, they give a lot of thought to "how, when, and in what context [the illness] will occur" (Hawk, 2007, p. 663).

Disclosure often is used to gain social support (Almeleh, 2006; Norman, Chopra, & Kadiyala, 2007; Slade, O'Neil, Simpson, & Lashen, 2007). Social support can mitigate the difficulties related to living with a stigmatized health condition by encouraging that person's sense of worth, value, esteem, or connectedness to a support network

(Albrecht & Adelman, 1984; Cobb, 1976). Social support also can help individuals with stigmatized conditions to manage the uncertainties they may have about their illness (e.g., managing the symptoms of a psychotic illness in public). In a study about social support and uncertainty management for people living with HIV or AIDS, support providers assisted with "information seeking and avoiding, providing instrumental support, facilitation skill development, giving acceptance or validation, allowing ventilation, and encouraging perspective shifts" (Brashers, Neidig, & Goldsmith, 2004, p. 323).

The benefits of disclosure may not be enough to encourage someone to disclose one's mental condition (Paxton, 2002), especially since there are many reasons to conceal one's condition. Hinshaw (2005) stated that mental illness stigma "is increasingly recognized as a central issue, if not *the* central issue, for the entire mental health field" (p. 714). The next section will discuss the risks of disclosing one's mental illness, further emphasizing the importance of this research.

Mental Illness Stigma and Disclosure

Seeking treatment presents many obstacles for people living with a stigmatized condition. Experiencing mental illness stigma can make it more difficult for people to disclose to seek support or continue treatment (Alvidrez, Snowden, & Kaiser, 2008; Ayalon & Alvidrez, 2007; Sirey et al., 2001; Weiss et al., 2006). For instance, someone may assume a person has a mental illness if he or she is seen leaving a treatment facility (Corrigan & O'Shaughnessy, 2007). Corrigan and colleagues (Corrigan & Rüsch, 2002; Corrigan, Edwards, Green, Diwan, & Penn, 2001) found that many people see those with mental illness as violent, childlike, incompetent, and easy targets for blame. Others avoid those with mental illnesses because they fear that they are violent and unpredictable (Crisp, Gelder, Rix, Meltzer, & Rowlands, 2000; González-Torres et al., 2007). A cross-sectional study about mental illness stigma was conducted with 196 people living with a mental illness (Lundberg, Hansson, Wentz, & Björkman, 2007). Over half of the respondents indicated that they believed their diagnosis would keep them from getting hired for a job (73%) and caused them to be viewed as untrustworthy (67%) and unintelligent (56%). These individuals also reported being treated differently by others, as well as being denied access to live in certain apartments after being released from a mental hospital.

Although mental illness stigma can be experienced in every area of life, such as "employment, occupational advancement, income, housing, education, and medical care" (Major, 2006, p. 193–194), identifying issues related to stigmatized conditions is especially helpful in settings where individuals with stigmatized conditions receive treatment and seek support (e.g., interpersonal relationships, hospitals, churches). The family is one of those settings and is the focus of this chapter. The following section will look at disclosing one's mental illness within the context of the family.

Family, Mental Illness, and Disclosure

Regardless of the reason for making one's mental illness known to others, one group of people commonly disclosed to are family members, who often play an important role in that person's treatment (Awad & Voruganit, 2008; Kohn-Wood & Wilson, 2005; Kreisman & Joy, 1974). For many families, caring for a person with a mental illness can be stressful, burdensome, and overwhelming due to a lack of support from the medical community (Saunders, 2003; Hinshaw, 2005). One could argue that these same issues would exist when caring for someone with any number of the health issues; however, not all health issues are considered stigmatized conditions (e.g., broken bones, the flu, chicken pox). In fact, families dealing with the mental illness of an offspring or relative often contend with the field's predominant view that mental disorders emanate from faulty parental discipline or socialization (Hinshaw, 2005).

Much of the research about families and mental illness stigma has focused on the stigmatization of family members because of their relation to a person living with a mental illness (Hinshaw, 2005; Perlick et al., 2007; Phelan, Bromet, & Link, 1998; Zauszniewski, Bekhet, & Suresky, 2008). This type of stigma also is known as courtesy stigma (Goffman, 1990/1963), which may be "related more closely to the presence of specific symptoms or behaviors of the mentally ill person than to the actual diagnosis" (Zauszniewski, Bekhet, & Suresky, 2008, p. 132). These symptoms or behaviors increase the visibility of the illness making family members more vulnerable to experiencing courtesy stigma.

A study by Gonzalez and colleagues (2007) about mental illness stigma among people ($N = 500$) caring for a family member with bipolar disorder found that a number of factors influenced the family members' perceptions of being stigmatized. These family members were identified as primary caregivers by the person with bipolar disorder. Information from both groups was gathered for the study. The results indicated that being diagnosed at an early age, hospitalized multiple times, and diagnosed with a more severe form of the disorder increased the caregivers' perceptions of being stigmatized.

In another study, González-Torres, Oraa, Arístegui, Férnandez-Rivas, and Guimon (2007) explored stigma experiences related to schizophrenia. Six focus groups ($N = 44$) were conducted with people with schizophrenia and family members who assisted in caring for these individuals. The researchers were interested in the stigma experiences of both groups. The stigma experienced by the family members was grouped into three categories. The first category consisted of experiences of guilt and isolation. One respondent was quoted saying, "They see you at the supermarket and they avoid you, they don't speak to you anymore. My own family says that it is because I spoiled him…" (p. 20). Family members were blamed for their loved one's illness and then alienated. The second category consisted of negative experiences with health care professionals. The respondents felt ignored and excluded in treatment decisions concerning their loved one, despite their experiences of caring for these individuals regularly. The last category was about the shame family members often felt that lead to them keeping the illness from others.

Some studies also have explored mental illness stigma among family members of a person living with a mental illness (Freeman, 1961; Phelan, Bromet, & Link, 1998). These stigmatizing attitudes have been observed at times when family members attempt to explain the behavior of the person with a mental illness, "…attributing the behavior to character weakness, physical ailments, or situational factors" rather than a mental illness (Kreisman & Joy, 1974, p. 36). Some family members ignore relatives with mental illnesses (Schulze & Angermeyer, 2003), others feel ashamed (Kreisman & Joy, 1974), guilty (Corrigan, Watson, & Miller, 2006), or embarrassed (Hinshaw, 2005), which has resulted in the person with the mental illness being avoided or rejected by his or her family (Corrigan et al., 2006; Kreisman & Joy, 1974).

Researchers conducted a study to understand the experiences of people diagnosed with bipolar and found that, for some, disclosing the illness to family members sometimes resulted in a loss of relationships and, for others, family members became overly-involved in the bipolar individual's life, resulting in a loss of independence (Michalak, Yatham, Kolesar, & Lam, 2006). Williams and Healy (2001) found that individuals who disclosed their mental illness felt they were regarded by others as weak, lacking self-control, and unable to deal with the realities of life. Focus groups conducted with 23 individuals living with depression found that most of the participants had not disclosed to family members for fear of negative responses (Barney, Griffiths, Christenson, & Jorm, 2009). One person did not disclose because depression "...is usually misinterpreted in a negative way, either through presuming someone to be stupid or presuming someone to be weak..." (Barney et al., p. 11).

Family members often play a crucial role in caring for a relative with a mental illness (Kohn-Wood & Wilson, 2005). Research on mental illness stigma and families primarily has focused on issues of courtesy stigma and coping (Hinshaw, 2005; Perlick et al., 2007; Phelan, et al., 1998; Zauszniewski et al., 2008). Disclosing one's mental illness to family can result in increased social support, stronger relationships (Michalak et al., 2006), and understanding (Williams & Healy, 2001); however, given the risks in disclosing information about a mental illness, it is not difficult to see why this disclosure is not an appealing choice for people living with this condition.

Is It Worth the Risk?
A Study about Family Disclosure Patterns of Bipolar Disorder

To investigate disclosure of mental illness in the family context, I chose to address a specific mental illness: Bipolar disorder. Bipolar disorder is a stigmatized mental illness and exhibits a genetic pattern (NIMH, 2009). The goal of the study reported in the remainder of this chapter was to examine the results of disclosing one's bipolarity to family members. This investigation was exploratory, but enriches the literature on family disclosure, stigma, and mental illness in three ways. First, unlike much of the current mental illness stigma literature (Hinshaw, 2005), this study focused on stigma experiences within one's family versus the courtesy stigma experienced as a result of being associated with a family member with a mental illness. Second, it focused on an illness that is under-researched. Proudfoot and colleagues (2009) stated that "...there is a shortage of research on living with bipolar disorder" (p. 121). Third, this study included a sample of people living with bipolar disorder. As Lundberg and colleagues (Lundberg et al., 2007) stated, "in contrast to attitudes in the general population, there are relatively few studies investigating the way people with mental illnesses themselves experience adverse reactions by others..." (p. 295).

Bipolar Disorder

Bipolar disorder, commonly referred to as manic-depressive illness, is a chemical imbalance in the brain "that causes unusual shifts in a person's mood, energy, and ability to function" (NIMH, 2001, p. 3). These shifts, or episodes of mania and depression, last for varying periods with normal moods in between. The exact cause of the illness is unknown; however, the disorder tends to run in families (NIMH, 2009). Illnesses that can be passed to other family members complicate the relationship between stigma and disclosure because nondisclosure can have devastating effects on others. Additionally, individuals with illnesses that exhibit a genetic pattern are typically held responsible for disclosing this information to other family members at risk (Forrest, van Teijlingen, McKee, Miedzybrodzka, & Simpson, 2009).

To study the results of disclosing one's bipolarity to family members, I collected data using an online survey. I focused on data that were part of a larger data set concerning family disclosure and bipolar disorder. The larger study was designed to explore the disclosure patterns of people affected, directly or indirectly, by bipolar disorder. For the present study, I specifically focused on the demographic data and responses to the following three open–ended questions:

1. What are the disadvantages of disclosing bipolarity to one's family?

2. What are the advantages of disclosing bipolarity to one's family?

3. What impact has knowing or not knowing of a bipolar presence in their family had on participants' own health?

Participants

I recruited participants through online support groups for people with bipolar disorder and/or their loved ones. The support groups were located by conducting a simple web search using the words "bipolar support groups" as search terms. The webmaster of each support group chosen was emailed asking if he or she would be willing to post a link to the survey on their support group webpage. This allowed access to people who participated in these groups. To access the survey, a person first had to access an online bipolar support group, then locate and click the link to the study. Each person who clicked on the link was greeted with a page explaining my role as the researcher and the goal of the study. The reader then needed to click on a tab that read "click here to enter the survey" at the bottom of the page to access the survey itself and then click a tab entitled "submit" to deliver the data.

Because many support sites provide support options for both people living with an illness and their loved ones, it was important to know each participant's connection to bipolar disorder. This was done using a survey-item asking each participant to self-identify by clicking on one of eight options. These options included statements such as *I am bipolar, I am the child of a bipolar parent*, and *I am the bipolar parent of a bipolar child*. An *other* option was also provided along with a blank space for the participants to fill in with their own relationship, if the ones listed did not apply to them.

Of the 125 total participants, 104 were female and 21 were male. Eighty-nine percent of the participants were Caucasian. The participants indicated that (a) they themselves had bipolar (30.6%); (b) they suspected a parent(s) had bipolar and they had bipolar (15.3%); or (c) they were a parent with bipolar (10.5%). Fifty-nine participants indicated that they were offspring of parents with bipolar, and 54 (43.2%) of the participants knew or suspected a sibling to have bipolar disorder. Forty percent of the participants were between the ages of 19 and

30, and 49.6% were between the ages of 31 and 50; these two groups accounted for 89.6% of participants. Forty-eight percent of the participants had biological children.

Method

A constant comparative analysis was performed to examine the data. According to Corbin and Strauss (2008), this type of analysis involves examining the data by breaking it down into smaller components to make comparisons within the data to understand how these components operate as a whole. The similarities and differences identified within the data represent the dimensions and properties of the data. In this case, these dimensions and properties reflect the advantages, disadvantages, and impact of disclosing one's bipolar disorder to family members. This analytic approach allowed me to break down each individual experience into its constitutive parts and then connect these parts with like experiences of the other participants. In the end, this allowed me to construct a larger picture of what occurs when disclosing one's bipolarity to family members. This analytic process is guided by the data in an inductive manner, rather than by theory in a deductive manner.

In the analysis, the responses to the three open-ended questions were reduced to individual codes before comparisons could be made. Coding entailed looking at the responses of each of the three research questions for each person and labeling each meaningful unit of their response. For example, if a response to the first open-ended question contained three different disadvantages, each disadvantage would be identified as a meaningful unit and labeled accordingly. The goal was to represent the data as clearly as possible to have a complete picture of what was experienced by participants as disadvantages, advantages, and impactful. After identifying and labeling individual codes in the responses, these codes were then grouped together into categories based on their similarities and differences (see Tables 7.1- 7.3 below for samples of these categories).

Table 7.1 Sample Categories of Disadvantages

Category	Conceptual Definition	Sample Comments
None	No disadvantages	I haven't had any disadvantages. *(male with bipolar)* I don't see any. *(female with bipolar)*
Stigma	Disclosers experienced stigmatizing behaviors	Ostracism, rejection... *(female with bipolar & daughter of parent with bipolar)* They would think I was crazy. *(female with bipolar & daughter of parent with bipolar)*
Negative Affective Responses	Disclosers experienced negative emotional responses	They will... always worry. *(female with bipolar)* It would only upset them, because of their denial. *(female with bipolar & daughter of two parents with bipolar)*
Illness as Scapegoat	Behaviors were attributed to the illness that should not have been	Sometimes people cannot differentiate between the illness and the person. *(male with bipolar)* Every mood you have is "part of the condition." *(parent with bipolar)*
Boundary Violations	Information disclosed was shared with others without consent	...Being talked about behind my back... *(female with bipolar)* Gossip *(female with bipolar, daughter of parent with bipolar, & mother of child with bipolar)*
Loss of Credibility	Disclosers treated as incompetent or untrustworthy	...They stop trusting me. *(female with bipolar & grandchild of grandparents with bipolar)* I think I will be looked upon as less capable. *(female parent with bipolar)*
Denial/ Lack of Understand ing from Others	Family members denied the existence of the illness or did not understand what it meant	They wouldn't understand my plight... *(female with bipolar)* It's hard to cope with parents that don't believe in mental illness...*(female with bipolar)*
Used as a Weapon	The illness was used against the person with bipolar	...my family uses it against me saying that I'm "unstable and crazy." *(mother with bipolar)* Insensitivity and name calling. *(mother of child with bipolar)*
Alienation	Disclosers were abandoned	Potential for alienation. *(daughter of parent suspected of having bipolar)* Some avoid us completely. *(female parent of bipolar child)*
Blame Discourse	The illness was seen as the fault of the discloser	They have a pick yourself up and get over it attitude. *(mother with bipolar)* Had one family member tell me to "think my way out of it"! *(female with bipolar)*
Family Turmoil	Poor relationships with family reduced likelihood of disclosing	Don't want to talk to parents because of bad relationships and mistrust. *(father with bipolar)* Sometimes strained relations, especially when I'm ill. *(male with bipolar)*

Table 7.2 Sample Categories of Advantages

Category	Conceptual Definition	Sample Comments
None	No advantages	None at present time. *(female with bipolar & daughter of parent with bipolar)*
Under-standing	Increased under-standing about the illness	It gives them a chance to understand why I do what I do while bipolar. *(male with bipolar)* So they can understand what is going on with me. *(female with bipolar)*
Social Support	Increased social support	They have known me all my life, recognize danger signs and care enough to help me. *(female with bipolar)* Continued support from family. *(male with bipolar)*
Diagnosis Accuracy	Increased ability of others to receive an accurate diagnosis	I want them to… recognize symptoms in case they have them. *(mother with bipolar)*

Table 7.3 Sample Categories of Impact

Category	Conceptual Definition	Sample Comments
None	No impact	Not really impacted. *(male with bipolar)*
Delayed Diagnosis	Timing of diagnosis negatively impacted by lack of knowledge	I wish I had known sooner. I was misdiagnosed for many years. *(mother with bipolar)* I could have been diagnosed sooner. *(mother with bipolar)*
Preparation	Preparation upon diagnosis positively impacted by knowledge	It has made me more aware to watch for/identify symptoms in [my]self… *(daughter of parent suspected to have bipolar)* It enabled me to see what was going on before I did any serious harm to myself... *(mother with bipolar & daughter of parent with bipolar)*
Diagnosis of Another Person	Ability to diagnose others positively impacted by knowledge	I knew as soon as I was diagnosed that my mother was bipolar also. *(female with bipolar & daughter of parent with bipolar)* I suspect my mom has bipolar, but she'll never see it herself and it's not worth trying to point it out to her. *(female with bipolar)*
Emotional Health	Emotional health of the person with bipolar impacted by knowledge or lack thereof	It has made me more comfortable with my illness… *(mother with bipolar of a child with bipolar)* It's a relief to know that I'm not going through this alone. *(male with bipolar)*
Support	Support positively impacted by knowledge	The impact of better support was great. *(female with bipolar, daughter of parent with bipolar, & mother of child with bipolar)* Disclosure and discussion has sped my recovery and strengthened my remission. *(male with bipolar)*

These categories were then examined for themes that cut across respondents. Finally, from the emergent themes, a model was constructed to offer a tentative explanation.

Findings

Disadvantages of Disclosing Bipolarity

Out of 127 participants, 112 commented on the disadvantages of disclosing one's bipolarity. Fifteen participants left the response box blank. The responses were divided into 11 categories that are discussed below: (a) stigma, (b) negative affective responses, (c) the illness as a scapegoat, (d) boundary violations, (e) loss of credibility, (f) denial or lack of understanding from others, (g) use as a weapon, (h) alienation, (i) blame discourse, (j) family turmoil and (k) none. The frequencies of each category are presented next to their titles in parentheses.

Stigma (36). Issues related to being stigmatized because of the disorder also were described. One woman with bipolar disorder shared her frustration saying, "Disadvantages…the public stigma, I have a mental disorder, therefore I must be crazy. I hate that. HATE it. But it is something that I have to deal with." Another woman with bipolar pointed out that both her mother and sister labeled her as "…unstable and crazy." Another female participant with bipolar wrote, "They look at you odd and don't understand. They treat you oddly and say discriminatory stuff."

Negative affective responses (9). Sometimes the news of a bipolar diagnosis evoked negative emotional responses (e.g., worry, anxiety, sadness) from loved ones. A father with bipolar disorder commented on the possibility of causing guilt and being watched too closely, "[They] may feel guilt at having passed the disorder on to you… " A mother with bipolar said "…trying to share experiences with my kids who were in their early teens [about] my diagnosis 'freaked' them out and they are not comfortable discussing it with me…" A woman with bipolar spoke of difficulties created when loved ones over-involved themselves in caring for her. "They often overreact and worry needlessly during cycling periods when I am medicated and under the supervision of a doctor."

Using the illness as a scapegoat (10). A frustration expressed by the respondents was the use of the disorder as a scapegoat. Behaviors that typically would be considered "normal" prior to the diagnosis now were attributed to the disorder. A woman with bipolar said, "Sometimes my behavior is over-analyzed by certain family members and immediately cast-off as 'just a bipolar thing.'" One mother with bipolar who also had children with bipolar shared the following experience:

> The disadvantage comes with family as well as ANY level of relationship. It's all too easy for others to blame the bipolar person(s) for things that aren't related to bipolar at all, such as REAL stressors that are life problems and NOT "episodes" or relapse. ... "You're manic!" I'll be accused of when I'm simply "up" and happy; "You're depressed!" I'll hear when something that is REALLY HAPPENING makes me stressed and even a bit "blue" for even just an hour or so; it's rare that I'm thought of as having "normal" times, it's almost always just assumed that I'm in one episode or another.

Boundary violations (7). Boundary violations were conflicts that arose when people's expectations of how information should be handled were not met (Petronio, 2002). An example of this was expressed by a woman with bipolar who stated, "They told other family members and friends about my diagnosis, without my permission." Another woman with bipolar stated that her family had a tendency "...to intrude and try to control me (particularly at affected times), loss of rights[,] of privacy[,] and self-determination." Another woman simply wrote "Gossip." She identified as a person with three generations of bipolar disorder including a parent, herself, and her child.

Loss of credibility (10). In some cases, individuals felt as if they were taken less seriously after their diagnosis. They were treated as less capable or competent. Three women with bipolar disorder shared the following statements: "You lose some sort of credibility and authority over your children—also, you are viewed as unstable." "I feel as if they see me as a weaker person." "I don't want everything I've ever said or done discounted and written off to bp."

Denial and lack of understanding from others (37). The largest category dealt with some sort of denial. Either the family denied the existence of mental illness, of bipolarity being in the family genes, or that the symptoms, behaviors, exhibited by the person with bipolar had anything to do with an illness at all. One woman with bipolar wrote about the difficulty of dealing with parents in denial, "It's hard to cope with parents [who] don't believe in mental illness." A lack of understanding also contributed to difficulties experienced in disclosing one's bipolarity. Another woman with bipolar said it "causes some problems with some members of the family because they don't understand that it is an illness." Lastly, a woman with bipolar whose parents also had bipolar said, "[I]t would only upset them because of their denial."

Used as a weapon against them (10). In times of conflict, one's bipolarity also was used as a weapon against the person. A woman with bipolar reported, "If you try to tell them about it, when they get angry they will throw it in your face later." Another person stated that it "gives terrible ammunition for arguments." Another said, "My family uses it against me."

Alienation (8). Alienation was another barrier that was identified in the responses of the participants. The significance of this barrier lies in the fact that disclosing is a crucial step and for many a first step in building social support. "Ostracism, rejection, [and] abandonment" were three words used by a woman with bipolar to describe the negative impact of disclosing to other family members. An adoptive parent of a bipolar child said, "[s]ome people... avoid us completely." A woman with bipolar said, "They can...stop talking to you all together."

Blame discourse (12). Family members who believed that the problem was a matter of will blamed the person with the disorder for symptoms of the illness. This belief seemed to be rooted in ignorance or denial about mental illness. This discourse appealed to the inner strength of the individual to help him or herself; a "pull yourself up by the bootstraps" mentality. A mother with bipolar said her family had a "pick yourself up and get over it attitude." A mother of a bipolar child said that other family members "...see it as a...matter of will." A woman with bipolar said she "had one family member tell me to 'think my way out of it'!"

Family relational turmoil (8). The state of family relationships prior to diagnosis also was an important component that many considered. All people with bipolar may not be at a place relationally to disclose such vulnerable information. For instance, a man with bipolar explained that he "[did not] want to talk to his parents because of bad relationships and mistrust." A parent with bipolar said, "Not all family members believe in psychiatric help. Some are not in a position of helping you due to their own issues or are part of the problem."

None (14). Some respondents indicated that there were no disadvantages to disclosing. A woman with bipolar said, "My parents are nurses, so I have no problem talking to them about it..." A woman of a parent with bipolar, who has bipolar herself said, "None, unless I talk too much about it, which could cause them to become 'deaf' to the information."

Advantages of Disclosing Bipolarity

Out of the 127 participants, 110 responded when asked about advantages of disclosing their bipolarity. The four categories emerging from these responses are discussed in the following sections: (a) understanding, (b) social support, (c) diagnosis accuracy and (d) none.

Understanding (55). A common advantage of disclosing the diagnosis that respondents reported was gaining understanding of how the illness affected them. Sometimes understanding was linked to reducing stigma. The respondents reflected a desire to be known within the context of the disorder, giving them a greater level of freedom to discuss the disorder more casually. One of the participants with bipolar responded that disclosure would enhance her family's understanding of her behavior, "They need to understand the reason why I have acted the way I have and done things and why behavior is the way it is." A woman with bipolar said, "So they will understand some of my behaviors at times. My ups and downs, need for meds, difficulties during a med change. Why I may withdrawal at times. That they haven't done anything." A daughter with bipolar of a bipolar parent stated, "It may help them understand what I am going through and how bad it hurts when people really don't care or want to understand that part of me."

Social support (53). A popular advantage of disclosure dealt with gaining social support. Many responses did not indicate what kind of support was being provided. Some respondents mentioned that family members were able to aid in issues related to caring for the person with bipolar disorder. One woman with bipolar described a team approach to the illness within her family stating that "Working to achieve understanding as a unit to be able to work together as a team to combat the illness and achieve stability, thereby forming a strong support group that will last throughout life." A mother with bipolar said, "Your family should be your primary support system…" A woman with bipolar said, "They have known me all my life, recognize danger signs and care enough to help me."

Diagnosis accuracy (18). Another category that emerged dealt with improving diagnosis accuracy through disclosure. Participants wanted to help others identify bipolar symptoms in themselves and others so that a proper diagnosis could be acquired in a timely fashion. A woman with bipolar who suspected her mother and siblings were bipolar said, "It [disclosing] helps me to be open about my life and my behavior, and if any of my siblings develop the symptoms then it's more acceptable for all of us." A parent of a child with bipolar stated that "[an advantage was] knowing to look for the signs and symptoms of it in other family members so that a diagnosis could be made sooner if applicable." A woman with bipolar disorder said, "If I can share info when I'm stable they might remember something about it if/when they are diagnosed and/or it may help them toward diagnosis."

None (11). Some respondents felt there were no advantages to disclosing. A mother with bipolar disorder who also was an offspring of a parent with the disorder said that denial keeps disclosure from being a productive communicative act:

> None. My mother hides her illness, as does my oldest brother who is a therapist. My other older brother thinks he's perfectly fine, and my father thinks all mental illnesses are fake. My husband is also bipolar, so our kids are screwed. We talk about it every once in a while, but it mainly comes out when we're pissed at each other.

Impact

The final open-ended question asked about how knowing or not knowing of one's own or a family member's bipolar disorder impacted personal health. Out of the 127 participants, 102 responded to this question. The responses were both positive and negative due to the broad nature of the question, and are divided into six categories: (a) delayed diagnosis, (b) preparation, (c) diagnosis of another person, (d) emotional health, (e) support, and (f) no impact.

Delayed diagnosis (22). Many respondents reported that the knowledge of a bipolar presence in their family would have led to an earlier diagnosis. A man with bipolar shared the effects of a delayed diagnosis in his own life: "Severe depression, suicide attempts, and uncontrolled mood swings. Having knowledge of these effects would have led me to get help earlier. Now I just have to cope and have wasted the last 15 years." Both his parents and siblings also had bipolar. Others felt they were misdiagnosed as a result of not knowing, which is common for this disorder because its symptomology overlaps with many other illnesses (alcoholism, depression, borderline personality disorder, etc.). One person with bipolar described how the delayed diagnosis negatively impacted her health, slowing her progress in coping with the illness.

> I wish I had known sooner—I was misdiagnosed for many years. If I had known sooner, I could have come to terms with it sooner, been medicated sooner, and so on. I would be so much further down the road than I am now.

Preparation (8). Participants also linked the knowledge of a bipolar presence with being better prepared to deal with their own diagnosis, or the diagnosis of another. A mother with bipolar of a child with bipolar said knowing about a bipolar presence in her family "has made me more aware to watch for [and] identify symptoms in self and others in family." Another mother with bipolar of a child with bipolar said, " It enabled me to see what was going on before I did any serious harm to myself, and to go in and get the help that probably has saved my life a dozen times over already."

Diagnosis of another person (6). In some cases, the impact of knowing of a bipolar presence in the family led to the participant's own diagnosis, or the unofficial diagnosis of another family member. For the purposes of this study, an unofficial diagnosis means that symptoms of bipolar were observable by other family members or loved ones without an actual diagnosis by a health care professional. Seeing the symptoms in another family member did not always lead to an official diagnosis and did not mean that the individual exhibiting these symptoms wanted to seek help. One woman with bipolar said, "I suspect my mom has bipolar, but she'll never see it herself and it's not worth trying to point it out to her." A mother with bipolar said the following:

> I suspect my paternal grandmother may have been bipolar too, based on my Dad's descriptions. There's a lot of depression on that side of the family, some of it may be connected to bipolar and we just don't know about it. I was in my late 30s before I succumbed to depression, in my early 40s before it was dx'd as bipolar. Before that, I just thought I was crazy—like the rest of my Dad's family.

Emotional health (32). The disclosure of bipolar disorder also can affect one's emotional health. For some, this effect was negative. One woman with bipolar shared, "It has been very stressful when people don't understand and don't try to understand to the point that I get very depressed." A mother of a child with bipolar stated that "As his mother, I have a lot of stress and exhaustion from dealing with it on a daily basis." A woman with bipolar stated that "Not having the knowledge created great strain and stress."

For others, this effect was positive. One woman with the disorder said, "I am thankful for being diagnosed so I finally know what has been wrong with me for all these years." A woman with bipolar, also the offspring of a parent with bipolar wrote, "I was glad to know I was not alone." A woman with bipolar who also had a parent with bipolar said, "I'm able to understand why things happen. It doesn't make it any less [difficult] to deal with, but at least I have an understanding."

Support (16). Others saw the disclosure as an aid in building social support. Support can take on many forms, physically and emotionally. Disclosure allowed one woman with bipolar to create an environment of freedom: "I don't feel I have to hide the fact I take medication."

The disclosure also allowed some to connect with other family members also diagnosed with the disorder. One woman with bipolar shared about this experience, "I had my cousin to talk to who completely understood...before she passed away. She and I talked a lot. Leaned on each other."

None (16). Finally, respondents said that they experienced no impact related to knowing or not knowing of a bipolar presence in their family. Many of these responses were very brief and indicated that the respondent was not sure of any impact.

Discussion

This study explored family disclosure of bipolar disorder, a stigmatized mental illness with a genetic pattern (NIMH, 2009). This study expands what is currently known about the disclosure of stigmatized health conditions in three ways—it focused on issues that emerged within the family as a result of the disclosure, it explored an illness that is under-researched, and it included people living with the disorder in the study.

This study analyzed three open-ended questions using qualitative methods (Corbin & Strauss, 2008) to unpack the responses to three specific survey questions, which also served as the research questions for this study. First, what are the disadvantages to disclosing one's bipolarity? Second, what are the advantages to disclosing one's bipolarity? Third, what impact has knowing or not knowing of a bipolar presence in their family had on participants' own health? Using constant comparative analysis (Corbin & Strauss, 2008), these questions were coded based on their similarities and differences, categorized, and then reconstructed collectively to paint a broader picture of the results.

Disadvantages of Disclosing

The primary disadvantages of disclosing were related to stigma, denial of mental illness, and relationship harm (negative affect and family turmoil). As discussed by Link and Phelan (2001) stigma is rooted in the attitudes and beliefs held about a certain issue, group of people, etc. The respondents who wrote about denial talked about how their family members denied the existence of the illness. As one woman with bipolar disorder stated, "My family, except my oldest brother, wouldn't understand. They think I'm crazy or faking. Or I'm just spoiled." In this case, as well as others, denial was related to understanding. Those who wrote about stigma often referred to it explicitly, using the word in their actual response. The remaining categories, with the exception of three, were either related to stigmatizing beliefs (e.g., loss of credibility) or stigmatizing behaviors (e.g., using the illness as a scapegoat).

Negative affect and family turmoil dealt with relational issues within the family. Negative affect responses often had to do with people overly caring for or about the person with the disorder, which are related to social support. For example, one woman with the disorder stated, "They worry too much sometimes and get in my face when I want to be alone." Family turmoil had to do with the inverse relationship between disclosure and poor relationships with one's family members.

Advantages of Disclosing

The advantages of disclosing one's bipolarity were all related to quality of life. The primary advantages included increased understanding and securing social support. The third category included enhancing accuracy of the diagnosis. The respondents valued the understanding and support of others in their lives. As one woman with bipolar disorder disclosed, "To help them understand and coordinate care for me better. To help them stereotype less. To help them understand problems they too may have."

The barriers to increased understanding, social support, and diagnosis accuracy are related to the disadvantages of stigma and relationship harm. Understanding bipolar disorder can be difficult when people deny the existence of the disorder or stigmatize it. Why would someone be motivated to understand an illness he or she does not believe exists in the first place? Social support is often complicated by poor relationships or poor responses by those with whom the discloser is in relationship (Coyne, Ellard, & Smith, 1990). Lastly, diagnosis accuracy is related to stigma because an unwillingness to accept bipolar disorder as an illness would prevent individuals from acknowledging symptoms or seeking treatment. Reducing the stigma of mental illness would ideally open the door for others living with the disorder undiagnosed to get help.

Impact of Disclosure on Health

Guided by research suggesting that bipolar disorder exhibits a genetic pattern (NIMH, 2009), the impact of disclosure was examined. Participants were asked, "What impact has knowing or not knowing of a bipolar presence in their family had on participants' own health?"[1]

The responses to this question could be divided into two groups—physical and emotional impacts. Excluding those who indicated "no impact," three of the five categories were related to physical outcomes—delayed diagnosis, preparation, and diagnosis of another person. Essentially, not having genetic information related to a family history of bipolar illness increased the amount of time it took to receive the proper diagnosis, decreased the ability to be prepared to deal with the illness, and hindered the ability to help others. On the other hand, having the information allowed individuals to receive the appropriate diagnosis in a timely manner, better prepared them to adjust to the illness and equipped them with the knowledge to help others receive help. These issues

1 Having a bipolar presence in one's family means that others with a similar genetic makeup (e.g., family members) could develop the disorder. The closer someone is genetically to a person with bipolar, the more likely he or she is to be affected (National Alliance on Mental Illness, 2008).

are important because bipolar disorder is an illness whose symptoms are not readily recognizable. Misdiagnosis of the illness is high, and in some cases deadly if it results in suicide (National Alliance on Mental Illness, 2008).

Two categories of impacts were related to emotional outcomes—emotional health and social support. The emotional health category contained many responses expressing how others' understanding of symptoms released the bipolar individual from negative emotions such as shame, guilt, stress, etc. One woman stated that "It has made me more understanding that this is a genetic disease, not a personal fault of my own." Not having the knowledge, however, resulted in being burdened by negative emotions. One man said he felt "loneliness & despair" resulting from not knowing about the genetic history in his family.

Broadly speaking, the impacts of disclosing can be linked to those advantages of disclosing identified by participants. If the advantages of disclosing include greater understanding, enhanced social support, and increased diagnosis accuracy, it is logical that these require an actual disclosure about bipolar disorder. That is, if a person was not aware of a bipolar presence, he or she would have a harder time receiving a timely diagnosis, being prepared upon diagnosis, helping others experiencing similar symptoms, achieving emotional health, or receiving adequate social support.

Collectively, these findings paint a broad picture of disclosure of stigmatized health conditions within families. The results of this study suggest that the disclosure of bipolar disorder, within families, can improve the quality of life and diagnosis accuracy of both people with bipolar disorder and their family members. These findings reveal that when barriers to disclosure are overcome, the advantages are *increased understanding, increased social support*, and *diagnosis accuracy*. Among these advantages, understanding seems to be foundational for both support and diagnosis accuracy. As one woman with bipolar stated, understanding allowed her family to better "...coordinate care for me. To help them stereotype less. To help them understand problems they too may have." A basic understanding of the illness may allow a family member to better support the person with the disorder and identify the symptoms in others. Securing social support and increasing diagnosis accuracy also have direct implications for emotional and physical health; specifically, preventing delayed diagnosis, enhancing preparation, diagnosing another person, and enhancing emotional health.

If understanding is the key advantage because it potentially enhances support and increased diagnosis accuracy, then the disadvantages might be viewed as barriers to understanding, support and diagnosis accuracy. Barriers such as stigma and denial can prevent disclosure of bipolar disorder, hindering social support efforts and diagnosis accuracy, and negatively affecting the impact categories generated from question three. In Figure 7.1 I present an explanatory model of stigma communication including the advantages, disadvantages, and impacts of mental illness disclosure.

Model of Stigma Communication

Increasing access to the advantages and positive impact of disclosing stigmatized health conditions means understanding and addressing the disadvantages, or barriers to this access. Two overarching themes regarding disadvantages of disclosing emerged in the data when comparing responses across cases. One recurrent theme focused on the state of the relationship between the person with bipolar and his or her family members prior to the diagnosis. People with bipolar disorder who did not have good relationships with their family prior to the diagnosis did not find the diagnosis itself to be a motivator for making interpersonal improvements. The categories of statements addressing *the use of the illness as a weapon, blame discourse,* and *family relational turmoil* reveal relational contexts in which disclosure increases personal risk. In these instances, loved ones simply acquired more ammunition for their personal arsenals. In times of conflict, or as a result of dislike, the illness could be used simply to derogate the person with bipolar. In these cases, disclosure would do more harm than good. This conceptualization highlights the importance of choosing disclosure targets wisely, especially when dealing with such a heavily stigmatized illness as bipolar disorder. This notion of selectivity is highlighted in this statement by a woman with bipolar, "It can be counter-productive to share with family members that you KNOW will not be supportive or understanding."

Another recurrent theme was rooted in the stigma surrounding the disorder, affecting how the person with bipolar is treated post-diagnosis. A family's ability to handle the disclosure of the illness by a loved one depends on their understanding of the illness, which was hindered by issues related to stigma (e.g., denial). Some categories of responses supporting this notion include *stigma, negative affective responses, using the illness as a scapegoat, boundary turbulence, loss of credibility, denial or lack of understanding,* and *alienation.* Each of these categories of responses pertained to the disadvantages of disclosure. What these categories have in common is that they are rooted in misunderstandings about the illness and the misapplication of the illness to the person's identity. Once the diagnosis is made known, family members tend to respond by making attribution errors about the individual's behavior, perhaps overinvolving themselves in social support, or increasing their social distance from that person. An example of an attribution error can be seen in this woman's statement, "They can hold it against you, blame you for things that are totally out of your control, and even stop talking to you all together." Being overly involved in providing social support is referred to as miscarried support and refers to support providers acting in unhelpful ways towards the person in need of support (Coyne & DeLongis, 1986). In a study about social support and AIDS, many respondents described their relatives as overly "mothering" or "babying" towards them (Hays, Chauncey, & Tobey, 1990, p. 382).

The choice to disclose and the level, or depth, of the disclosure, seems to depend on the family's orientation to bipolar disorder and the health of their relationship with the person with the disorder. Stated broadly, the decision to disclose is determined by the interaction between the relational intimacy with the target as well as by the target's orientation, or perceived orientation, to the topic.

See this model represented in Figure 7.1.

Figure 7.1 A Conceptual Model for Understanding Disclosure of Stigmatized Topics

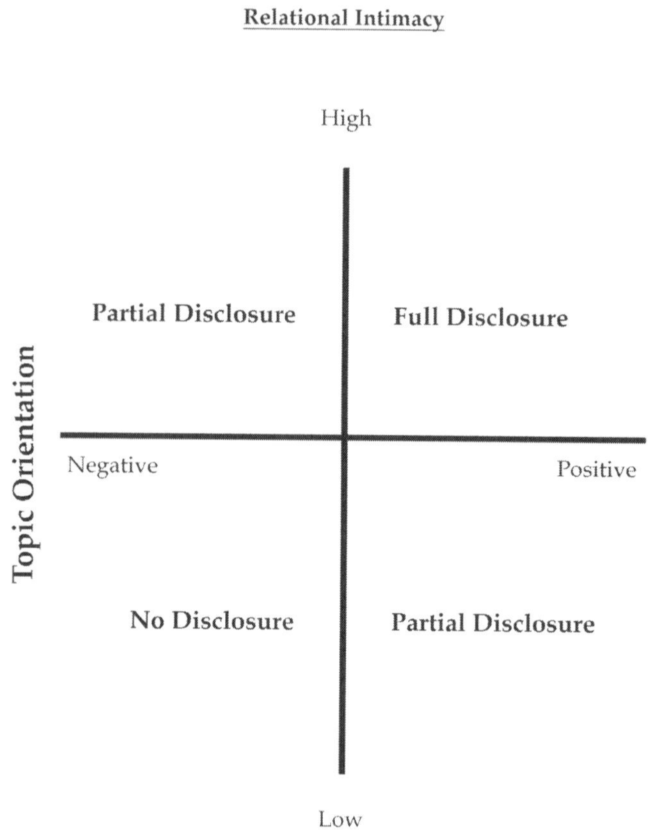

Figure 7.1 presents a conceptual model of stigma disclosure and displays possible outcomes of the interaction between the two constructs. The y-axis represents the level of relational intimacy; the x-axis represents one's orientation to the topic, positive or negative. It is hypothesized that high relational intimacy and a positive topic orientation will produce the highest level of disclosure. However, variations in either axis will reduce the level of disclosure from full to partial or to no disclosure at all. This can be seen using another stigmatized issue—abortion. A person who has had an abortion likely will engage in this disclosure assessment to make decisions about whether and to whom she discloses. If the desired target for her disclosure is a close friend who is pro-life, this person is less likely to ful-

ly disclose. If her close friend is pro-choice, that friend is more likely to receive a full disclosure.

This model attempts to explain how disclosure patterns may be altered by relationship quality and topic orientation. Based on the results of the study reported in this chapter, a person with bipolar disorder is least likely to disclose to family members with whom he or she has a poor relationship, or with members who hold a negative topic orientation. Poor relationships generally are not characterized by in-depth disclosures (Roloff, 1987), so it would follow that one would not disclose a mental illness if he or she is not disclosing other sensitive information. A negative topic orientation can result from holding stigmatized attitudes about the illness like those described as disadvantages.

Reducing stigma requires a "multifaceted and multilevel" approach according to Link and Phelan (2001), who stated that interventions should be aimed at producing "...fundamental changes in attitudes and beliefs...or the power relations that underlie the ability of dominant groups to act on their attitudes and beliefs" (p. 381). Their suggestions, however, do not address stigma experienced interpersonally. Duggan (2006), on the other hand, does take an interpersonal approach to stigma and stated:

> To understand dyadic communication patterns between romantic partners or family members, a researcher must consider the stage of development of the relationship, the point at which the health issue became a key component of the relationship, the types of strategies romantic partners or family members use to help their loved one cope with the illness, and the ways roles within the relationship change during the course of illness. (p.98)

This process, however, does not consider the family members' orientation to, or understanding of, the illness at hand, which may or may not be heavily stigmatized. This model combines both prescriptions to assess both the interpersonal and topical relationships. Using the model prescriptively, one would need to assess what changes are needed to achieve the desired result. If a full disclosure is desired, what barriers are preventing it—a topical one or a relational one? If it is topical, then efforts need to be targeted in such a way to reduce stigma attitudes to attain a positive topic orientation. If it is relational, meaning that the discloser has a poor relationship with someone with a positive topic orientation, then the person would need to perform a cost-benefit analysis of some sort to determine if disclosing was worth the risk. It also is an option for the discloser to take steps to improve the relationship if that was desired.

Duggan (2006) concluded the article stating that the next decade of interpersonal health communication research would need to "...take into account perspectives of multiple family members" (p. 101). This study does just this by looking at the relationships that potential disclosers have with their family members, in addition to these members' views about the illness. This model could be used by mental health care professionals to better help people living with stigmatizing conditions to improve their quality of life through increasing understanding, which in turn, increases social support and diagnosis accuracy.

Limitations

Several issues limit the generalizability of the research findings. Because the study was conducted on the Internet, only people who had access to a computer were able to participate. This would have prevented a number of people from lower socioeconomic brackets from participating in the study. Additionally, bipolar patients who are housed in special facilities were not included in the study. Moreover, since 82% of participants were female and 88.5% of the participants were between the ages of 19 and 49, this limits the transferability of the findings.

Conclusion

There are a wide range of emotions and responses felt when a loved one is diagnosed with a life-changing illness. This chapter highlighted both the role of disclosure in transitioning from being unaware to being aware of bipolar disorder in one's family and the difficulties presented by this awareness. Ideally, family members would respond positively to a disclosure of mental illness; realistically, this is not always the case. Although much of the family stigma literature concerns courtesy stigma, or stigma experienced by family members for being associated with a person with a stigmatized illness, the reality is that stigmatized attitudes toward the ill individual are also endorsed by family members.

The literature reviewed in this chapter and the findings of the current study contributed to the development of a model of stigma communication. This model offers an explanation of how disclosure of a stigmatized illness is affected by the family member's orientation to the illness (positive or negative) and the member's relationship with the person with a stigmatized illness (high intimacy or low intimacy). The model indicates that an interaction of these two concepts determines the disclosure. For example, low relational intimacy and a negative topic orientation likely would result in a nondisclosure. Although we would like to believe that crises bring people together, this chapter suggests otherwise. Essentially, families will be more willing to go through a health transition together, if they were "together" from the beginning and if they are open to the reality of the health condition with which they are faced.

References

Albrecht, T. L., & Adelman, M. B. (1984). Social support and life stress: New directions for communication research. *Human Communication Research, 11,* 3-32.

Alvidrez, J., Snowden, L. R., & Kaiser, D. M. (2008). The experience of stigma among Black mental health consumers. *Journal of Health Care for the Poor and Underserved, 19,* 874-893.

Almeleh, C. (2006). Why do people disclose their HIV status? Qualitative evidence from a group of activist women in Khayelitsha. *Social Dynamics, 32,* 136-169.

Ayalon, L., & Alvidrez, J. (2007). The experience of black consumers in the mental health system: Identifying barriers to and facilitators of mental health treatment using the consumers' perspective, *Issues in Mental Health Nursing, 28,* 1323-1340.

Awad, A. G., & Voruganti, L. N. P. (2008). The burden of schizophrenia on caregivers: A review. *PharmacoEconomics, 26,* 149-162.

Barney, L. J., Griffiths, K. M., Christenson, H., & Jorm, A. F. (2009). Exploring the nature of stigmatising beliefs about depression and help-seeking: Implications for reducing stigma. *BMC Public Health, 9,* 1-11.

Baxter, L. A., & Montgomery, B. M. (1996). *Relating: Dialogues and dialects.* New York: Guilford Press.

Brashers, D. E., Neidig, J. L., Goldsmith, D. J. (2004). Social support and the management of uncertainty for people living with HIV or AIDS. *Health Communication, 16,* 305-331.

Chaikin, A. L., & Derlega, V. J. (1974). Liking for the norm-breaker in self-disclosure. *Journal of Personality, 42*, 117-129.

Cobb, S. (1976). Social support as a moderator of life stress. *Psychosomatic Medicine, 38*, 300-314.

Corbin, J., & Strauss, A. (2008). *Basics of qualitative research* (3rd ed.). Los Angeles: Sage.

Corrigan, P. W., & O'Shaughnessy, J. R. (2007). Changing mental illness stigma as it exists in the real world. *Australian Psychology, 42*, 90-97.

Corrigan, P. W., & Rüsch, N. (2002). Mental illness stereotypes and clinical care: Do people avoid treatment because of stigma? *Psychiatric Rehabilitation Skills, 6*, 312-334.

Corrigan, P. W., Watson, A. C., & Miller, F. E. (2006). Blame, shame, and contamination: The impact of mental illness and drug dependence stigma on family members. *Journal of FamilyPsychology, 20*, 239-246.

Corrigan, P. W., Edwards, A. B., Green, A., Diwan, S. L., & Penn, D. L. (2001). Familiarity with and social distance from people who have serious mental illness. *Psychiatric Services, 52*, 953-958.

Coyne, J. C., & DeLongis, A. (1986). Going beyond social support: The role of social relationships in adaptation. *Journal of Consulting and Clinical Psychology, 54*, 454-460.

Coyne, J. C., Ellard, J. H., & Smith, D. A. (1990). Social support, interdependence, and the dilemmas of helping. In B. R. Sarason, I. G. Sarason, & G. R. Sarason (Eds.), *Social Support: An interactional view* (pp. 129-149). New York: Wiley.

Crisp, A. H., Gelder, M. G., Rix, S. M., Meltzer, H. I., & Rowlands, O. J. (2000). Stigmatisation of people with mental illnesses. *British Journal of Psychiatry, 177*, 4-7.

Derlega, V., Winstead, B., Wong, P., & Greenspan, M. (1987). Self-disclosure and relationship development: An attributional analysis. In M. E. Roloff & G. R. Miller (Eds.), *Interpersonal processes: New directions in communication research* (pp. 172-187). Thousand Oaks, CA: Sage.

Dindia, K. (2000). Self-disclosure, identity, and relationship development: A dialectical perspective. In K. Dindia & S. Duck, (Eds.), *Communication in personal relationships* (pp. 147-162). Chichester, England: Wiley.

Duggan, A. (2006). Understanding interpersonal communication processes across health contexts: Advances in the last decade and challenges for the next decade. *Journal of Health Communication, 11*, 93-108.

Elmore, K. (2006). Southern discomfort: AIDS stigmatization in Wilmington, North Carolina. *Southeastern Geographer, 46*, 215-230.

Forrest Keenan, K., van Teijlingen, E., McKee, L., Miedzybrodzka, Z., & Simpson, S. A. (2009). How young people find out about their family history of Huntington's disease, *Social Science and Medicine, 68*, 1892-1900.

Freeman, H. E. (1961). Attitudes toward mental illness among relatives of former patients. *American Sociological Review, 26,* 56–66.

Goffman, E. (1990/1963). *Stigma: Notes on the management of spoiled identity.* London: Penguin Books.

González-Torres, M. A., Oraa, R., Arístegui, M., Fernández-Rivas, A., & Guimon, J. (2007). Stigma and discrimination towards people with schizophrenia and their family members: A qualitative study with focus groups. *Social Psychiatry and Psychiatric Epidemiology, 42,* 14-23.

Gonzalez, J. M., Perlick, D. A., Miklowitz, D. J., Kaczynski, R., Hernandez, M., Rosenheck, R. A.,...Patel, J. (2007). Factors associated with stigma among caregivers of patients with bipolar disorder in the STEP-BD study, *Psychiatric Services, 58,* 41-48.

Gray, A. J. (2002). Stigma in psychiatry. *Journal of the Royal Society of Medicine, 95,* 72-76.

Hawk, S. T. (2007). Disclosures of maternal HIV infection to seronegative children: A literature review. *Journal of Social and Personal Relationships, 24,* 657-673.

Hays, R. B., Chauncey, S., & Tobey, L. A. (1990). The social support networks of gay men with AIDS. *Journal of Community Psychology, 18,* 374-385.

Herek, G. M. (2002). Thinking about AIDS and stigma: A psychologist's perspective. *Journal of Law, Medicine & Ethics, 30,* 594-607.

Hinshaw, S. P. (2005). The stigmatization of mental illness in children and parents:

Developmental issues, family concerns, and research needs, *Journal of Child Psychology and Psychiatry and Allied Disciplines, 46,* 714-734.

Jourard, S. M. (1959). Health personality and self-disclosure. *Mental Hygiene, 43,* 499-507.

Kreisman, D. E., & Joy, V. D. (1974). Family response to the mental illness of a relative: a review of the literature. *Schizophrenia bulletin, 10,* 34-57.

Kohn-Wood, L. P., & Wilson, M. N. (2005). The context of caretaking in rural areas: Family factors influencing the level of functioning of seriously mentally ill patients living at home, *American Journal of Community Psychology, 36,* 1-13.

Link, B. G., & Phelan, J. C. (2001). Conceptualizing stigma. *Annual Review of Sociology, 27,* 363-385.

Lundberg, B., Hansson, L., Wentz, E., & Björkman, T. (2007). Sociodemographic and clinical factors related to devaluation/discrimination and rejection experiences among users of mental health services. *Social Psychiatry and Psychiatric Epidemiology, 42,* 295-300.

Major, B. (2006). New perspectives on stigma and psychological well-being. In S. Levin & C. Van Laar (Eds.), *Stigma and group inequality: Social psychological perspectives* (pp. 193-210). New York: Routledge.

Michalak, E. E., Yatham, L. N., Kolesar, S., & Lam, R. W. (2006). Bipolar disorder and quality of life: A patient-centered perspective, *Quality of Life Research, 15,* 25-37.

Miller, L. C. (1990). Intimacy and liking: Mutual influence and the role of unique relationships. *Journal of Personality and Social Psychology, 59,* 321-331.

National Alliance on Mentally Illness (2008). Understanding bipolar disorder and recovery: Everything you need to know about this medical illness. Retrieved from http://www.nami.org/Template.cfm?Section=By_Illness&template=/Content Management/ContentDisplay.cfm&ContentID=67728

National Institute of Mental Health. (2001). *Bipolar disorder* (NIH Publication No. 08-3679). Washington, DC: Author. Available from http://www.nimh.nih.gov/ health/publications

National Institute of Mental Health. (2008). *The numbers count: Mental disorders in America* (NIH Publication No. 06-4584). Washington, DC: Author.

National Institute of Mental Health (2009). *Schizophrenia and bipolar disorder share genetic roots: Chromosomal hotspot of immunity/gene expression regulation implicated.* Retrieved from http://www.nimh.nih.gov/science-news/2009/schizophrenia-and-bipolar-disorder-share-genetic-roots.shtml

Norman, A., Chopra, M., & Kadiyala, S. (2007). Factors related to HIV disclosure in 2 South African Communities. *American Journal of Public Health, 97,* 1775-1781.

Parker, R., & Aggleton, P. (2003). HIV and AIDS-related stigma and discrimination: A conceptual framework and implications for action. *Social Science and Medicine, 57,* 13-24.

Paxton, S. (2002). The paradox of public HIV disclosure. *AIDS Care, 14,* 559-567.

Perlick, D. A., Miklowitz, D. J., Link, B. G., Struening, E., Kaczynski, R., Gonzalez, J., ...Rosenheck, R. A. (2007) Perceived stigma and depression among caregivers of patients with bipolar disorder. *British Journal of Psychiatry, 190,* 535-536.

Petronio, S. (2002). *Boundaries of privacy: Dialectics of disclosure.* Albany: State University of New York Press.

Phelan, J. C., Bromet, E. J., & Link, B. G. (1998). Psychiatric illness and family stigma. *Schizophrenia Bulletin, 24,* 115-126.

Proudfoot, J. G., Parker, G. B., Benoit, M., Manicavasagar, V., Smith, M., & Gaved, A. (2009). What happens after diagnosis? Understanding the experiences of patients with newly-diagnosed bipolar disorder. *Health Expectations, 12,* 120-129.

Roloff, M. E. (1987). Communication and reciprocity within intimate relationships. In M. E. Miller (Ed.), *Interpersonal processes: New directions in communication research* (p. 11-38). Beverly Hills, CA: Sage.

Rüsch, N., Angermeyer, M. C., & Corrigan, P. W. (2005). Mental illness stigma: Concepts, consequences, and initiatives to reduce stigma. *European Psychiatry, 20,* 529-539.

Saunders, J. C. (2003). Families living with severe mental illness: A literature review. *Issues in Mental Health Nursing, 24,* 175-198.

Schulze, B., & Angermeyer, M. C. (2003). Subjective experiences of stigma. A focus group study of schizophrenic patients, their relatives and mental health professionals. *Social Science and Medicine. 56,* 299-312.

Sirey, J., Bruce, M., Alexopoulos, G., Perlick, D., Raue, P., Friedman, S., et al. (2001). Perceived stigma as a predictor of treatment discontinuation in young and older outpatients. *American Journal of Psychiatry, 158,* 479-481.

Slade, P., O'Neil, C., Simpson, A. J., & Lashen, H. (2007). The relationship between perceived stigma, disclosure patterns, support and distress in new attendees at an infertility clinic. *Human Reproduction, 22,* 2309-2317.

Stiles, W. B. (1978). *Manual for a taxonomy of verbal response modes.* Chapel Hill: University of North Carolina, Chapel Hill Institute for Research in Social Science.

Weiss, M. G., Ramakrishna, J., & Somma, D. (2006). Health-related stigma: Rethinking concepts and interventions. *Psychology, Health and Medicine, 11,* 277-287.

Williams, B., & Healy, D. (2001). Disclosure of minor mental health problems: An exploratory theoretical study. *Journal of Advanced Nursing, 35,* 108-116.

Zauszniewski, J. A., Bekhet, A. K., & Suresky, M. J. (2008). Factors associated with perceived burden, resourcefulness, and quality of life in female family members of adults with serious mental illness. *Journal of the American Psychiatric Nurses Association, 14,* 125-135.

PART 3

Living with Invisible Illness

CHAPTER 8

Serenity, Courage, and Wisdom: Life with an Invisible Disability

Emily Bowlby

I have a disability. I'm not in a wheelchair, I do not use a cane or crutches and I don't have a seeing-eye dog. In fact, just looking at me you would have no idea that I'm disabled. That's because I have an invisible disability. I may look healthy the majority of the time, but in reality I have a serious health condition that affects almost every decision I make, every day of my life.

There are, according to a 2001 estimate, 56 million Americans with a disability (Brueggemann, White, Dunn, Heifferon, & Cheu, 2001), but this number is far from accurate for two reasons. First, there is no precise or universally accepted definition of disability (Jung, 2002). Even within the disability rights movement, inclusion and exclusion criteria for what constitutes a disability are in dispute (Davis, 1999). Davis reports that even if sufficient delimiters were established, any estimate would be amorphous because boundaries between disabled and not disabled would be permeable. He further argues that anyone can become disabled and, in fact, most people will develop impairments with age. As Brueggemann et al. pointed out, "If we all live long enough, we'll all be disabled. We are all TABs—temporarily able-bodied" (2001, p. 369). Additionally, there are millions of Americans who have invisible disabilities (IDs) and invisible chronic illnesses (ICIs); that is, illnesses that are not readily apparent because their symptoms are not manifest in ways that are visible. Grumbach (2003) suggests that, while largely unrecognized, invisible "chronic conditions, not acute ailments, are now the most common problems in health care" (p. 4). The Partnership for Solutions, which is led by Johns Hopkins University and the Robert Wood Johnson Foundation, found in 2001 that one in three people have at least one chronic health condition, approximately 60 million live with multiple chronic conditions, and more than 3 million live with five or more (Schestok, 2005).

These conditions compound the already complex situation of acknowledging and addressing the concept of disability.

The characteristics IDs and ICIs share in common are that they are "chronic and incurable, that they exacerbate and remit, that they resist diagnosis, that they pose a constant threat to physical well-being, and that, while they often leave the sufferer looking well, they exact a physical and psychological toll" (Donoghue & Siegel, 1992, p. 40). IDs and ICIs are "often characterized by pain, fatigue, inflammation, limitation in mobility, and inability to perform the activities of daily living" (Jung, 2002, p. 180). Further complicating these symptoms is that they are not only "non-observable, but also typically immeasurable. They are subjective experiences"(Donoghue & Siegel, 1992, p. 7).

There is very little research available to help understand the experiences of individuals with IDs and the challenges they face in the various aspects of their lives; school, work, and social networking to name a few. There is even less research on family communication in connection with nonvisible disabilities; though we know that family members often play an integral (and sometimes dominant) role in the management of chronic illness (Grumbach, 2003). It is natural for family members to resist and struggle with the adjustment of accommodating a loved one as they shift from able-bodied to disabled because the shift directly affects the identities and daily activities of every member. The introduction of an ID further complicates the situation because it is easier to reject and ignore that which is unseen and often unverifiable. More research on this topic is necessary. As a start, this chapter will discuss some of the unique complications posed by IDs and ICIs and provide a brief autoethnographic account of my ID and its impact on my familial relationships; specifically my relationship with my father. To accomplish this, I layer alternating voices of my two personas: the writer/researcher and the once-able-bodied, youngest-child and only daughter of my divorced parents.

When I was 16 years old, a conflict with my father escalated to a point where he and I were estranged for nearly a year. It took less than two months after this separation began for my body to start physically mirroring the emotional turmoil I was experiencing and I succumbed to a condition the doctors say I've probably had all of my life. I lost ten pounds of muscle and quickly went from being an energetic athlete to an underweight and scared young woman experiencing random and unpredictable fainting spells three or four times a week.

There is something taboo about sharing one's personal life with the world. My father has always taught me that "our business is our business" and in writing this chapter there is a serious possibility that I am literally writing myself out of my family. There is an inherent risk in sharing personal experiences, but it is a risk I share with other autoethnographers and one I take because I am resigned to the idea that sharing personal experiences helps people break through the social barriers holding them down. I believe, as Dow (1997) states, "the personal is political" (p. 248), and autoethnography exposes the personal. I value this method and agree with Olson (2004) who explains: "Like other autoethnographers, I offer this personal story not in an attempt to make myself the center of attention, but in hope that, through my voice, candor, and self-absorption, we can all better understand…" (p. 7).

I am a woman who has lived with an ID for almost 10 years; through high school, college, graduate school and now in the corporate world. I am a woman who knows the value of familial support in the management of an ID, and a woman who knows how to survive without it. It is my hope that my story is instructive for those with IDs and ICIs and the people who are close to them.

Everyone assumed I had an eating disorder. I was told I could not return to high school until I had met with a specialist, but even after being cleared by the doctor, the administration asked me to withdraw. I refused, and opted instead to teach myself the material and attend classes only when I had an exam. I lost my driver's licens,e and one by one my friends disappeared, each accusing me of intentionally causing my spells refusing to be associated with the "girl who passes out." I saw doctor after doctor and endured a battery of tests, but a diagnosis never came. I continued to lose consciousness without warning and injured myself several times as a result; I fell down stairs, tumbled down football bleachers, and slammed my head against tables and into the ground. Still wary of their liability concerning my school attendance, the administration decided the separation from my father was causing me to spiral into a self-destructive state of depression and required the two of us to attend therapy sessions. There had been no communication between us since the day I walked out of the house and was told I was no longer a part of the family; but the school-mandated therapy finally broke the silence.

Invisibility Is in the Eye of the Beholder

Society has been conditioned to presume disability is something that can be visually affirmed and verified, and is absolute. Individuals with IDs challenge all three of these assumptions and, as a result, are often met with skepticism, disbelief, and even hostility. First, IDs and ICIs lack visual affirmation because in remission we look just like everyone else; we are able to pass as normal. However, when we experience "flares" and "bad days" the state of our health changes while our visual appearance does not. This fluctuation from healthy to impaired can happen often and very suddenly. Unfortunately, "[t]here is great suspicion of claims that one cannot do something when there is no clear physical sign of inability or disability" (Davis, 2006, p. 58). Cal Montgomery (2001) explains, "[t]he person who challenges the particular expectations of disability that other people have is suspect. 'I can't see what's wrong with him,' people say, meaning, 'He's not acting the way I think he should'" (¶8).

> *My dad doesn't believe I have a legitimate medical condition. He says my episodes are "all in my head" and desperate cries for attention. I had no medical proof to offer him in my defense. His explanation was the only answer anyone was giving me, so I started to believe him. I convinced myself that I could control my spells if I only tried hard enough. Every time I felt ill I would try to pretend like nothing was wrong, but ignoring the symptoms only led to more falls. Afterwards I would berate myself for not trying hard enough.*

Second, "[t]here is no set of well-defined, objectively identifiable physical factors or bodily changes that can be identified as 'causing' the symptoms that contribute to or comprise [some of] the disabling conditions" (Davis, 2006, p. 204)·. There is no possibility of making an objective diagnosis that disregards—or is independent of—the person's reported experiences (Davis, 2006). As such, a diagnosis of an ID or ICI may depend heavily on the presumption of the truthfulness of the person who reports his or her experiences. This not only opens an individual with an ID up to accusations of exaggeration and lying from members of society, but from medical personnel as well. The term "symptom magnification"—implying exaggeration on the part of the patient—is often used in medical documentation to explain pain and behaviors with no physical findings (Grady, 2004, ¶31). This skepticism and disregard for the patient's experiences only perpetuates more pain and suffering and encourages lay persons to question the credibility of the sick individual. Fibromyalgia (FM) is an example of this sort of controversial ICI. Conditions like FM are diagnosed based on a set of predefined but unverifiable indicators. "The mandatory symptom is widespread pain not explained by an inflammatory or degenerative musculoskeletal disorder. There are no objective markers of [the] disease" and no valid instruments are able to assess the severity of the condition (Goldenberg, 1999, p. 777). Many doctors are unwilling to make a diagnosis of FM—often citing symptom magnification—and those doctors that are willing, exhaust all possible alternative explanations for the ailments before doing so. As a result "[m]ost patients with FM have had symptoms for 5 to 7 years before a diagnosis is made" (Goldenberg, 1999, p. 782).

I needed the services of ambulances more than 30 times before a doctor could diagnose me. Some of my fainting episodes were fairly straightforward; I would fall, someone would elevate my feet, I would wake, talk with the paramedics—who I grew to know quite well—and then I would restore my energy level with food, water, and bed rest. The incidents became less alarming and almost routine for those around me. On occasion, however, the episodes were not so simple and predictable; some were accompanied by severe convulsions and extended periods of unconsciousness, and sometimes I would stop breathing and required CPR.

After many years of fruitless testing, the doctors finally, FINALLY, found something—vasovagal syndrome. I have an autonomic dysfunction that causes my blood vessels to expand and blood to pool in my feet and lower legs. The pooling causes my blood pressure to drop suddenly and drastically and this deprives the brain of oxygen, thus triggering a fainting episode. There were medications I could take. There was an answer. There was relief.

Unfortunately, the relief was short-lived.

A few weeks later I had one of my worst episodes. I was unconscious and convulsing when the paramedics arrived and transported me to the ER. I was tachycardic, which means my heart was beating at an abnormally fast and life-threatening rate. Seconds before the ER doctor was going to correct the rhythm with an electric defibrillator, my heartbeat returned to normal. We now knew the problem was more complex than vasovagal syndrome. We were missing something.

As individuals with IDs and ICIs wait for a medical diagnosis—that may or may never come—they often conduct their own searches for the cause of their maladies. Psychologists Donoghue and Siegel in their book *Sick and Tired of Feeling Sick and Tired: Living with Invisible Chronic Illness* explain that, "[t]ypically, people with ICIs suffer from symptoms such as nausea, or headaches, or fatigue—all common ailments, generally caused by overeating or drinking or overwork or stress…These symptoms in healthy people are usually self-inflicted and self-treated" (1992, p. 69). It is human nature to seek explanation for the struggles and suffering we must endure. When there is little or no medical support for symptoms, accusations of self-infliction and/or an unwillingness to prevent said symptoms are not uncommon. Sufferers are conditioned, like all of us, to feel responsible for being sick. Unfortunately, they are unable to correct their problems with behavior modification like healthy people. This inability can have serious psychological impacts. "Without an objective explanation of her ailments, the suffering person is terribly vulnerable to the notion that she is suffering from psychosomatic illness or that she is depressed, neurotic, or hysterical" (p. 47).

People's understanding of illness is based mostly on acute conditions, but disability is not an absolute. In *Living in the Gap,* Grady (2004) explains:

> We understand a cold or a broken leg. People are either sick or healthy. The sick and healthy roles are well understood. …But what about the role of someone with a chronic condition that is not totally disabling? Someone who can go for walks, for example, and do some errands, but has limited capacity. This role is not so well defined in our culture (¶19).

Montgomery (2001) illustrates the same issue in *A Hard Look at Invisible Disability*. He offers the example of the person who uses a wheelchair to get into the library stacks, but then stands up to reach a book on a high shelf. *Normals* witnessing the unexpected sight begin to question such an individual. Thoughts of "perhaps he's just lazy," "maybe he's trying to draw disability from the government," "it's people like that who cause problems for those who are truly disabled," or "he just wants attention" shape their assumptions. Strangers do not realize that while the individual they are judging may in fact be capable of walking in and out of the library at that point in time, the stress of the exertion may have a severe impact on the body and symptoms may not manifest until later. While not all of the physical symptoms we experience are preventable, for the individual in the library, the use of the wheelchair may allow him to avoid hours of future pain caused by what most people would view as a mundane task. Those of us with IDs and ICIs do not find pleasure in taking the accommodations we need, but we are forced to decide if the pain we feel as a result of not taking them is worth the trade of the stigma we face if we do. Grady (2004) cautions, "there is a cost for letting other people's opinions keep you from activities that give you health....Your illness then becomes the focus of your life and takes away more and more of the quality of life you have left. That is the price you pay" (¶27).

The episodes continued, and so did the doctor's probing of my body. For almost a year I tried different medications and endured more tests. I even had a heart monitor surgically implanted. About the size of a cigarette lighter, the recorder protruded from the center of my chest. As a young woman I was mortified. But the horror ended up being the answer to my prayers—more answers. In this case, heart pauses. My heart was flat-lining at random intervals, the longest of which lasted thirteen seconds. My doctor called it neuro-cardiogenic syncope. I was having adrenaline-induced heart pauses and was told I needed a pacemaker immediately. Feeling vindicated and relieved at finally having an answer, I underwent the surgery at age 17. Soon thereafter, I began to experience physical warnings before my spells and was thus able to secure a driver's license again. The fainting episodes—while decreasing in frequency—continued to occur, and have never stopped.

If My Family Doesn't Understand...Who Will?

Although those with chronic conditions often suffer discrimination from society in general, it is commonly assumed that family members will form an individual's support network through the long and arduous process of diagnosis and disease management without question (Samuels, 2003). Unfortunately, this may not be the case. After conducting a series of interviews with individuals with IDs, Rocco (1997) concluded that, "[t]here is less opportunity for family support and understanding of the participants with invisible disabilities...Family members may react with disbelief, just as society at large does" (¶21). For most people, their identity has been shaped by the family they were raised with, and conversely, families take on their own identity based on a conglomeration of the characteristics of their participating members. The sudden introduction of a disability severely alters an individual's identity and therefore his or her familial identity as well. However, once the adjustment has been made to the new circumstances, the identities of all involved individuals stabilize once again. This is not true for those with IDs and ICIs. As Donoghue and Siegel eloquently explain:

> Like those who are healthy, she experiences very few limitations, has little physical discomfort, is not dependent on others, and needs no contact with the medical world. Her self-image is active, independent, even vigorous and attractive . . . When the illness is acute, the patient is back in doctors' offices, back in the hospital, back leaning on others, back feeling hopeless. Adjusting to such contrasting states can lead the person to feel as if she has a split personality. (1992, p. 66)

These alternating states are not only trying for the suffering individual, but they put inconsistent demands on family members, and as a result, many find the burden of supporting someone with an ID or ICI to be quite unbearable. McKenna and Seidman (2005) expound on this idea and explain that those around the individual in need of support quickly become weighed down with their own emotional responses and so wish to avoid reminders of the subject. "Friends and family members may begin to ignore or avoid the sufferer in an effort to avoid dealing with the issue" (p. 92). This avoidance leaves individuals with chronic conditions to cope on their own.

> *With my health improving and my emotional well-being stabilizing, I was convinced the relationship with my father could now be repaired. After all, I had the monitor strips showing my heartbeat flat lining; I had evidence that I wasn't just being dramatic. It didn't matter. He maintained the pacemaker was just another ploy for attention. I remember clearly the therapy session when I tried explaining that I had sought out the medical opinions of three different specialists who all concluded the pacemaker was imperative and that no doctor would operate on someone—especially someone so young—and give them a pacemaker if they didn't really need one. His response?*
>
> *"That's bullshit, you don't really need that thing!"*

Depression is 15—20 percent higher for the chronically ill than for the average person (Rifkin, 1992). Add on the stress of abandonment felt when family and friends do not trust reported symptoms or are unable to physically and emotionally support you, and individuals with IDs and ICIs are likely to become extremely depressed or even self-destructive. Schestok (2005) elucidates that isolation commonly accompanies the existence of an ID and ICI and explains that this segregation is what often leads people into depressive states. Isolation from society can cause this despair, but the separation from family members can impede the disabled person's identity development and serve as a relational transgression.

> *The year after my pacemaker surgery, my dad and step-mother announced they had an idea for an annual family vacation—a ski trip. I explained—what I was sure they already knew—that while skiing would be fun for all of THEM, my heart stops and I lose consciousness when my system floods with adrenaline, so perhaps skiing was not a good idea. I provided several alternative suggestions, but no one changed their minds. Motivated by guilt, I joined them and sat in a crowded and dirty cafeteria while the rest of my family skied. I sometimes wonder if he would have let me ski if I had tried. Would he really risk my life? I almost wish I had tested him, but I was—and am—scared that he would have let me go against my doctor's recommendation and participate. I still feel a strong sense of heartbreak and uneasiness when I try to process this idea. What if his harsh accusations are not just posturing? What if he is not just masking his fear and illustrating his denial? What if he truly believes I am faking my medical condition?*
>
> *The fact that I cannot answer these questions with certainty may forever give me pause.*

This Is Who I Am

My narrative accounts woven throughout this chapter are provided so that readers can better understand the challenges of having an ID. One of the most significant challenges for me, as well as for others, is establishing a positive ID identity. The following recollection is an illustration of what, for me, was a turning point in my emotional and cognitive journey to accept my identity as a person with an ID. This account is intended to be instructive because it represents the interdependence of family, disability, identity, and communication.

In between graduate school and finding permanent employment I moved back home with my father and served as a substitute teacher at the grade school I attended as a child, and where my father currently served as president of the school board.

I made sure the women I worked with were aware of my condition and I left my medical information on file with the main office in case there was ever a problem. I also made friends with another teacher, Anna, who had a sister who suffered from occasional fainting episodes. She assured me should anything happen she would be comfortable helping me.

One day, while my students were taking a vocabulary test, it started. My head grew heavy and my eyelids started fluttering. Suddenly my center of balance was shifting to the left and I planted my feet firmly to prevent the inevitable. I felt the familiar tug of something trying to pull my eyes through the back of my head. My balance shifted to the right and I grasped blindly for the countertop behind me. I slid my back down the cabinet and sat on the ground counting each deep breath as I had been taught; in through the nose, out through the mouth. I knew this process well, and I knew I had to get help. I swallowed and forced my eyes open long enough to see a student out of the corner of my right eye and I signaled to her. I knew the words sounded muddled, but she must have understood because she ran from the room. I rested my head back against the counter and focused on my breathing again. Help was on the way. The force was still pulling at my eyes, forcing them deeper and deeper down my throat…into my stomach…I fought it. The darkness crept at me from all sides. I was determined not to completely pass out, but I was paralyzed.

Suddenly I felt Anna's warmth on my arm and I heard the comforting murmur of her indistinguishable words. I was placed on my back, my feet were elevated and in a couple of seconds the grip the force had on me began to weaken. It let go of my eyes and they drifted up through my throat…back to my head…the darkness melted away…I started to understand what Anna was saying…I felt the cool of a wet cloth on my forehead…I smiled. It hadn't been a *good* spell, but I hadn't completely lost consciousness either. For me, it was a victory.

Although I was very shaky, after some food and water I was given a ride home and I was able to get myself in the house without any assistance. I made sure to call my father and let him know what happened before I laid down to rest; I knew it would be better if he heard it from me rather than someone else. Surprisingly, the conversation went well. I let out a sigh of relief. Maybe things really had changed.

Wishful thinking.

I didn't feel 100% the next morning so I took the necessary precautions and stayed home from work. I was there when my father called: *"You want to tell me what really happened yesterday?"*

Uh oh, I knew that tone. I was in trouble for something.

"What do you mean? I did tell you."

"Well apparently it was more serious than you let on."

"No it wasn't, I didn't even completely pass out."

His volume increased: *"Well everyone up there is really worried and they were asking about it!"* There was the anger I knew so well.

"They're concerned dad, that's normal." I was rolling my eyes and attempted to stifle my sarcasm and exasperation. We weren't REALLY going to fight over this were we? Was he ACTUALLY upset because there were people worried about me?

"Emily…we can't have this."

"We can't have what?"

"You can't be up there causing problems. You're distracting people from doing their jobs and scaring the kids and we just can't have it."

"What? How did I do that? You mean because I got sick? Dad, I didn't even pass out!"

"Well that's not what I heard."

All I could think was: *not again. I've come too far to let him treat me like this.*

"Dad, I don't know what you heard but that's what happened and it's fine. The kids are fine and the teachers are fine."

"Well you can't go back there."

"What? What do you mean?" Oh no…I knew even before he answered what he wanted. I felt the dread in the pit of my stomach.

"I mean that you need to quit."

I couldn't believe it. This was extreme even for him. I sprang up from my chair.

"Quit? Because I got dizzy? Are you kidding?"

"No. I'm not."

I knew the tears were coming. Pain and anger boiled inside of me. This was absolutely ridiculous. "What am I supposed to do dad? Quit every job I have if I get dizzy while I'm at work? I'll never have permanent employment!"

"Well maybe you can find somewhere to go at your next job where you can have your little episodes."

The dismissive emphasis on *episodes* brought on the tears; tears of sadness, anger, and disappointment. I thought he had changed. He'd been so supportive and helpful and now THIS? Again? Then it hit me. He had been understanding because there had been nothing to understand. I had been healthy and flare free since returning home. I had been normal. Years of repressed anger and resentment erupted from me. *"My little episodes? What, do you think that I can schedule these things? That I can say,'Oh, sorry guys, it's 2:00, I have to go pass out but I'll be back in a few!'"*

The sarcasm was thick. He didn't appreciate it either. There was a flash of anger. He was practically yelling now.

"I don't care what you do THEN, but for NOW you have to quit."

"Dad, they were fine! Everyone was fine! It wasn't a big deal!"

There was a pleading tone to my voice as I responded and this only increased my anger. I was pacing and coaching myself inside my head: *"Don't beg Emily. You knew this day might come and you know what you want to say to him. Don't you DARE beg!"*

"Well it sure sounds like it was!"

"Look, I don't know who you talked to, but I'm telling you it wasn't even a full episode! Besides Dad, this is me! This is what happens to me! Welcome to what I've been dealing with since I was 16!"

"Yeah…right."

There he was. With two little words he illustrated his disgust with me. The way he disregarded everything that I had been through sent a surge of electricity through me. This was it, this was everything I had been writing about and working on playing out right in front of me. It was almost surreal. I exploded.

"I CAN'T BELIEVE THIS! Do you hear yourself? Do you have any idea how ridiculous this is? How ridiculous you are? You're what I write about! And you're the reason people read what I write! Normal people can't believe people like you exist!"

Just like that I had changed the course of our relationship forever. I had referenced my graduate thesis, an autoethnography on IDs and ICIs that referenced him several times. It was something he knew about but never acknowledged and I knew I had done the unthinkable in bringing it up. I didn't care. I was tired of being silent. The release gave me a sense of empowerment. I was proud of myself. I was still crying, but I was standing up to him. I was 25. He couldn't MAKE me quit. I didn't have to be ashamed of myself or scared of him any longer.

"Look, if you don't quit I'm going to have to use my position as President of the School Board to have you fired!"

I felt sick that the man saying these hateful things was my own father, but I refused to buckle.

"Do whatever you have to do! I'm NOT quitting!" I hung up the phone and threw it into the chair next to me. I screamed. My hands went to my temples and I squeezed, pulling my hair as I made indistinguishable noises of frustration. I was sobbing and heaving and struggling to control myself. My own father was going to get me fired? This was outrageous even for him. He couldn't do this to me! But I knew he could and I knew he would. My only chance was to get to the decision makers at school before he did.

I showered, dressed, put on makeup—a weak attempt to hide my swollen eyes—and I walked to the school. There was a slight feeling of betrayal biting at me as I sat down with the principal and told her that she may receive a call from my father and explained how he would be asking her not to have me substitute for the school any longer. I almost started crying again when I heard her reassurance that she had no intention of letting me go regardless of what my father said.

I prepared myself for another fight and waited anxiously for the confrontation, but it never came. He refused to acknowledge my presence at home but he never went forward with his threat. The relationship between the two of us disintegrated even more but I was—and am—finally content with myself while in his presence. After years of pain and shame I finally believed in myself enough to call his bluff, and it worked.

It has been more than ten years since the symptoms of my ID first manifested. During that time I have had three concussions, two pacemakers, four surgical procedures, a pinched nerve causing the loss of feeling in my left arm, and more hospital visits than I can count. I have borne the stares of bystanders as I emerge from my parked car in a handicapped parking space and the whispers of strangers when I board an airplane early. I endured professors who accused me of drug use and "faking" episodes to get out of taking tests, and the guilt of knowing how much my ID—and my difficulty accepting it—has worried and frustrated those closest to me. But the pain from all of these experiences together is still nothing compared to the pain of knowing my own father doesn't accept my disability—that he doesn't accept me as I am.

Conclusion: Finding Serenity, Courage, and Wisdom

For those dealing with IDs and ICIs, there is a growing number of Internet chat rooms and websites you can visit to find others with similar conditions and experiences. These resources can be extremely valuable, not only because of the emotional comfort you can find knowing that you are not alone in your trials, but because until there is a greater understanding of invisible illnesses among sanctioning groups such as medical professionals, family members are likely to be confused about IDs and ICIs and the assistance they can provide. The support group you have always found in your family members—however you define your family—will be tested when your ID or ICI manifests and as you cope with a new identity and new approach to life. It will be extremely difficult for you and for everyone that loves you. Finding another source of comfort is not a betrayal to those you love, it is a survival skill that can promote healthy living and reduce the stress levels of all involved. What we must all work to understand is that family members play a pivotal role in the management of IDs and ICIs. We have to continuously remind ourselves that each member of a family contributes to the overall familial identity. When one member is suffering, the rest do as well.

I will never claim it is easy to be encouraging and not to question the motives or to doubt the reliability of a loved one's report of symptoms. I will fully admit—although I am embarrassed by the undeniable hypocrisy—that I find myself wondering if others I meet are magnifying their symptoms. I wonder if people who look normal but who are using handicapped parking decals are simply taking advantage of a loved one's disability to get a better parking spot, or if they really need the accommodation. The issue is extremely complex, and there really is no one correct way to handle it. This is why the conversation about IDs is necessary.

My stepfather's favorite prayer is Niebuhr's Serenity: "God, grant me the serenity to accept the things I cannot change, the courage to change the things I can, and the wisdom to know the difference" (Brown, 1987). This prayer has hung on the wall in my home for years, but it wasn't until last year that I realized its significance and that it was exactly what I have been striving for since my symptoms first started.

It took me until graduate school to find serenity with my health and to accept that I cannot always change the way my body responds to its environment. Sadly, there are days I still grapple with the many medical unknowns; the doctors still cannot tell my why my heartbeat was ever abnormally fast, why I had—and have—seizure-like convulsions, or why I stopped breathing so many times. I'm still learning daily to accept serenity with my family, and that I can neither change my father nor force him to realize his behavior is irrational and his words harmful. I found the courage to change my approach to life over the years as I studied invisible illness and disability, but truly found it as I stood up to my father. As for wisdom, well...wisdom is the process of balancing all of the emotional and physical challenges every day. Wisdom is choosing my battles. In response to my father's threat, I embraced my identity, I called his bluff, and I won. I didn't win against him. I never will. I'll never change his beliefs, but I won that particular battle because I resisted succumbing to his negative image of me. I won, I think, because I struck a balance between serenity, courage, and wisdom.

References

Brown, R. M. (Ed.) (1987). *The Essential Reinhold Niebuhr: Selected Essays and Addresses.* New Haven, CT: Yale University Press.

Brueggemann, B. J., White, L. F., Dunn, P. A., Heifferon, B. A., & Cheu, J. (2001). Becoming visible: Lessons in disability. *College Composition and Communication, 52,* 368-398.

Davis, L. J. (1999). Crips strike back: The rise of disability studies. *American Literary History, 11,* 500-512.

Davis, N. A. (2006). Invisible disability. *Ethics, 116,* 153-213.

Donoghue, P. J., & Siegel, M. E. (1992). *Sick and tired of feeling sick and tired: Living with invisible chronic illness.* New York: W.W. Norton & Company.

Dow, B. J. (1997). Politicizing voice. *Western Journal of Communication, 61,* 243-251.

Goldenberg, D. L. (1999). Fibromyalgia syndrome a decade later: What have we learned? *Arch Intern Medicine, 159,* 777-785.

Grady, B. (2004). Living in the gap. *The Invisible Disabilities Advocate.* Retrieved from www.MyIDA.org.

Grumbach, K. (2003). Chronic illness, comorbidities, and the need for medical generalism. *Annals of Family Medicine, 1,* 4-7.

Jung, K. E. (2002). Chronic illness and educational equity: The politics of visibility. *NWSA Journal, 14,* 178-200.

McKenna, K. Y. A., & Seidman, G. (2005). Social identity and the self: Getting connected online. In W. R. Walker and D. J. Herrmann (Eds.), *Creative technology: Essays on the transformation of thought and society* (pp. 89-110). Jefferson, NC: McFarland & Company, Inc.

Montgomery, C. (2001). A hard look at invisible disability. *Ragged Edge, 2.*

Olson, L. N. (2004). The role of voice in the (Re)construction of a battered woman'sidentity: An autoethnography of one woman's experiences of abuse. *Women's Studies in Communication, 27,* 1-33.

Rifkin, A. (1992). Depression in physically ill patients: Don't dismiss it as "understandable." *Postgraduate Medicine, 92,* 147-154.

Rocco, T. S. (1997) Hesitating to disclose: Adult students with invisible disabilities and their experience with understanding and articulating disability. In S. J. Levine (Ed.), *Proceedings of the 16h Annual Midwest Research-to-Practice Conference in Adult, Continuing, and Community Education* (pp. 157-163). Lansing: Michigan State University.

Samuels, E. (2003). My body, my closet: Invisible disability and the limits of coming-out discourse. *GLQ: A Journal of Lesbian and Gay Studies, 9,* 233-255.

Schestok, J. (2005). A Call for Awareness. *Advance Newsmagazines: Advance for Audiologists.* Retrieved from http://audiology.advanceweb.com/article/a-call-for-awareness.aspx

CHAPTER 9

In Sickness and in Health: Coping with Chronic Illness While Transitioning into Marriage

Jonathan Pettigrew and Breanne Pettigrew

THE PENNSYLVANIA STATE UNIVERSITY

Jonathan's Account: A Muffin-Run Story

One morning in 2009, I woke up to the sound of my wife moaning softly in pain. I groggily asked what was wrong. She groaned about being hungry and being exhausted. I pulled myself out of bed, clumsily slipped my feet into sandals, and stumbled downstairs to fetch some muffins. On the way out of our bedroom I checked the time on my cell phone: 2:43 am.

As I descended the narrow staircase I reflected on the fact that scenes like this were commonplace in our household. Breanne's sleeplessness resulted from something like a migraine headache accompanied by a searing pain. She had experienced these headaches since January 2005—as long as I had known her. The headaches were daily, incessant, and sometimes overpowering. They influenced every dimension of our relationship.

Breanne's Account: A Sleepless Night Story

I drowsily came in and out of nightmares as I tried to shake off the pain that sent chills throughout my body. How I wished for someone to sit with me and lighten that dreadful night. Frustrated, hurt, and lonely, I gently shook my husband's shoulder. No response. So I pulled myself up to sweetly kiss his cheek. Still he slumbered. As the night waged on, I began to wonder if Jonathan even cared about me. I could hardly believe that I was in bed with so much pain, and yet there he lay, slumbering in his peacefully oblivious state. Tossing and turning, I finally decided to take action. Digging out a lost pillow from the twisted heap of covers, I mischievously tossed the pillow onto the floor, hoping to cause enough commotion to wake my sleeping husband.

The room was suddenly filled with noise as I accidentally knocked over items on our dresser top. There, that should wake him now! Yes, there was a new sound coming from his snoozing body—a loud SNORE. Ah well, at least I had a reason to get up for a while—what a mess to clean up. I couldn't help but chuckle and quietly supposed that he must have needed this night's rest.

There were times when Jonathan really did meet my needs—like 2 am muffin runs. But there were other times, like this one, when he was oblivious. At such times, I was faced with a decision: Would I allow my headaches to provoke anger within me and direct the anger toward him? Would I let stress overshadow our commitment? In answer to my own musings, that evening I chose to put my relationship with Jonathan over my own needs and let it slide. I cleaned up my mess and sat awake through the remainder of the night. The next morning, when Jonathan finally awoke to his alarm, he gave me a smile as bright as the daybreak and asked, "Did you have a sweet sleep last night?" Such innocence.

I must confess that I was not always so generous with my own attitude. There were days when I was angered, frustrated, and hurt. Having an invisible illness sometimes made me feel invisible, even to my caring husband.

Overview

We were a family coping with an invisible chronic illness, which is "characterized by chronicity and symptoms that are not externally manifested" (Donoghue & Siegel, 2000, p. 4). To tell the story of a family coping with an invisible chronic illness, we offer this autoethnographic account; that is, this personal story presented in juxtaposition with social scientific information (Ellis, 2004). This approach "draws on many points of view and presents them to the reader as representations of lived experience" (Ronai, 1995, p. 396). Our goal in writing this chapter is to share our story of navigating through a new marriage while managing an invisible, unnamed, painful, and sometimes debilitating health condition. Consequently, our story fits somewhere between the lines of relational, family, and health communication research. In this chapter we hope to describe the experience of managing a chronic illness during our first eighteen months as a newlywed couple. Although the headaches did not end after eighteen months, we have limited our narratives to this time frame. Consequently, our stories are written in past tense, but the issues they highlight are struggles we continue to face, so the commentary and analysis we offer are written in the present tense. As of this publication, the headaches have not ceased. In telling our story we attempt to capture the essence of our lived experience, while linking that experience to research literature.

Although there is a plethora of communication constructs we could address when telling our story, we have chosen to discuss how stress (Hill, 1949) and privacy boundary management (Petronio, 2002) functioned in our daily lives during this time period. While our intention is to explicate these constructs through our autoethnographic account, our story necessarily incorporates myriad communication concepts into the narrative. Our lives—like the rest of social reality—do not fit neatly within one particular theory. Rather, the two areas we select serve to focus our narratives.

This chapter is organized into three sections. First we attempt to articulate what Breanne's health condition is and is not. This is not an easy task, as it has baffled a number of physicians. Next we explain how stress and privacy relate to the sickness. We conclude the chapter by offering four communication strategies we have used to cope with the illness: counseling, cuddle-time, crowding support, and confessing commitment.

As you read the analysis and stories we present in this chapter, particularly in the section on privacy management, you may wonder why you are being linked into our privacy network. After all, it seems inconsistent to say that headache-related information is secret and then to publish stories in a book chapter about our experiences! This is not a trivial concern and we are keenly aware of it. Only after much deliberation did we decided to submit our struggles and experiences for publication. Our decision rests on the position that there are more potential benefits to revealing our private information in this forum than there are to concealing the information. In sharing, we hope to impact both those who experience similar invisible and visible illnesses and those who interact with families that are coping with debilitating health conditions. To those for whom our story resonates because of personal experiences, we describe ways we have been able to not merely survive the illness as a family but to enjoy life *together* "in sickness and in health." To those who have never dealt with a health-related limitation similar to ours, we hope to evoke sympathy for others who do face an invisible illness. We seek to explain some of the challenges we've faced both relationally and communally as our lives have intersected with those in our social network. As an audience, we ask you to be judicious stewards of our story.

Breanne: What Is My Headache?

I described my illness quite simply: I had a walking migraine. While others could sleep in a cool, dark room and take the usual over-the-counter drugs, such remedies only exacerbated the pain in my head. Furthermore, my migraine was continuous. That is, a headache arrived one cloudy January afternoon in 2005, and became a thunderstorm that never rolled away. Some days and nights I was confined to bed, praying that the morning would bring relief; other days, I zealously took advantage of a lighter pain level. Nonetheless, my pain was unrelenting and experienced daily. On our wedding day, it had been over two and a half years since my senses were free from the oppression of a steady, dull ache. Although countless physicians and specialists had been consulted, my illness remained unnamed and undiagnosed.

In one sense I was quite functional, and I could carry out daily tasks and social interactions with no apparent uneasiness. Perhaps I masterfully disguised the inward turmoil of pain. I don't know. And honestly, some days were not as difficult as others. Again, my headache was steady but not always debilitating. Yet, my struggle was a weary one, affecting my stamina, diet, strength, schedule, and relationships. There were few areas which had been left untouched by this ongoing health crisis.

In many respects the illness Breanne is afflicted with can be considered an invisible chronic illness (Donoghue & Siegel, 2000). The sickness is not obvious to an observer. She looks like nothing was wrong with her. But, she carries with her an invisible strain. This strain has been constant, affecting every moment of her life. One important distinction between her illness and other types of invisible illnesses is that very little is known about the causes, mechanisms, or treatments for Breanne's affliction. Neurologists, dietitians, naturopathic practitioners, hematologists, chiropractors, and other specialists have not been able to identify cures for her ailment or remedies to alleviate her pain. Treating the illness requires adopting and testing various theories for what caused the headaches. Additionally, Breanne's illness is very uncommon. We have met only two or three others who were similarly afflicted.

What we do know is that, whatever the cause of Breanne's persistent headache, it has profoundly influenced our lives. Her illness is part of who we are as a couple. The physical ailment affects Breanne directly. While she has always experienced a baseline headache, its affects vary with the intensity of pain. Sometimes it is a struggle for her to get out of bed in the morning. Sometimes the headache impairs her ability to focus her attention or process information. Sometimes the pain makes her nauseous. But all of the time her symptoms are hidden.

In less obvious and sometimes indirect ways, the headaches influence our relationships with one another and others. Jonathan often is unable to provide all the comfort and support Breanne needs because of her headaches and sometimes Breanne is unable to encourage and support Jonathan. For example, if Breanne is exhausted from coping with pain all day and Jonathan's mind is debilitated from hours of writing papers, if we attempt to support one another—neither of us has much to offer. The headaches also affect the quantity and quality of time we spend interacting with others socially. Breanne's weary struggle requires rest, so we sometimes withdraw from potentially tiresome social engagements. One way to understand both the direct and indirect effects of Breanne's headaches is to consider family stress.

Stress

Despite the physical challenges posed by Breanne's pain, we eagerly anticipated our marriage and the adventure of starting our new life together. Some aspects of the events surrounding our wedding, however, were stressful. Stress comes from either negative or positive events and involves a physiological response to unusual stimuli (Afifi & Nussbaum, 2006). One pathway through which families encounter stress is novel experiences or life changes (e.g., marriage, relocation). Rubin Hill (1949) proposed the ABCX theory for understanding family stress. The theory involves three parts: the number and severity of stressors (A), environmental and individual coping resources available to a particular family (B), and perceptions or framing of the stress (C). Mismanaged stress can result in a family crisis (X) (Afifi & Nussbaum).

Stressors: Forming a Family

According to a number of stress theories, including ABCX, stress is cumulative. For instance, if a family relocates across the country to start a new job at Christmas time, they experience the combined effect of all three stressors. Because stress is cumulative, the summer we married we topped the charts. We both graduated from a university in May. I finished my master's thesis and participated in an oral defense after returning from our honeymoon. Breanne completed an honors bachelor of arts degree. We were both under a number of pressures to complete our degrees and arrange our graduation. In addition to these responsibilities, we prepared for our wedding ceremony.

We were married on June 24, 2007. After a week's honeymoon, we returned to Indianapolis and for the first time lived together in one household. We occupied a small, two-room, basement apartment. Although it wasn't fancy, it was livable, affordable, and safe. And it was temporary. We relocated to Pennsylvania within thirty-five days of our wedding ceremony. In our new location, Breanne searched for employment in a saturated job market and I started a rigorous PhD program. We knew no one in the area. Two months after settling into our new home, we were delighted to learn we were expecting our first child who was born a month shy of our first wedding anniversary.

Utilizing Holmes and Rahe's (1967) classic stress scale we were subject to an incredible amount of stress just from life events. Pervasive during all of these life events was Breanne's head pain. It was relentless, permeated our everyday activities, and increased our total level of stress (see Table 9.1). Our cumulative stress score of 249 was practically two and a half times more than the most stressful event on the scale: the death of a spouse. Compounding these stressors from life events was the stress of living with an invisible illness. Breanne's illness was potentially stigmatizing. Young people are assumed to be healthy. Healthy people are expected to work, either outside or within the home. Yet, this invisible illness forced us to be flexible in our family roles and to frequently renegotiate our responsibilities.

Table 9.1 Life Event Stressor Scores

Category	Description	Score
Personal Injury or Illness	Bre's Headaches	53
Marriage	June 24, 2007	50
Change in responsibilities	New Work/Start PhD program	29
Beginning or ending school	Graduation	26
Change in residence	Relocation to Pennsylvania	20
Change in social activities	New Friends	18
Vacation	Honeymoon	13
Pregnancy	August 2007-May 2008	40
TOTAL		249

Breanne: Wishing to Be an Ideal Housewife

It had been a productive day, as I had successfully cleaned the kitchen, picked up the living room, cleared away the baby toys, folded laundry, and stocked up on groceries. Like a picturesque housewife of the 1950s, I had fresh bread baking and dinner on the table. With deep satisfaction, I imagined Jonathan's face when he came home from work. He would know immediately that I had a "good head day," as he so plainly described it. Indeed, I took full advantage of the window of health that brightened my day. This is how I dreamed of fulfilling my role as a wife.

Now, I realized that this scenario is idyllic. Even if my headaches departed immediately, I couldn't hope to orchestrate this theme of orderliness on a daily basis. Is this not what marital counseling encouraged couples to recognize? Pinpointing unrealistic expectations that seeped into our minds? But I felt trapped. This scene might not be so unrealistic were it not for my headaches. And my dream was to keep a clean, orderly, nurturing home—something I felt physically unable to offer my husband.

Housekeeping was one area that illustrated the daily impact of my illness. For days, weeks, and sometimes months, I managed household duties. Even when the pain level rose, I endeavored to selflessly handle my responsibilities. Love is, in part, the pursuit of another's well-being. But all too often, I suffered a rough headache spell, and many daily chores fell to Jonathan. While I desired to be the "Supermom" who cooked, cleaned, exercised, cared for and played with the kids, and dazzled my husband continuously, I had to recognize my limitations. Jonathan learned to be very understanding and was willing to help where needed. I was constantly humbled by his readiness to pick up my share of the load—usually without any complaint. His assistance was praiseworthy but did not diminish my desire to fulfill my own familial responsibilities.

Breanne's headaches which are invisible to all but the two of us require us to adapt our household roles and responsibilities. The amount of assistance Breanne needs changes daily because of the unpredictable nature of her headaches. At times, we establish a routine for tasks and chores that lasts a few weeks. But, in the end, it proves difficult for us to follow our ideal social scripts for household chores. Instead, we negotiate our responsibilities based on the needs of the day.

Applying the ABCX model, given the large number and the severity of our stressors (A), from both life events and social expectations, we were primed for a family crisis (X). However, the coping resources we have learned to employ (B) and how we continue to frame our stress (C) helps us maintain family health. Issues related to framing are discussed next.

Framing: Situational Stress

One way of accounting for the immense load of stress we experienced during the first months of our marriage, in particular, was to redefine what we labeled as stressful. Breanne's headaches altered the baseline for what we considered stressful. In other words, our norm was for Breanne to have a headache. Stress then fluctuated from that new baseline. If Breanne ever had a "good head day" it meant that we are very well equipped to deal with whatever novel situations we experienced that day. Conversely on a "bad head day," or when other stressors surpassed a typical load, we had more difficulty dealing with stress. Particularly on bad days, we found it very important to identify the source of our stress. During those periods, relatively minor events often ruptured into conflict due to the accumulation of headache-related stress.

Jonathan: Journaling a Reaction to Stress

My heart pounded quickly as my mind cooled. I was angry. Not at my wife, but I was angry at my own helplessness. I wanted to fix the problem and couldn't, although I'm not even sure I knew what the problem was. I was frustrated that mundane, surface arguments crescendo so quickly, until the pitch was so loud, so sustained, and so shrill that the issue triggering our tiff was muted, overwhelmed by the noise. In these situations I felt unable to express my thoughts or intentions to her.

I feared that stress orchestrated these episodes; stress from my impatience, withdrawal, and uninsightful reactions. When would I get it through my thick skull that getting defensive didn't help anything and that Breanne's reactions to me were only partially reflective of her feelings and thoughts? I knew that there was another dynamic at play in her body. The cumulative force of our stress quickened the tempo, strained our typical harmony, and altered our daily rhythm. But I know we weren't reacting to the immediate issue when we argued, but to something outside our relationship. On bad days, we were primed for quarrels and triggered by "situational stress."

Situational stress is the cumulative force of external pressures on our relationship. Situational stress often manifests in marital conflict

(McCubbin & Patterson, 1983). Conflict resulting from situational stress, however, is different from conflict caused by pressures within the relationship. Markman, Stanley, and Blumberg (1994) depict conflict resulting from internal relational stress as geysers. Frustrating daily events trigger the geyser's eruption. The geyser is fed by core issues (e.g., relational control, recognition, commitment, acceptance), which supply more surface issues (e.g., relatives, careers, money, sex, religion). Pressure builds in one of the core issues, and surface issues erupt creating conflict. From their view, *relational stress* accumulates because of pressures internal to the relationship. Conversely, *situational stress* is the accumulation of pressures external to the relationship, such as a move or an invisible chronic illness.

Every marital relationship, including ours, deals with both relational and situational pressures. Because of the pervasive external pressures we faced during our first 18 months of marriage, it became important for us to recognize when situational stress was impinging on our relationship. Detecting situational stress required us to vigilantly monitor the source of our frustrations. The stress of Breanne's ongoing illness manifests itself in many ways—some of which we have yet to discover. Nevertheless, making an explicit effort to differentiate between the types of stress influencing us is one way we have managed to reframe and understand our stressors.

Coping: Posture of Love

A final component of ABCX theory is the coping resources available to a family. These coping resources help avert crisis. Although this particular theory focuses on rather static environmental resources (e.g., wealth, employment, education, length of relationship), in our experience we found community and communication to be important resources. Regardless of whether our stress was situational or relational, communicating with one another and maintaining a posture of love toward one another was crucial. Doing so required time, diligent observation, and dedication. The following examples demonstrate how we have come to identify and account for situational stress by choosing to maintain a loving disposition toward one another.

Breanne: Loving When Overbooked and Underappreciated

One week, Jonathan scheduled several social engagements that we both anticipated eagerly. It was a new week, and I was freshly enthusiastic to engage socially with friends. However, by the time Thursday arrived, my strength was waning and I much preferred a quiet evening at home. Nevertheless, situations were such that our social engagements needed to be honored. Longing to retreat from the demands of polite company, my wandering mind began questioning, why did we spend so much time with his friends? Why not postpone these meetings? While Jonathan wanted to keep the appointments, I felt my preferences ignored. Why didn't he care about me?

Upon further consideration, I realized that I wasn't necessarily disappointed with Jonathan. Indeed, together we decided to keep our engagements. Certainly, Jonathan had not wronged me; instead, I was disappointed by my own lack of stamina. I had inappropriately projected my frustration and weariness onto Jonathan's conduct, rather than identifying the source of my underlying disappointment. Once identified, we were better positioned to correctly address the situational stress.

Jonathan also has been frustrated by my headache; and, situational stress caused him to misplace his response. For example, one rainy afternoon Jonathan commented angrily that the laundry had been piling up and that he was too tired to attend to it. He was annoyed that it had been left unhandled for several days. This complaint was offered during a time when my headache had been debilitating enough to keep me in bed for several days. At first, I was hurt by the remark, interpreting it as, "I know you're sick in bed, but can't you try to keep house?" Later discussion revealed that Jonathan was frustrated with pain, rather than the specific issue of laundry. He was angry that I had to endure this illness and that he was incapable of making it better for me.

In confronting stress, it was imperative that Jonathan and I dedicated ourselves to maintaining a posture of love. Such a posture was not riddled with accusations; instead, it sought to correctly address any frustration with the goal of reconciliation. In this instance, as in many others, our relationship overcame situational stress when we lovingly sought to handle it in a way that showed respect and concern for one another.

Jonathan: "An excellent wife, who can find?" (Proverbs 31)

I have been constantly amazed at how gracious Breanne has been toward me. She has wrestled with her headache every moment of every day—even when it has been just a minor annoyance. What I found incredible was that she rarely let it affect her attitude or disposition toward me. And she has done her best to manage our growing household. Even while pregnant and in the sleepless weeks following our eldest's birth, she managed her condition with grace. The fact that she has not been more reactive or impatient is nothing short of admirable. If I had such continuous, unceasing headache, I would not be nearly as polite, kind, warm, patient, or respectful as she. "Her worth is far more than jewels!"(Proverbs 31)

In addition to dealing with stress caused by the headache, we have had to learn to manage and negotiate when and what to disclose to others about Breanne's illness. Because it is invisible, only those we told knew about her illness.

Privacy

Communication privacy management theory (CPM; Petronio, 2002) provides a vocabulary for understanding some of the issues we experience related to privacy. CPM posits that people utilize three management processes to coordinate when they reveal or conceal information. First, rules are acquired and developed based on several factors (e.g., gender and culture). Rules for managing private information are subject to change as needs, situations, or goals. For example, transitioning from single to married life stimulated a change in our privacy rules. Second, boundary coordination involves boundary permeability (how secure or how tightly guarded is the private information), boundary linkage (who becomes privy to private information), and boundary ownership (the felt responsibility to maintain private information by those who are linked to it). The third broad concept of CPM is boundary turbulence. Petronio (2000, 2002) and colleagues (Petronio, Ellemers, Giles, & Gallois, 1998) describe that boundaries are not perfectly managed. When there is some violation of a privacy rule, turbulence results.

The first major family transition for us related to privacy boundaries was when Breanne shared information about her headaches with me. Then, as a couple we had to decide what information to share with whom. Several researchers point out that there is a stigma attached with having a chronic illness and afflicted persons face a dilemma in deciding whether or not to disclose the illness (Joachim & Acorn, 2000; Lonardi, 2007). Revealing information about the illness may result in stigma and concealing may prevent needed social support. For us, learning to maintain privacy in social situations on bad head days required me to learn how to read Breanne's subtle, often nonverbal social cues.

Just the Two of Us: Sharing the Burden by Disclosing Medical History

Given that Breanne had struggled with her headache for over two years before our marriage, it proved to be quite a task for her to reveal information about her medical history to me. Our family formation not only altered each of our individual privacy rules but also required boundary coordination. I needed to be informed of the nuances that accompanied her illness, so that I could share her burden. This information was tightly guarded knowledge and the boundaries around this information were fairly impermeable, so disclosure was a difficult process. Revealing this information to me before our marriage required that Breanne disclose personal information to me, but she also had to communicate her desire that the information remain private (boundary ownership). Ultimately, making me privy to information about her headache provided a boundary linkage.

Breanne: Giving the Facts

In the task of briefing Jonathan, he received support from those who knew my illness best. Before our marriage, I lived at home and was greatly aided by my parents who witnessed my illness from the beginning. Thus, they were aware of the daily challenges that I faced. My parents tried to paint a realistic picture for Jonathan, as our life together would have additional trials that were outside the realm of premarital counseling. Moreover, my parents assisted in describing my illness, giving a background of all the treatments that had been attempted. For example, my mom walked Jonathan through my health records, described my past treatments, and offered suggestions for future medical actions. My dad cautioned Jonathan to consider my illness a lifelong struggle, as we had little evidence to suggest that the illness would soon be healed.

Social Stigma: Dilemma of Privacy

Once I was apprised of her illness, together we had to negotiate when to tell, whom to tell, and how much information to share with others. Selecting who to tell, however, was not quite a straightforward process. Based on our experience, we can affirm that there certainly is a stigma attached to people who struggle with a chronic, invisible illness.

Breanne: Disclosure Can Provoke Varied Responses

I couldn't go to the hospital and come home better. I couldn't fill a prescription and say that my symptoms were relieved. I couldn't even go through a treatment and say that it was completed. Yet, I found most people assumed that a doctor, prescription, or treatment could "fix" my problem. People didn't really know how to react to a condition that was ongoing and lacking a familiar method of treatment consisting of a beginning and an end. The stigma I experienced regarding my health condition was not due to intentional malfeasance. Rather, stigma arose from uncertainty and labeling me—or being unable to label me—and not knowing how to react to the nature of my illness. Some acquaintances continually inquired "Are you feeling better?" hoping that I had improved. I disappointed them repeatedly when I didn't have much progress to report. Others shied away from addressing the issues altogether, afraid that I would find their questions too personal or prying.

My dad once remarked that people would better understand my health condition if I walked around in a full body cast. There are days when it was tough, and I was desperate for some recognition and support. Yet, there were other days when I wanted to be regarded as normal as possible. I wanted the consideration of being thought of as more than a sickly person—someone who had joys, concerns, frustrations, achievements, and worries outside of my health. Such is the dilemma I faced; while I desired to be cared for and understood fully as a chronic illness sufferer, I also wanted to be treated normally. Both were not possible, but a true friend would try to "live the tension" with me.

We did not believe that people we met intentionally cast a stigma onto Breanne. Instead, they oversimplified her condition and reacted to her in one of two extremes: treating her as someone who was ill or, conversely, as a normally functioning person. For some, her illness overtook her identity; she was to them a walking migraine. When these people talked with Breanne, their conversation was dominated by health-related questioning. When people first learned about the condition, this was a common reaction. For others, the illness was not only invisible but also ignored. Breanne was normal to them, and they did not quite empathize or accommodate her illness-induced limitations. These people did not inquire about how Breanne's headaches were or even ask about what treatments we were trying. No one got it right all the time; some came closer than others. Friends and family who "got it" perceived when everything was alright and when some extra encouragement was needed.

Social Settings: Managing Boundaries by Reading Cues

Dealing with the issues of privacy was a challenging task, especially given the stigma attached to revealing an invisible chronic illness. We were careful to choose who we linked as co-owners of information about Breanne's illness because some people did not respect our desire to keep the information private. Consequently, when we went out in public, maintaining secure privacy boundaries—that is, keeping Breanne's illness a secret—required extra attention.

Jonathan: Cards, Coffee, and Cues

After we were married, I felt in some way that it was my responsibility to watch out for my wife in order to help her when she was hurting. The problem with her invisible illness, however, was that it was, well, invisible. I couldn't see when she was unwell. So, when we were out in public, with friends, or even at home, I couldn't easily discern when she was really hurting and when she was feeling okay. In a sense, I needed to learn to see the invisible. It was my responsibility to pick up on subtle cues. Unfortunately I missed much more than I saw. Sometimes I did poorly and other times I did well. Two stories illustrate.

The setting for my first story is at our friends' house. We had joined them for dessert and games. En route to their place, Breanne and I talked about how her head was feeling and whether or not she was up to the evening's engagement. She wasn't feeling great but wanted to enjoy the evening anyway. Sometimes we set up a codeword or a signal so I could know when she was ready to leave. I don't remember if we had done so this particular evening. Anyway, the night went smoothly. We enjoyed our dessert. The games passed the time. At one point, we got into a riveting discussion of theology. Breanne reached over and took my hand, squeezing it lightly. I felt warm and proud knowing she agreed with my brilliant observation! It wasn't until we left about an hour later that Breanne informed me she was really signaling that we should leave when she took my hand. She was in a lot of pain and felt like she was about to black out. Finally hoping to get my attention, she squeezed my hand. I missed the cue.

Other times I have done much better discerning how Breanne was feeling and what she needed. For example, a family from our church invited us to dine at their house one evening. We had not spent much time with them and they did not know about Breanne's headaches. After a relaxing outdoor cookout we joined the family for des-

sert and coffee. I noticed that Breanne seemed to be processing information slower than usual and even had slurred a few words, which often signals a bad head day. As we were served dessert, I covertly asked how she was feeling. "Not too good."

With Breanne's head flaring, coffee was a bad choice. It sometimes triggered a painful reaction. The problem was that we had already each been given a cup of coffee. Because Breanne had a strong sense of propriety, I knew she would try to empty her coffee cup. She wouldn't want our hosts to think the dessert or coffee were anything less than splendid. She often put politeness over her own comfort. I felt I should intervene but without drawing attention to Breanne's condition since our hosts didn't know about her headaches. So, I quickly finished my cup of coffee and casually reached over and began drinking hers.

These stories illustrate at least two dynamics of revealing and concealing information about Breanne's headaches. First, seeing the invisible illness, that is, picking up on Breanne's subtle cues, afforded the opportunity to manage the dilemma created by maintaining a privacy boundary and acquiring needed support. Covert nonverbal or verbal codes communicated what was needed without disclosing why it was needed. Moreover, shared codes were relationship-specific and unrecognizable to an outside observer. Using codes has helped us to maintain privacy boundaries during social encounters.

Secondly, co-ownership of secret information required shared rules for revealing and concealing. It was very important to negotiate privacy rules and communicate what and how much information was acceptable to share with whom. Because we relocated to a new community in a different part of the country, we had to decide how much information to share with our acquaintances and new friends. Mostly through a process of trial and error I learned what Breanne believed was appropriate and inappropriate to disclose. Similarly, Breanne learned about my expectations regarding privacy. We were able to successfully establish our own privacy rules, adapting both our prior rule systems and forming safeguards around our privacy behavior. For example, we both agreed that if I wished to share information about her illness with a particular confidant, I would ask Breanne before I spoke with that person. In sum, we learned the importance of negotiating privacy boundaries.

Four Cs of Coping

Dealing with Breanne's illness while forming a new family has not been easy. The added stress of an invisible illness atop the normative events of family formation presents unique challenges. We have learned how to manage household responsibilities as well as coordinate information about Breanne's condition. Our experiences have taught us at least two important lessons. First, coping with an invisible illness requires community. Second, coping with an invisible illness requires an open flow of information—communication.

Coping with the invisible illness requires community. Stable, supportive relationships are key to well-being (Moore & Zaff, 2002). Indeed, relationships are fundamental to being human, much more to coping with human experience. We have learned that to go through this together we must rely not only on each other but also on a network of others who have supported, listened to, empathized with, and encouraged us. From Breanne's parents to friends who can read the subtle cues of her illness, our community provides needed emotional and instrumental support.

Coping with this invisible illness also requires communication. In this final section, we detail four specific communication coping strategies we find helpful. First, we describe how *counseling* in a safe haven allows us to vent our frustrations. Second, we relate how *cuddle time* is tremendously reviving. Thirdly, we explain the benefits of taking time to *crowd ourselves with support*. Finally, *confessing our commitment* to one another refocuses our perspective, reminding us that there is more to life than our immediate health status.

Counseling

Finding a safe place to release headache-related pressure has been important. It is tremendously helpful to vent in a safe environment. It keeps our frustrations from exploding toward each other. Likewise, it prevents anxiety from imploding. While counseling may be one situation described as a safe haven, it does not necessarily mean that we are seeking advice. We do not expect or seek solutions, corrections, strategies, or even practical suggestions. We simply need listening ears and sympathetic voices, encouraging us to keep pressing forward in our love and regard for one another.

Breanne: Venting Frustrations

I am reminded of a particularly difficult week, when my headache pricked our relationship into soreness. We were not angry, disappointed, or frustrated with each other; nevertheless, the strain caused by my pain level was emotionally exhausting. While Jonathan struggled to maintain his support, I felt the heaviness of my ongoing burden.

One night, the relational pressure was finally intense enough to seek an outlet. After a prayer meeting at our church, which itself often provided us an outlet, our pastor and his wife asked us how we were doing. With loving concern, they allowed us to release our inward struggles. Jonathan and I mostly just talked. We shared our frustrations. We vented our failings. We expressed our commitment. We confessed our fears, the unknown future and the final implications of my headaches. Because our pastor and his wife already knew about my headaches, we did not feel the need to justify ourselves, or even provide lengthy explanations. We were indeed grateful to have discovered the emotional release provided by a safe haven.

Cuddle Time

Sometimes, listening ears are not even necessary. In such times, we simply need to cuddle. Rabbi Abraham J. Heschel (1951) poetically mused: "In the tempestuous ocean of time and toil there are islands of stillness where man may enter a harbor and reclaim his dignity." (p. 29). When Breanne is having a difficult day (or sometimes on the very best head days) it is a great coping mechanism to take pleasure in our relationship by being together—communicating presence. We might hold hands during a walk or cuddle together on the couch while watching a movie. We may or may not talk. We simply enjoy each other's company. We find refreshment for ourselves and our relationship in time together. We take the time to let our relationship exist, without the pressure of important discussions, social obligations, or constant status reports on Breanne's headache.

It is through these mundane, everyday encounters that our relationship is strengthened. As Duck (1995) would put it, these interactive moments constitute and recreate our relationship. Modifying his thesis, we think these encounters accrue for us shared experiences and relational inertia. We made space for our relationship to be rejuvenated. Each encounter is not absolutely novel; we bring history and memories, perceptions, expectations, and goals into our encounters. In this sense, we do not re-create our relationship; rather, we continued it. We share positive experiences and, most importantly, we share time when our relationship can be nourished. It is these cuddle times that amass substance to outweigh the stress, difficulties, or disagreements we face.

Comforting Environment

Support offered from family and friends is helpful, and their love and attention is particularly refreshing. We enjoy retreating from the stress of life by crowding ourselves with loved ones who understand our difficulties. For example, we spent one Thanksgiving week with Breanne's parents and siblings. While the business of the holiday set a different pace and tone, it was indeed beneficial to be couched in the family who best knew our situation. We were freed from the ongoing task of explaining our trials. We reasoned that Breanne's family understood our experiences, since they had dealt with it for two and a half years before we married and they continued to assist in our efforts to find treatments and a cure. It is not just in the presence of Breanne's family that we find support. People often acknowledge Breanne's illness, support us, but simultaneously treat the illness as a non-issue. In many ways, crowding ourselves with support serves to erect another safe haven where we can rest and just be.

Confessing Commitment

A final tactic we use to cope with the invisible chronic illness is to remind one another of our commitment to our marriage and to each other.

Jonathan: Rephrasing Wedding Vows

In a church before our God, our family, and our friends we vowed to forsake all others and be loyal only to one another as long as we both shall live. We try to find novel and creative ways to restate this commitment to one another again and again. Sometimes I'll paraphrase the classic wedding vow and tell Breanne she's "stuck with me until we're both dead." I'll remind her I'm not going anywhere or quote a line from a poem significant to our relationship. Breanne tells me that she loves me or that she's glad she married me. It's like we've developed verbal shorthand, or ways of conveying a lot of meaning with just a few symbolic phrases or gestures.

Articulating our commitment to one another is an important way for us to minimize worry about our relationship. Building from a program of research on intimacy in dating relationships (e.g., Knobloch & Solomon, 2005; Solomon & Knobloch, 2004), Knobloch, Miller, Bond, and Mannone (2007) examined the effects of uncertainty in marital relationships. They found that when married couples experience relational uncertainty, the way they interpret messages is affected. Even when taking into account marital satisfaction, those experiencing uncertainty about their relationship perceived their spouse's messages to contain less affiliation (liking, solidarity), more dominance (control, power), and less involvement (engagement, intensity). In addition, after controlling for satisfaction, those experiencing uncertainty were more likely to perceive conversations as threatening to themselves and their marriage. Given these negative effects on information processing, it has been useful for us to reaffirm our commitment to one another. By articulating our commitment we lessen relational uncertainty and thereby increase our chances of overcoming a pessimism bias in our conversations. Combating pessimism has not been something we attempted just in order to better process messages, but also in order to better our general outlook on our relationship.

Jonathan: The Best Is Yet to Come

About five years before I was married, a friend invited me to eat pizza with some of our classmates and his parents who were visiting from out of town. I remember that evening, going around the room and sharing something we had learned—some important life lesson. When we got to his parents, they shared a motto they adopted early in their marriage: The best is yet to come. They explained that at the very best and in the most trying times of their 30+ years of marriage, this motto was a constant reminder to remain optimistic. I was impressed by their testimony and their marital relationship. I desired to have a similar perspective in my own marriage. So, when Breanne and I were engaged, I shared this story and motto with her. We agreed to incorporate their motto as our own, so in whatever we experienced, we shared this hope. It pointed us toward a life of new experiences together. It gave us something to look towards, in this life or the one to come. It kept us optimistic in the face of our difficulties.

Each of these four strategies has helped us cope with Breanne's invisible illness. Adopting these strategies has enabled relational growth and stability. Recognizing that we both handle our frustrations imperfectly, these coping strategies have helped ensure that we continue to display love and concern to each other. These strategies help us maintain a posture of love.

Conclusion

To conclude our chapter, we would like to offer one of Shakespeare's (1964) most famous sonnets for consideration. We have decided to fix our aim on love, which is "a perfect determination of the will to further the true good of another person" (Budziszewski, 1997, p. 72). Even though this view of love is lofty, perhaps unattainable, for us it is not a philosophical abstract. Instead, love is a tangible work. Sometimes it materializes as muffin runs at 2:43 am, putting Breanne's well-being above my own. Other times it means Breanne's suffering alone so I can sleep.

We have certainly witnessed changes in this illness—sometimes for the better, other times for the worse. Life brings its alterations. Although we admit impediments of pain, struggles, and sacrifice, we will surely not be shaken by their tempest. Whether or not this thunderstorm passes, we will say with confidence that our love and commitment is an ever-fixed mark and a perfect determination, in sickness and in health.

Sonnet 116 (Shakespeare, 1964)

Let me not to the marriage of true minds
Admit impediments. Love is not love
Which alters when it alteration finds,
Or bends with the remover to remove.
O no, it is an ever-fixèd mark
That looks on tempests and is never shaken,
It is the star to every wand'ring bark,
Whose worth's unknown, although his height be taken.
Love's not time's fool, though rosy lips and cheeks
Within his bending sickle's compass come:
Love alters not with his brief hours and weeks,
But bears it out even to the edge of doom.
If this be error and upon me proved,
I never writ, nor no man ever loved.

References

Afifi, T. D. & Nussbaum, J. F. (2006). Stress and adaptation theories: Families across the lifespan. In D. O. Braithwaite & L. A. Baxter (Eds.), *Engaging theories in family communication: Multiple perspectives* (pp. 276-292). Thousand Oaks, CA: Sage.

Budziszewski, J. (1997). Why we kill the weak. *Human Life Review, 23,* 67-96.

Donoghue, P. J., & Siegel, M. E. (2000). *Sick and tired of feeling sick and tired: Living with invisible chronic illness.* New York: W. W. Norton & Company.

Duck, S. (1995). Talking relationships into being. *Journal of Social and Personal Relationships, 12,* 535-540.

Heschel, A. J. (1951). *The Sabbath: Its meaning for modern man.* New York: Farrar, Straus and Young.

Hill, R. (1949). *Families under stress.* New York: Harper.

Holmes, T., & Rahe, R. (1967). The social readjustment rating scale. *Journal of Psychosomatic Research, 11,* 213-218.

Joachim, G., & Acorn, S. (2000). Stigma of visible and invisible chronic conditions. *Journal of Advanced Nursing, 32,* 243-248.

Knobloch, L. K., Miller, L. E., Bond, B. J., & Mannone, S. E. (2007). Relational uncertainty and message processing in marriage. *Communication Monographs, 74,* 154-180.

Knobloch, L. K., & Solomon, D. H. (2005). Relational uncertainty and relational information processing: Questions without answers? *Communication Research, 32,* 349-388.

Lonardi, C. (2007). The passing dilemma in socially invisible diseases: Narratives on chronic headache. *Social Science & Medicine, 65,* 1619-1629.

Markman, H., Stanley, S., & Blumberg, S. L. (1994). *Fighting for your marriage: Positive steps for preventing divorce and preserving a lasting love.* San Francisco, CA: Jossey-Bass.

McCubbin, H. I., & Patterson, J. M. (1983). The family stress process: The double ABCX model of adjustment and adaptation (pp. 7-37). In H. I. McCubbin, M. B. Sussman, and J. M. Patterson (Eds.) *Social stress and the family: advances and developments in family stress theory and research.* Binghamton, NY: Haworth Press.

Moore, K., & Zaff, J. (2002). *Building a better teenager: A summary of "what works" in adolescent development.* Washington, DC: Child Trends Research Brief.

Petronio, S. (2000). The boundaries of disclosure: Praxis of everyday life. In S. Petronio (Ed.), *Balancing the secrets of private disclosures* (pp. 37-49). Mahwah, NJ: Lawrence Erlbaum.

Petronio, S. (2002). *Boundaries of privacy: Dialectics of disclosure.* Albany, NY: SUNY Press.

Petronio, S., Ellemers, N., Giles, H., & Gallois, C. (1998). (Mis)communicating across boundaries: Interpersonal and intergroup consideration. *Communication Research, 25,* 571-595.

Rambo, C. R. (1995). Multiple reflections of child abuse: An argument for a layered account. *Journal of Contemporary Ethnography, 23*(4), 395-426.

Shakespeare, W. (1964). *Sonnet* CXVI. Worcester, England: Stanbrook Abbey Press.

Solomon, D. H., & Knobloch, L. K. (2004). A model of relational turbulance: The role of intimacy, relational uncertainty, and interference from partners in appraisals of irritations. *Journal of Social and Personal Relationships, 21,* 795-816.

PART 4

Interfacing with Others

CHAPTER 10

Medical Disclosure in Oncology among Families, Patients, and Providers: A Communication Privacy Management Perspective

Sandra Petronio and Shannon Sweeney-Lewis

INDIANA UNIVERSITY-PURDUE UNIVERSITY INDIANAPOLIS

During the life-course of an illness such as cancer, there are numerous times that patients, their families, and providers encounter situations of medical disclosure (e.g., Gordon & Daugherty, 2003; Mack, Wolfe, Grier, Cleary, & Weeks, 2006). From an initial diagnosis, to discussions of the prognosis, through the trajectory of care post-treatment, and to hospice and end-of-life, there is interplay of decisions to reveal information, temptations to conceal information, reactions to unexpected disclosures, and digestion of desired and unwanted information. The phenomenon of medical disclosure has been discussed in numerous ways, though unsystematically. Typically, medical disclosure tends to be viewed in terms of four domains in the medical literature. These domains include discussions on truth-telling, perspectives of full and honest disclosure, breaking bad news, and disclosure deliberations (e. g., Barnett, Fisher, Cooke, James, & Dale, 2007; Collis, 2006; Gordon & Daugherty, 2003; McDaniel, Beckman, Morse, Silberman, Seaburn, & Epstein, 2007). In this chapter, we explore how medical disclosure plays a part in patient care of individuals with cancer. While this is not an exhaustive review, we look at the way that communication privacy management theory helps frame the issues to gain new insights into a difficult issue. We consider the way patients and their families come to grips with the stages of cancer and how providers traverse the terrain of disclosures to their patients and families. Although much of the disclosure process found in medical care is not specific to cancer as a disease, we focus on cancer because the research literature is more extensive and the issues appear more evident than with some other diseases.

While research examining disclosure in medical care of cancer patients exists, it tends to be atheoretical. Thus, to better understand the dynamics involved with medical disclosure, we use the communication privacy management (CPM) theory to understand these disclosure episodes in a more systematic fashion (Petronio, 2002; Petronio & Durham, 2008). CPM is an evidence-based theory that explains the management of revealing (disclosure) and concealing private information. The chapter is framed in three sections that follow the life-course of cancer care, including (1) disclosure issues surrounding diagnosis and prognosis, (2) disclosure through trajectory of care post-treatment, and (3) hospice and end-of-life disclosure events.

Communication Privacy Management

CPM Theory Overview

Six fundamental principles help define the parameters of privacy management according to CPM. These include:

1. CPM theory considers that privacy and disclosure (or access) are in a dialectical tension where both must be recognized for the relationship they have to each other and cannot be considered separately to fully comprehend the nature of privacy management.

2. CPM defines the nature of private information as something that people believe they own and therefore want to control, as illustrated by thinking about this information within a boundary that people give access to or protect from intrusion depending on the degree of openness or privacy individuals desire.

3. In order to control the flow of private information, people develop privacy rules. These rules are derived from decision criteria for giving or denying access to the information. They include, motivational reasons to tell or not to tell medical information, cultural and gender issues upon which rules are based, risk-benefit judgments about revealing or concealing private information that de-

termine the kind of privacy rules a person uses, and situational criteria that often serve as a catalyst for changing a given rule.

4. Co-owners (shareholders, stakeholders, or guardians) of the information are created when private information is shared with others. The creation of co-owners results in the formulation of a separate privacy boundary dedicated to the shared information that can be thought of as independent cells collectively regulated by the original owner and those people given co-ownership status.

5. Because it is presumed that co-owners of the private information have a level of responsibility to care for the information, there is an expectation that privacy rules used to make decisions about access and third party disclosures are negotiated and coordinated between the original owner and the co-owners.

6. Although there are often expectations that the parties will recognize and respect the rules that have been collectively devised and negotiated to manage the co-owned private information, at times there are intentional or unintentional breaches of those rules resulting in boundary turbulence (Petronio, 2002). These instances lead to privacy violations, privacy dilemmas, privacy intrusions, and privacy misunderstandings (Petronio, & Jones, 2006; Petronio, Jones, & Morr, 2003).

This brief explanation of the main concepts in communication privacy management sets the stage for our understanding of how patients, their families, and providers regulate the disclosure process. CPM theory allows us not only to grasp the issues surrounding choice making from the perspective of the discloser, it also lends insights into the way the disclosure process impacts the recipients. In this chapter, we utilize CPM to unpack the complexities of medical disclosure among and between patients, providers, and the patient's families. We also conduct this exploration across three turning points of cancer care; the initial diagnosis and prognosis stage, the trajectory of care post-treatment, and hospice, end-of-life phase of the cancer journey.

Within cancer care, three categories of people tend to intersect in this journey, (patient, families, and providers). Thinking about the way disclosure and privacy function is more accurate and useful when framed in terms of the boundary formations around private information for these people, the privacy rule regulations they use to reveal or conceal, and the assumption that privacy turbulence will erupt among and between patient, patient families, and providers[1]. Thus, understanding the way privacy boundaries are established and managed for provider-families relationships, patient-family relationships, patient-provider relationships, and more specific cases of a child in patient-parents-provider relationships, affords a grasp on the dynamics of the way that medical disclosure takes place and the complexities that patients, their families, and providers face over the course of cancer care. In this chapter, we integrate the lens of CPM into the different turning points of the cancer journey across patients, families, and providers.

Disclosure in Diagnosis and Prognosis of Cancer

Disclosure plays a prominent role during diagnosis and prognosis in cancer care (Gordon & Daugherty, 2003; Sankar & Jones, 2005). In general, research on medical disclosure during the initial diagnosis and prognosis of cancer suggests that disclosure is often considered a place for "truth-telling" from the perspective of the provider, which in turn, tends to be equated with honesty (Miyata, Takahashi, Saito, Tachimori, & Kai, 2005). Thus, in CPM terms, truth-telling, defined as "honest communication," implies that the providers consider the boundaries protecting the diagnostic and prognostic information as highly permeable. To be "honest," therefore, all medical information should be told in an uncensored fashion (Hancock et al., 2007). In doing so, providers often endeavor to produce messages they believe convey the reliability of their information and have the optimal ability to be perceived as credible by the patients and their families. How-

1 We recognize that using the concept of "providers" reflects a generic label that encompasses physicians, nurses, social workers, and other health care workers. Where possible, we identify the professional role of a healthcare worker in the chapter.

ever, at times, providers may withhold relevant information because they are not ready to tell. The tests may not be conclusive or the providers might not feel confident enough about the issues to initially disclose particular aspects of the condition. Nevertheless, providers who desire to be open and honest with patients have the task of telling information in a way that "does not appear to hide the truth" and that suggests they are offering their best judgment. These goals are likely to drive the kinds of privacy rules that providers tend to use when telling patients medical information about their condition. Although providers largely endorse this trend, enacting disclosure represents a paradigmatic shift for the medical community. Thus, engaging in "full disclosures" reflects changing from a tendency to restrict access about diagnostic and prognostic information to an expectation of disclosing the complete details of a patient's condition (Parsons et al., 2007).

Provider Disclosure Predicaments

The tension that providers experience surrounds ethical judgments of beneficence on one hand and respecting patient autonomy on the other. This tension impacts the boundary rules that providers use to reveal or conceal and underscores the difficulty they face in balancing these dual needs regarding patient care. Thus, choices not to reveal information concerning diagnosis, test results, or long-term prognoses are motivated, in part, by acts of beneficence—protecting patients' well-being (Parsons et al., 2007). While it is clear that beneficence still carries weight for providers, they also recognize the patient's right to autonomy that may change the privacy rule used toward a decision to reveal information (Parsons et al., 2007).

Despite the fact that healthcare teams are legally obligated to share the prognosis of cancer with patients, the way in which they convey the information can vary from direct to vague (Sheu, Huang, Tang, & Huang, 2006). Oncologists may feel a reluctance to make a direct disclosure about prognostic information because they project the impact factor of receiving the information for the patient (Gordon & Daugherty, 2003). Receiving a poor prognosis, for instance, especially if it is unanticipated, is likely to produce psychological stress for the patient (Fallowfield et al., 1994; McHugh et al., 1995). Studies on disclosure of bad news recognize the need to present information clearly and effectively (Fujimori, Akechi, Morita et al., 2007; Back, Anderson, Bunch, Marr et al., 2008).

Although the literature on the effective methods of delivering bad news advocate reliance on clear messages communicating the news, the disclosed information may be blocked out and therefore possibly misunderstood or forgotten by the patient (e.g., Beadle et al., 2004). This is especially true in emotionally charged situations. When individuals are highly aroused in terms of emotionality, they find it difficult to process disclosed information (Pennebaker, 1995; Petronio, 2002). In these cases, the patients and their families are likely to close down their privacy boundary to the incoming information as a protective device (Petronio, 2002). To overcome these barriers, providers need to take into account how the information is presented, the timing, content, and factor in the possibility of patients needing several sessions to "digest" the information disclosed (Ptacek, Ptacek, & Ellison, 2001).

The motivations behind the physician's decision to explicitly and completely disclose or to remain indirect are not always evident (Ptacek, & Eberhardt, 1996; Robinson et al., 2008). Yet, some studies suggest that the choice of communicative strategy can be associated with the level of uncertainty providers feel about the initial diagnosis and resulting prognosis (Amir, 1987; Epstein & Street, 2008; Gordon & Daughtery, 2003). Complicating these ambiguities, physicians may feel uncomfortable about whether patients desire complete disclosure and, if so, how they will be able to comprehend and cope with such information (Amir, 1987; Eggly, Penner, Albrecht, Cling, Foster, Naughton, Person, & Ruckdeschel, 2006). Concern about "hitting them over the head" with the information may also drive some of the uncertainty about disclosure (Hancock et al., 2007). In addition, discussions regarding hope and prognostic disclosures create further hurdles for physicians (Clayton, Hancock, Parker et al., 2008; Helft, 2006; Mack, Wolfe, Cook, Grier, Cleary & Weeks, 2007).

The ability to communicate a prognosis effectively, yet deliver the information in a way that does not convey "false hope" or ambiguous technical information is a challenge. Helft (2006) argues that with advanced cancer patients, for example, a collaborative strategy is useful to balance hope with disclosure of prognosis because it "ultimately relies on a series of conversations, during which…forecasting is used to bring about incremental awareness of the ultimate course and outcomes of the disease, and on careful and honest maintenance of hope" (p. 119). These factors illustrate the way that providers regulate the boundary around a patient's diagnostic and prognostic information. The motives providers have for revealing or concealing patient information in these situations influence the rules that guide choices of communicative strategies adopted when telling or guarding this information. Besides a provider's motivations, other decision criteria such as risk-benefit calculations may also influence judgments about which privacy rules to use when considering revealing or concealing diagnostic and prognostic information to the patient.

From the research literature that focuses on the provider disclosures to patients about the diagnosis and prognosis, it appears that providers feel a sense of ownership over the information even though they know the diagnostic and prognostic information belongs to the patient (e.g., Butow, Dowsett, Hagerty, & Tattersall, 2002; Fallowfield, Jenkins, & Beveridge, 2002; Gattellari, Butow, Tattersall, Dun, & MacLeod, 1999). While truth-telling is expected, a difficulty lies in the sense of ownership providers have over the diagnostic and prognostic information. The ensuing tension that evolves out of ownership issues for the patient, patient's family, and for the providers often leads to a sense of ambiguity that all parties feel with regard to decision making. However, CPM research predicts that when patients and providers directly and openly negotiate how private medical information will be managed, establishing privacy rules regulating access and protection, these tensions are reduced. Working to come to agreements about information management helps patients, their families, and providers more effectively receive and provide care. Through these private medical information negotiations, the expectations for maintaining control by the owner are met and the co-owners are clear about how the patient wants information handled.

Managing Co-ownership of Medical Information

There are two dimensions that define medical information co-ownership. The first often functions as a catalyst for the second to prevail. First, the provider gains access to private information about the patient's medical condition by the patient directly telling the provider. In other words, the patient discloses symptoms and behaviors that are used to describe the patient's condition. Second, there is an expectation that once this disclosure takes place, inherent expectations emerge for the provider that define his or her professional role regarding confidentiality. The patient assumes there will be confidentiality and the provider feels an obligation toward maintaining that confidentiality. Thus, the characteristics of maintaining a confidential relationship are marked by the unconstrained access to all of the patient's medical information (e.g., test results, labs, etc.), with the assumption, however, that the provider has been granted guardianship over his or her information (Petronio & Kovach, 1997; Petronio & Reierson, 2009).

Patient-provider information co-ownership. The intersection between original owner (patient) and co-owner (provider) of private medical information characterizes a dimension of the patient-provider relationship, though it is not often recognized as such. However, the co-owner or guardianship role that the provider plays has an added dimension that complicates the way that this role is understood. For the provider, a large portion of medical information about the patient is known without direct disclosures from the patient. Because providers are granted access rights to a large category of information (having to do with the medical condition) that does not require step-by-step permission when new information about a patient's condition becomes known, the kinds of ownership parameters that providers have are substantively different than in many other situations (Petronio & Reierson, 2009). Providers, as co-owners, serve as guardians of the patient's information. In a sense, they play three integrated roles. They are: (1) the interpreters of the message, (2) the carriers of the message about information such as test results, and (3) the deliverers of the message. Thus, providers may feel ownership toward the information without necessarily accounting for or recognizing the way the patients define their rights to the content. This assumption about ownership of the patient's medical information may account for some tensions that patients experience during decision-making interactions with providers (Beadle et al., 2004). Ownership rights often extend to family members. Clearly, families and caregivers are profoundly affected by their loved ones' illnesses (Grinyer, 2006). Although the diagnostic information may be unsetting, the family still wants to know the outcome (Mack et al., 2006). Patient-provider confidentiality laws prevent physicians from disclosing medical information to their families without signed consent. Thus, for confidentiality reasons and other issues that arise about sharing medical information, there are many possible tensions among patients, families, and providers.

Family, patient, and provider information co-ownership. The patient has a personal opinion about how the diagnosis and prognosis should be conveyed and sustained (Miyata, Takahashi, Saito, Tachimori, & Kai, 2005). While there is no doubt that the provider is aware of these personal opinions, each party in the patient, family, and provider triad may not be aware of the struggle that can evolve regarding sharing private medical information. Because families develop privacy orientations that represent concretized rules (i.e., long-held and enacted rules agreed upon by all members) members ascribe to, the family, as a unit, also has expectations about the way medical information concerning a member "should" be disclosed (Petronio, 2002; Serewicz & Canary, 2008). The intersection of family assumptions about medical disclosure further complicates the way that information about diagnosis and prognosis is managed.

Families regulate both external privacy boundaries that represent the flow of information outward to those not part of the immediate family and internal privacy boundaries that regulate privacy among and between those internal to the family structure (e.g., Petronio, 2002). Knowing that both types of privacy boundaries exist for families is helpful in discerning the multiple layers of issues that often prevail when a member has a medical problem that is likely to be salient for the whole family. Thus, certain family members may have built alliances protecting specific information and assume that because of their alliances, they would be more privileged to know information that is private to the patient. They may also feel that they have more ownership rights than the patient might assume. The family members may, therefore, assume that they would be involved in making decisions about treatment. This happens with parents, for example, when they leave their adult children out of the decision-making loop regarding treatment options. Parents with younger children who are ill make assumptions that they have complete control over decisions and may leave the child out of the disclosures about the disease (Beale, Baile, & Aaron, 2005; Duggan & Petronio, 2009).

Controlling private information to those outside the external family privacy boundary also has the possibility of restricting family information that could have a bearing on the medical aspects of the patient's case. Families may enact rules that limit disclosure about issues such as child sexual abuse or other behaviors that may be viewed negatively by outsiders. Family members may not feel able to disclose, even when it would be helpful in determining a productive course of care for the patient. In all, good judgment about care issues may depend on seeking as much pertinent information from family members, yet, might be hampered by privacy rules the family members hold. Consequently, better understanding the basis for the privacy rules protecting information is helpful for the providers and patient care.

Patients' expectations for ownership of medical information. Although the provider wants to balance beneficence and patient autonomy, and in advanced cases, preserve hope, in determining revealing or concealing information about diagnosis and prognosis, there remains the extent to which the patient defines the parameters of control over his or her medical information. Much of the research focuses on the provider's disclosure, but less considers how the patient defines his or her role as the original owner of the information. Contemporary oncology patients desire a higher level of involvement in the treatment process than patients of the past (Beadle et al., 2004). This desire for involvement and control is coupled with their desire to be fully informed of the diagnosis, prognosis, and treatment process (Brown, Dunn, & Butow, 1997). Clearly, patients report that in order to make informed, autonomous decisions about moving forward with the appropriate treatment, they need to be informed of the full diagnosis (Harris, Winship, & Spriggs, 2005). Thus, this feeling of ownership over the information leads them to believe they have a right to give or deny permission to providers to proceed with treatment. If the provider is unaware of the patient's desire for and often expectations of ownership control, a type of power struggle can ensue.

While the patient desires to exercise the right control choices, paradoxically, patients also want the information to be co-owned with the provider (e.g., Back, Anderson, Bunch, Marr et al., 2008). They do not simply want to have complete control over the information; they expect it to be shared. They desire the boundaries around the information to include patient, provider, and often family members. In an attempt to enlighten palliative care nurses about the importance of communicative elements in the nurse-patient relationship, for example, Dunne (2005) stresses that patients often desire an equal amount of input in the communication process. When dealing with any serious illness, patients often define the act of granting access as something they have given to the providers because they believe they are worthy of sharing information ownership. However, even for those patients whose providers perceive them as particularly dependent on them and willingly giving control over the information, it is likely these patients still feel they should be recognized as having control over the information. For some patients, a level of trust is a key catalyst for granting co-ownership status. For other patients, trust may be less of an impetus for giving over control; instead, it may be the level of vulnerability that drives the willingness to give up complete control and put their faith in the provider without question.

Considering the magnitude of disclosing a cancer diagnosis, countless patients express frustration over the way that bad news is delivered or are unhappy with the lack of information disclosed (Rodriguez, Gambino, Butow et al., 2008; Salander, 2002). When physicians are forthcoming about the diagnosis and prognosis and express interest in the patients' overall well-being, patients are more likely to be satisfied with the patient-physician interaction (Brown, Dunn, & Butow, 1997). This, in turn, encourages the patient to be more open with the physician and confident about the diagnosis. From a communication privacy management perspective, it is possible that patients feel an increased sense of ownership over the treatment process because they must take responsibility for managing medications and arranging treatment appointments, and therefore feel like they have a certain partnership standing with the physician and medical team.

Yet, at times, patients may encounter a certain degree of resistance concerning the depth and breadth of control granted by the medical team, leading to a certain level of dissatisfaction with the communication. Unfortunately, when patients are dissatisfied with consultations they tend to withdraw from treatment plans, seek other physicians' opinions, and even lodge complaints about their healthcare team (Brown, Dunn, & Butow, 1997). In these cases patients may feel they have little control over the information and seek other avenues of influence.

Disclosure Trajectory and Process of Care

Patients' Privacy Management Strategies

Despite the fact that providers accurately disclose test results and treatment progress to the patients, the time period in which the patient must wait to receive the information can cause stress. Based on a CPM perspective, the difficulty stems from patients having to give up some control over the information about their condition to "outsiders" (lab technicians, administrative assistants, etc.). Because the provider is their liaison with the other medical personnel, as a designated co-owner/stakeholder, patients believe the providers should keep them in the informational loop and become frustrated when they do not notify them about the progress of acquiring results or check in to see how they are doing. While both providers and patients are often dissatisfied with the delay in receiving test results, effective communication with the primary physician is vital for the patient and family (Farguhar et al., 2005; Maguire, Faulkner, Booth, Elliott, & Hillier, 1996). Patients suffering from cancer need unambiguous and clear information about their disease delivered in a timely manner (Van der Kam et al., 1998). Perhaps, these feelings are the result of the patient's desire to have some control over the process and regulation of information disclosed by the medical team. Therefore, the delay in delivery of the information increases the anxiety the patient may already be feeling about the disease.

One of the ways patients manage their private information concerning a cancer diagnosis and ensuing treatment is to deny the information altogether. Doing so is a protective device for the patient that controls the information by keeping it outside their informational privacy boundary and therefore disclaims "rightful" ownership. Often there is a conscious element of denial in which patients refute information expressed to them by their physicians in order to calm fears and anxieties (Rabinowitz & Peirson, 2006; Weisman & Hackett, 1961). Denial is used to defend against threatening thoughts, feelings, and doubts (Rabinowitz & Peirson, 2006). Early in the process, in some cases, patients are willing to accept the information disclosed to them by their providers, but denial emerges later in the treatment process. When treatment does not proceed as hoped and impending death is inevitable, patients may use denial as a defense mechanism to counteract fears of death. In these situations, denial may manifest itself as refusing to acknowledge ownership of the information. In outwardly rejecting custody of the information and refusing to admit the claim of ownership, patients disown and divest themselves of its burden. In other situations, manifestations of denial may lead patients to restrict access to the information about their condition or new symptoms that arise from the healthcare team and family. For example, a woman recently confessed to her adult daughter that she had a lump growing in her breast for twenty years. At the point the tumor burst through her skin and could not longer remain hidden, the woman had to reveal the secret she had been keeping about her health for all these years. However, she protected the information within her privacy boundary for as long as she was physically able.

Even though the woman in the above example worked to keep her condition secret, many patients wish to disclose their health condition to family members. However, when patients want to reveal to their families, they typically want to control how, when, and to what extent the information is disclosed. As we find generally in high stress situations, people often want to modulate and monitor the flow of private information, especially when the content of the messages may directly impact someone for whom they care (Petronio, 2000, 2002; Petronio, Reeder, Hecht, & Ros-Mon't Mendoza, 1996). Thus, patients often are concerned about the way medical information is disclosed to family members because they are apprehensive about the impact diagnostic and prognostic information might have on the family (Rabinowitz & Peirson, 2006). When patients anticipate that the medical information about their disease would make their loved ones frightened or anxious, they are more likely to regulate their privacy boundaries more tightly. Some may even completely conceal the information such as the woman discussed above. In other cases, patients may regulate disclosure concerning this disease by minimizing obvious pain they experience in front of their family, offering excuses or justifications that have little to do with their actual disease (Rabinowitz & Peirson).

Families, Patients, Providers and Treatment Disclosures

The relationship among patients, their families, and the healthcare team is important throughout the cancer journey but seems particularly important where treatment is concerned. Often the family members are the caregivers during treatment and incorporating them as a legitimate part of the healthcare "team" is often in the best interest of the patient. To grant family caregivers membership on the "team," providers have to open up their boundaries around private medical information about the patient they have controlled and tell the family members all that they have been given permission to tell by the patient. Thus, communication and particularly disclosures that help the family deliver the best care become a vital component in interfacing families with the health care providers (Dunne, 2005).

While patients often experience a great deal of stress during their disease, their families also face considerable upheaval in their own lives (Kim & Given, 2008). When a family member is diagnosed with cancer, the whole family deals with an extraordinarily difficult phase (Houtzager et al., 2005). Yet, the patient's treatment produces a different kind of strain on the family, particularly those who are responsible for caregiving, and often children have a difficult time coping with their parents' illness. In addition, when children are diagnosed with cancer, there are many more complicated issues that families face (Rabineau, Mabe, & Vega, 2008). For the family as a whole, those directly involved with care, and for children, the family's life becomes refocused around coping with the emotional upheaval associated with illness (Barnes et al., 2000; Cappiello et al., 2007; Kristjanson et al., 2004; Last & Grootenhuis, 1998; Northhouse & Swain, 1987).

Parents as Guardians of Medical Information

The literature on children and cancer reflects two main themes: (1) examining issues that revolve around disclosure related to pediatric cancer; (2) disclosure about parental cancer to children (e.g., Houtzager, Grootenhuis, & Last, 1999; Hymovich, 1995; Kristjanson, Chalmers, & Woodgate, 2004; Parsons, Saiki-Craighill, Mayer et al., 2007; Patterson, Holm, & Gurney, 2004).

Disclosure surrounding children's cancer. Dealing with pediatric cancer is a painstaking and often lengthy process. Complicating the issues is the fact that depending on cognitive level, previous life experiences, and age, children tend to be naïve about illness and death (Hymovich, 1995). Afflicted children and their families are faced with a great deal of upheaval and distress throughout the experience (Patterson, Holm, & Gurney, 2004). Among many issues the parents face is the issue of disclosing the disease to the child and to others such as siblings or extended family members (Patenaude, & Kupst, 2005). There has been considerable debate over the amount that parents and providers should disclose with children about their disease and how to talk with children about their cancer diagnosis in general (e.g., Ranmal, Prictor, & Scott, 2008). Many providers, especially in the U.S. feel that it is essential to explicitly tell children about their disease (Parsons, Saiki-Craighhill et al., 2007). However, since parents believe that the information disclosed about a child's condition also belongs to them and the parents are mindful of how their child copes with issues, it is likely that the parents will want considerable control over how, when, where, and to what extent the child is told about a cancer diagnosis, prognosis and treatment plan (Levetown & Committee on Bioethics, 2008). Thus, in CPM terms, the parents view their role as guardians and co-owners of their child's medical information. While the information belongs to the child, the age, cognitive level, and cultural issues no doubt intervene in determining how influential the parents will be in controlling the flow of information to and from the child regarding the illness (Duggan & Petronio, 2009).

Possibly, the amount of influence the parents exercise may depend, in part, on the child's ability to comprehend issues surrounding the illness. Some research shows that children understand much more about their disease and its seriousness than is often assumed by the adults (Patenaude & Kupst, 2005; Spinetta, 1974). When the parents or providers chose to appropriate the control over the child's privacy boundary and dominate information flow to and from the child, the child may be left to cope with fears alone (Patenaude & Kupst, 2005).

The challenge for the parents (in conjunctions with discussions they have with the child) and the providers is to agree on a set of privacy rules that regulate the way information should flow to and from the child early in the detection of the disease. Doing so helps everyone, but particularly the child, receive information that is understandable, consistent with a cognitive level, age appropriate, and meaningful for the child. Engaging in a discussion about the best way to regulate information concerning the disease not only helps the child, it also makes obvious to the provider and parents the expectations for how information about the disease will be handled.

Disclosing about parental cancer. In relation to conveying information to children about a parent's cancer diagnosis, prognosis, and treatment, some evidence suggests that children adjust better to their parents' cancer when information is disclosed according to their level of cognitive development (Kristjanson et al., 2004; Hymovich, 1995; Northhouse & Swain, 1987). Northhouse and Swain (1987) point out that the process of sharing information may be more important than the content. Issues such as timing of the disclosure, the way in which the information is told, whether incremental disclosure is used, and the setting may be particularly important (Petronio, Reeder, Hecht, & Ros-Mon't Mendoza, 1996). In some cases, parents choose to keep the information from the children, often contributing to the child's sense of isolation, lack of control, and sometimes the feeling of insignificance in the scheme of dealing with their disease (Kristjanson et al., 2004). Children have been found to cope better when told the diagnosis and treatment plan for a parent (Levetown & Committee on Bioethics, 2008). Thus, incorporating the children into the privacy boundary surrounding the information about a parent's illness is likely to make them feel the same sense of ownership to the information involving their family as the other members.

Post-Treatment and End-of-Life Disclosure Events

With advances in detection, diagnosis, and treatment of cancer along with the dedication to healthier lifestyle choices, rates of cancer survivors have dramatically increased within the last few decades (Aziz, 2007; Chu et al., 1996; McKean et al., 2000; Tesauro, Rowland & Lustig, 2002). Many patients report they are satisfied with their quality of life overall after surviving the disease, yet studies report that residual psychological and physical symptoms can remain indefinitely and clearly have an impact on the family (Aziz, 2007; Gotay & Muroaka, 1998; Tesauro, Rowland, & Lustig, 2002). Challenges such as fatigue, cognitive changes, body image, and sexual functioning are often cited as issues for cancer survivors. Moreover, the fear of recurrence typically plagues most survivors and their families (Alfano & Rowland, 2006). For example, childhood cancer patients and their families face several lingering uncertainties and immediate as well as long-term complications after treatment is complete (Klassen, Raina, Reineking et al., 2007; Levi & Drotar, 1999). Even with the increasing knowledge of the long-term effects of cancer and methods of improving quality of life, there are still many questions regarding the care of cancer patients after they have completed the active treatment phase (Harrison, Young, Price, Butow, & Solomon, 2009).

Research suggests that much of the post-treatment phase shifts away from the patient, family, and provider triad to cancer support groups, dietary counseling, and other forms of rehabilitation (Tesauro et al., 2002). However, patients move away from reliance on providers to increased dependency on family and friends when in post-treatment. Curiously, the break from constant reminders of being ill, in terms of going to the hospital or clinic for treatment and frequent visits to the physician, may allow patients and their families to regain a sense of control over their lives. For patients in particular, control is regained through their ability to "take back" jurisdiction over their own private medical information (Petronio & Ostrom-Blonigen, 2008). For example, patients may perceive less need to share every detail of their bodily functions, pains, and so forth with family members. Consequently, while there may be unmet medically supportive care needs, there are other aspects of a patient's life that revert back to pre-cancer diagnosis such as claiming control over personal information that they would like to keep private but have not been able to because of their illness (Harrison, Young, Price, Butow, & Solomon, 2009).

Survivor Disclosure

A large base of research has focused on breast cancer survivors and the coping strategies they use after treatment is complete (e.g., Stewart et al., 2000; Thewes, Butow, Girgis & Pendlebury, 2004). While disclosure issues are not often the main focus of this research, there is information that helps discern some aspects of managing personal information about the illness. For example, in a study of factors affecting breast cancer survivors, Stewart et al. (2000) found that two-thirds of the women surveyed had disclosed their breast cancer to friends, family, siblings, children and partners. Thus, in selecting recipients to invite as co-owners of the information surrounding breast cancer diagnosis, individuals having close personal ties tended to be targets. However, other more functional choices of recipients were made by approximately half who disclosed to coworkers and bosses.

Many reasons were given by these respondents for not telling about their illness (Stewart et al., 2000). These reasons function as filters or privacy rules determining who is not invited into a privacy boundary. For instance, they did not tell when they feared they might embarrass someone. In other cases, these women felt they needed to protect the information from certain individuals because they thought it was too personal to tell them. They also regulated their privacy boundaries by protecting the information because they worried that it might negatively affect relationships or career prospects. Even though these women had cause to protect their privacy boundary and limit disclosure about their illness, when the conditions met their criteria for revealing and they did so, they felt that disclosing had a positive effect. Because these women regulated their privacy boundaries effectively, the outcome of the disclosure experience was viewed as positive and allowed for a more supportive environment. Due to the intimate and personal nature of breast cancer, some women tend to be guarded and private about their past struggle and survivorship. Thus, for many, the experience serves to create less permeable boundaries around this private information. Yet, others have a positive outlook on their cancer experience and they tend to be less guarded in sharing their survival of breast cancer. This information underscores the different ways that cancer survivors regulate the flow of information about their illness to others and the privacy rules they used to manage disclosure and protection.

One of the more trying aspects of cancer survival is observed in the difficulty many couples and partners have adjusting to all phases of the illness, including post-treatment (Hodgkinson et al., 2007). The family members, particularly partners, must adapt to economic shifts, to the physical demands of caregiving, and role changes (Alfano & Rowland, 2006). Partners tend to rely heavily on one another for support and encouragement, especially in the post-treatment phase because they no longer have an external, healthcare support team (Hodgkinson et al.). Thus, post-treatment is a time for survivors to re-center privacy boundaries around close friends and family. When family is a significant part of survivors' lives, they are often more resistant to depression, have improved quality of life, and viable relationship connections (Hodgkinson et al.; Thewes, Butow, Girgis, & Pendlebury, 2004). As a consequence, cancer survivors tend to have a significantly more positive adjustment when they have partners or family members with whom they feel not only open to granting co-ownership of their medical and personal information, but also feel comfortable relying on them for psychological support.

Families and Child Survivors

The research that relates to pediatric oncology and adjustment strategies shows that survivors and their parents adjust relatively well (Pantenaude & Kupst, 2005). Nevertheless, children and families often deal with many residual psychological and medical uncertainties, making adjustment to normalcy difficult (Levi & Drotar, 1999; Meadows & Silber, 1985). The move for some pediatric oncologists toward open communication about the child's disease has motivated providers to include psychological advisors in the treatment process (Beale, Baile, & Aaron, 2005). If treatment methods are not effective and death is imminent, social workers, psychiatrists, and psychologists are called in to help families and the child to cope. As a consequence, much of the access to private information regarding medical and emotional issues is permitted, not only to the patient, family, and primary provider, but also the mental health personnel (Patenaude & Kupst). CPM argues that often when there are functional needs met by individuals who are typically outside an established privacy boundary, those individuals are given temporary access to accomplish a goal, such as mental health personnel (Petronio, 2002). Although the mental health personnel are seen as primarily helping the children and their families, psychologists, for example, are equipped to educate providers about the emotional and developmental factors that may impact such issues as informed consent and final treatment options.

End-of-Life Disclosures

Disclosing bad news has always been a difficult issue for physicians, and when the results of treatment become bleak, breaking the news can become even more laborious (Kirk, Kirk, & Kristjanson, 2004). In these situations, providers must discuss with patients and their families issues such as recurrence of cancer, the spread of cancer, the failure of treatment to minimize cancer, the development of irreversible side effects, initiating hospice care, or that a treatment is no longer effective. Disclosing this type of bad news requires providers to take into account patients' emotional reactions and likewise attend to family members. Further, these kinds of disclosures must be accomplished in skillful ways to set the stage for making effective decisionns regarding patient care.

Discussions of end-of-life care necessitate a high level of communication skills including trust building, so that the disclosures needed by the provider to achieve good care goals can be met effectively. Again, the provider telling this news is carrying information that ultimately belongs to patients and their families. Respect for the ownership that patients and families will feel about that "private" medical information is critical to achieving the care goals. When information is disclosed inappropriately or situations are handled poorly, it can damage the patient-provider relationship. The Audit Commission (1993) found that one of the main reasons for litigation and complaint in the health care system is due to the poor communication between patients and healthcare professionals. The literature suggests patients desire a willingness from the physician to engage in open discussion about their disease and treatment (Hurwitz, Duncan, & Wolfe, 2004). While physicians are more apt to use explicit language regarding death, oncologists still tend to include implicit language in their delivery. This may be a means to mitigating the impact of the message (Rodriguez et al., 2007). During palliative care, patients and families desire a high level of disclosure from their healthcare team. A relationship of open disclosure between the patient, family, and physician, may lessen the psychological stress of the patient and family during end-of-life.

Conclusion

As this chapter illustrates, the nature of the disclosure process and privacy management as a whole for patients, their families, and providers who attend to them is often embedded in both the pragmatic conversations surrounding care and the emotional outcomes of going through the cancer journey. Understanding a multiplicity of issues involved with privacy management is essential to better communication, effective care, and handling illness. Consequently, we need to know that each member of the triad regulates the flow of information, makes choices about who knows and how they are told, makes conscious decisions about the amount of information disclosed, and encounters mistakes in communication where disclosure is concerned. As we argue, overlooking such a management process often results in confusion, conflicts, and misunderstandings increasing the stress that all parties involved experience. From the time patients learn they need medical testing for their symptoms and are diagnosed and provided treatment, through the end-of-life, understanding the way that information is regulated from the perspective of patients, families, and providers helps all concerned to better grasp strategies for more productive interactions and better patient care. However, this chapter points out the reasons why coming to an understanding of these processes is so difficult and why more work is needed to uncover ways to improve the communication involved in regulating revealing and concealing medical information.

The lens of CPM encourages us to think about disclosure as a complex process that is more involved than simply revealing medical information. To more accurately grasp the system and subsequent import of medical disclosure, we must first recognize that these interactions are between and among people, that each party makes a contribution, and that each party claims some degree of ownership and control over the information. Hence, the generator of messages and the recipient of messages coalesce to form a communicative relationship. In this case, disclosed medical information is technically viewed as the property of the patient and the provider treats the information as confidential; however, as this chapter demonstrates, there are many other aspects to understand.

Parents struggle to gather information from providers about their child's treatment options, children find out about their parent's illness through overhearing them discuss it with a friend, spouses serving as surrogate decision makers for their partners are told (disclosed) results of tests for their loved one and asked to decide on a treatment, patients tell providers information and restrict them from telling family members, family members try to coerce information about a loved one from providers, patients are surprised by disclosures of unexpected findings from their surgery, patients have to tell their family about a diagnosis, and providers have to decide on whether to tell information to patients that they are unsure is the right answer. In all of these situations, the balance between revealing and concealing looms large in the minds of those who hold the information. Because these are never easy choices, the path to understanding what drives some of the choice making has the potential to help patients, families, and providers reach a more productive outcome with both compassion and intelligence.

References

Alfano, C. M., & Rowland, J. H. (2006). Recovery issues in cancer survivorship: A new challenge for supportive care. *Cancer Journal, 12*, 432-443.

Amir, M. (1987). Considerations guiding physicians when informing cancer patients. *Social Science and Medicine, 24*, 741-748.

Audit Commission (1993). *What seems to be the matter?* HMSO, London as cited in Dunne, K. (2005) Effective communication in palliative care. *Nursing Standard, 20*, 57-64.

Aziz, N. M. (2007). Cancer survivorship research: State of knowledge, challenges, and opportunities. *Acta Oncologica, 46*, 417-432.

Back, A. L., Anderson, W. G., Bunch, L., Marr, L. A., Wallace, J. A., Yang, H. B., & Arnold, R. M. (2008). Communication about cancer near the end-of-life. *Cancer, 113, (7* supplement), 1897-1910.

Barnes, J., Kroll, L., Burke, O., Lee, J., Jones, A., & Stein, A. (2000). Qualitative interview study of communication between parents and children about maternal breast cancer. *The Western Journal of Medicine, 173,* 385-389.

Barnett, M. M., Fisher, J. D., Cook, H., James, P. R., & Dale, J. (2007). Breaking bad news: Consultants' experience, previous education and views on educational format and timing. *Medical Education, 41,* 947-956.

Beadle, G. F., Yates, P. M., Najman, J. M., Clavarino, A., Thomson, D., Williams, G., … Schlect, D. (2004). Beliefs and practices of patients with advanced cancer: Implications for communication. *British Journal of Cancer, 91,* 254-257.

Beale, E. A., Baile, W. F., & Aaron, J. (2005). Silence is not golden: Communicating with children dying from cancer. *Journal of Clinical Oncology, 23,* 3629-3631.

Brown, R., Dunn, S., & Butow, P. (1997). Meeting patient expectations in the cancer consultation. *Annals of Oncology, 8,* 877-882.

Butow, B. N., Dowsett, S., Hagerty, R., & Tattersall, M. H. (2002). Communicating prognosis to patients with metastatic disease: What do they really want to know? *Official Journal of the Multinational Association of Supportive Care in Cancer, 10,* 161-168.

Cappiello, M., Cunningham, R. S., Khobf, M. T., & Erdos, D. (2007). Breast cancer survivors. *Clinical Nursing Research, 16,* 278-293.

Chu, K. C., Tarone, R. E., Kessler, L. G., Ries, L. A. G., Hankey, B. F., Miller, B. A., & Edwards, B., K. (1996). Recent trends in U.S. breast cancer incidence, survival, and mortality rates. *Journal of the National Cancer Institute, 88,* 1571-1579.

Clayton, J. M., Hancock, K., Parker, S., Butow, P. N., Walder, S. W., Carrick, S., …Tattersall, M. H. N. (2008). Sustaining hope when communicating with terminally ill patients and their families: A systematic review. *Psycho-Oncology, 17,* 641-659.

Collis, S. P. (2006). The importance of truth-telling in health care. *Nursing Standard, 20,* 41-45.

Duggan, A., & Petronio, S. (2009). When your child is in crisis: Navigating medical needs with issues of privacy management (pp. 117-132). In T. Socha & G. Stamp (Eds.), *Parents, children and communication II: Interfacing Outside of Home.* Thousand Oaks, CA: Sage.

Dunne, K. (2005). Effective communication in palliative care. *Nursing Standard, 20,* 57-64.

Eggly, S., Penner, L., Albrecht, T., Cline, R., Foster, T., Naughton, M., Peterson, A., & Ruckdeschel, J. C. (2006). Discussing bad news in the outpatient oncology clinic: Rethinking current communication guidelines. *Journal of Clinical Oncology, 24,* 716-719.

Epstein, R. M., & Street, R. L. (2008). *Patient-centered communication in cancer care: Promoting healing and reducing suffering*. Washington, DC: U.S. Department of Health and Human Services, National Institute of Health, National Cancer Institute.

Fallowfield, L. J., Jenkins, V. A., & Beveridge, H. A. (2002). Truth may hurt but deceit hurts more: Communication in palliative care. *Palliative Medicine, 16*, 292-303.

Fallowfield, A. H., Maguire, P., Baum, M., & A'Hern, R. P. (1994). Psychological effects of being offered choice of surgery for breast cancer. *British Medical Journal, 309*, 448.

Farguhar, M. C., Barclay, S. I., Earl, H., Grande, G. E., Emery, J., & Crawford, R. A. (2005). Barriers to effective communication across the primary/secondary interface: Examples from the ovarian cancer patient journey (a qualitative study). *European Journal of Cancer Care, 14*, 359-66.

Fujimori, M., Akechi, T., Morita, T., Inagaki, M., Akizuki, N., Sakano, Y., & Uchitomi, Y. (2007). Preferences of cancer patients regarding the disclosure of bad news. *Psycho-Oncology, 16*, 573-581.

Gattellari, M., Butow, P. N., Tattersall, M. H., Dun, S. M., & MacLeod, C. A. (1999). Misunderstanding in cancer patients: Why shoot the messenger? *Annals of Oncology: Official Journey of the European Society for Medical Oncology, 10*, 39-46.

Gordon, E. J., & Daugherty, C. K. (2003). "Hitting you over the head": Oncologists' disclosure of prognosis to advanced cancer patients. *Bioethics, 17*, 142-168.

Gotay, C. C., & Muraoka, M. Y. (1998). Quality of life in long-term survivors of adult-onset cancer. *Journal of the National Cancer Institute, 90*, 656-667.

Grinyer, A. (2006). Caring for a young adult with cancer: The impact on mothers' health. *Health and Social Care in the Community, 14*, 311-318.

Hancock, K., Clayton, J. M., Parker, S. M., Walder, S., Butow, P. N., Carrick, S., ...Tattersall, M. H. N. (2007). Truth-telling in discussing prognosis in advanced life-limiting illnesses: A systematic review. *Palliative Medicine, 21*, 507-517.

Harris, M., Winship, I., & Spriggs, M. (2005). Controversies and ethical issues in cancer-genetics clinics. *Lancet Oncology, 6*, 301-310.

Harrison, J. D., Young, J. M., Price, M. A., Butow, P. N., & Solomon, M. J. (2009). What are the unmet supportive care needs of people with cancer? A systematic review. *Support Care Cancer, 17*, 1117-1128.

Helft, P. R. (2006). An intimate collaboration: Prognostic communication with advanced cancer patients. *The Journal of Clinical Ethics, 17*, 110-121.

Helft, P.R., & Petronio, S. (2007). Communication pitfalls with cancer patients: "Hit-and-run" deliveries of bad news. *Journal of the American College of Surgeons, 205*, 807-811.

Hodgkinson, K., Butow, P., Hunt, G. E., Wyse, R., Hobbs, K. M., & Wain, G. (2007). Life after cancer: Couples' and partners' psychological adjustment and supportive care needs. *Support Care Cancer, 15*, 405-415.

Houtzager, B. A., Grootenhuis, M. A., Hoekstra-Weebers, J. E. H. M., & Last, B. F. (2005). One month after diagnosis: Quality of life, coping and previous functioning in siblings of children with cancer. *Child: Care, Health, and Development, 31*, 75-87.

Houtzager, B. A., Grootenhuis, M. A., & Last, B. F. (1999). Adjustment of siblings to childhood cancer: A literature review. *Supportive Care in Cancer, 7*, 302-320.

Hurwitz, C. A., Duncan, J., & Wolfe, J. (2004). Caring for the child with cancer at the close of life: "There are people who make it, and I'm hoping I'm one of them." *Journal of the American Medical Association, 292*, 12141-12149.

Hymovich, D. P. (1995). The meaning of cancer to children. *Seminars in Oncology Nursing, 11*, 51-8.

Kim, Y., & Given, B. A. (2008). Quality of life of family caregivers of cancer survivors: Across the trajectory of illness. *Cancer, 112*, 2556-2568.

Kirk, P., Kirk, I., & Kristjanson, L. J. (2004). What do patients receiving palliative care for cancer and their families want to be told? A Canadian and Australian qualitative study. *Clinical Research Education, 328*, 1343.

Klassen, A., Raina, P., Reineking, S., Dix, D., Pritchard, S., & O'Donnell, M. (2007). Developing a literature base to understand the caregiving experience of parents of children with cancer: A systematic review of factors related to parental health and well-being. *Support Care Cancer, 15*, 807-818.

Kristjanson, L. J., Chalmers, K. I., & Woodgate, R. (2004). Information and support needs of adolescent children of women with breast cancer. *Oncology Nursing Forum, 31*, 111-119.

Last, B. F., & Grutenhuis, M. A. (1998). Emotions, coping and the need for support in families of children with cancer: A model for psychosocial care. *Parental Education and Counseling, 33*, 169-79.

Levetown, M., & Committee on Bioethics (2008). Communicating with children and families: From everyday interactions to skill in conveying distressing information. *Pediatrics, 121*, e1441-e1460.

Levi, R. B., & Drotar, D. (1999). Health-related quality of life in childhood cancer: Discrepancy in parent-child reports. *International Journal of Cancer, 12*, 58-64.

Mack, J. W., Wolfe, J., Grier, H. E., Cleary, P. D., & Weeks, J. C. (2006). Communication about prognosis between parents and physicians about children with cancer: parent preferences and the impact of prognostic information. *Journal of Clinical Oncology, 24*, 5265-5270.

Mack, J. W., Wolfe, J., Cook, E. F., Grier, H. E., Cleary, P. D., Weeks, J. C. (2007). Hope and prognostic disclosure. *Journal of Clinical Oncology, 25*, 5636-5642.

Maguire, P., Faulkner, A., Booth, K., Elliott, C., & Hillier, V. (1996). Helping cancer patients disclose their concerns. *European Journal of Cancer, 32A*, 78-81.

McDaniel, S. H., Beckman, H. B., Morse, D. S., Silberman, J., Seaburn, D. B., & Epstein, R. M. (2007). Physician self-disclosure in primary care visits: Enough about you, what about me? *Archives of Internal Medical, 167*, 1321-1326.

McHugh, H., Lewis, S., Ford, S., Kewkinds, E., Rustin, G. Coombes, C., Smith, D., O'Reilly, S., & Fallowfield, I. (1995). The efficacy of audiotapes in promoting psychological well-being in cancer patients: A randomized controlled trial. *British Journal of Cancer, 71*, 388-92.

McKean, R. C., Feigelson, H. S., & Ross, R. K. (2000). Declining cancer rates in the 1990s. *Journal of Clinical Oncology, 18*, 2258-2268.

Meadows, A. T., & Silber, J. (1985). Delayed consequences of therapy for childhood cancer. *A Cancer Journal for Clinicians, 35*, 271-286.

Miyata, H., Takahashi, M., Saito, T., Tachimori, H., & Kai, I. (2005). Disclosure preferences regarding cancer diagnosis and prognosis: To tell or not to tell? *Journal of Medical Ethics, 31*, 447-451.

Northouse, L. L., & Swain, M. A. (1987). Adjustment of patients and husbands to the initial impact of breast cancer. *Nursing Research, 36*, 221-225.

Parsons, S. K., Saiki-Craighill, S., Mayer, D. K., Sullivan, A. M., Jeruss, S., Terrin, N.,...Block, S. (2007). Telling children and adolescents about their cancer diagnosis: Cross-cultural comparisons between pediatric oncologists in the US and Japan. *Psycho-Oncology, 16*, 60-68.

Patenaude, A. F., & Kupst, M. J. (2005). Psychosocial functioning in pediatric cancer. *Journal of Pediatric Psychology, 30*, 9-27.

Patterson, J. M., Holm, K. E., & Gurney, J. G. (2004). The impact of childhood cancer on the family: A qualitative analysis of strains, resources, and coping behaviors. *Psycho-oncology, 13*, 390-407.

Pennebaker, J. W. (1995). *Emotion, disclosure, and health.* Washington, DC: American Psychological Association.

Petronio, S. (2000). *Balancing the secrets of private disclosures.* Mahwah, NJ: Lawrence Erlbaum Associates.

Petronio, S. (2002). *Boundaries of privacy: Dialectics of disclosure.* Albany, NY: SUNY Press.

Petronio, S., & Durham, W. (2008). Understanding and applying Communication Privacy Management theory. In L. A. Baxter & D. O. Braithwaite (Eds.), *Engaging theories in interpersonal communication* (pp. 309-322). Thousand Oaks, CA: Sage Publications.

Petronio, S., & Jones, S. M. (2006). When "friendly advice" becomes a privacy dilemma for pregnant couples: Applying CPM theory. In R. West & L. Turner (Eds.), *Family Communication: Sourcebook*, (pp. 201-218). Thousand Oaks, CA: Sage.

Petronio, S., Jones, S. M., & Morr, M. C. (2003). Family privacy dilemmas: Managing-communication boundaries within family groups. In L. Frey (Ed.), *Group commu-*

nication context: Studies of bona fide groups (pp. 23-56). Mahwah, NJ: LEA Publications.

Petronio, S., & Kovach, S. (1997). Managing privacy boundaries: Health providers' perceptions of resident care in Scottish nursing homes. *Journal of Applied Communication Research, 25,* 115-130.

Petronio, S., & Ostrom-Blonigen, J. (2008). *Family stress of managing privacy during cancer care.* Paper presented at the National Communication Association Meeting, San Diego, CA.

Petronio, S., Reeder, H., Hecht, M., & Mon't Ros-Mendoza, T. (1996). Disclosure of sexual abuse by children and adolescents. *Journal of Applied Communication Research, 24,* 181-199.

Petronio, S., & Reierson, J. (2009). Privacy of confidentiality: Grasping the complexities through Communication Privacy Management. In T. Afifi & W. Afifi (Eds.), *Uncertainty and information regulation in interpersonal contexts: Theories and application* (pp. 365-383). New York: Routledge.

Ptacek, J. T., Ptacek, J. J., & Ellison, N. M. (2001). "I'm sorry to tell you..." Physicians' reports of breaking bad news. *Journal of Behavioral Medicine, 24,* 205-17.

Ptacek, J. T., & Eberhardt, T. L. (1996). Breaking bad news. A review of the literature. *The Journal of the American Medical Association, 276,* 496-502.

Rabineau, K. M., Mabe, P. A., & Vega, R. A. (2008). Parenting stress in pediatric oncology populations. *Journal of Pediatric Hematology Oncology, 30,* 358-365.

Rabinowitz, T., & Peirson, R. (2006). "Nothing is wrong, doctor": Understanding and managing denial in patients with cancer. *Cancer Investigation, 24,* 68-76.

Ranmal, R., Prictor, M., & Scott, J. T. (2008). Interventions for improving communication with children and adolescents about their cancer. *Cochrane Database of systematic Reviews, 4,* (CD002969), 1-44.

Robinson, T. M., Alexander, S. C., Hays, M., Jeffreys, A. S., Olsen, M. K., Rodriguez, K. L., ...Tulsky, J. A. (2008). Patient-oncologist communication in advanced cancer: Predictors of patient perception of prognosis. *Support Care Cancer, 16,* 1049-1057.

Rodriguez, K. L., Gambino, F. J., Butow, R., Hagerty, R., & Arnold, R. M. (2007). Pushing up daisies: Implicit and explicit language in oncologist-patient communication about death. *Supportive Care in Cancer, 15* (2) 153-161.

Rodriguez, K. L., Gambino, F. J., Butow, R., Hagerty, R., & Arnold, R. M. (2008). "It's going to Shorten your life": Framing of oncologist-patient communication about prognosis. *Psycho-Oncology, 17,* 219-225.

Salander, P. (2002). Bad news from the patient's perspective: An analysis of the written narratives of newly diagnosed cancer patients. *Social Science and Medicine, 55,* 721-732.

Sankar, P., & Jones, N. L. (2005). To tell or not to tell: Primary care patients' disclosure deliberations. *Archive of Internal Medicine, 165,* 2378-2383.

Serewicz, M. C. M., & Canary, D. J. (2008). Assessments of disclosure from the in-laws: Links among disclosure topics, family privacy orientations, and relational quality. *Journal of Social and Personal Relationships, 25,* 333-358.

Sheu, S. J., Huang, S. H., Tang, F. I., & Huang, S. L. (2006). Ethical decision making on truth telling in terminal cancer: Medical students' choices between patient autonomy and family paternalism. *Medical Education, 40,* 590-598.

Spinetta, J. J. (1974). The dying child's awareness of death: A review. *Psychological Bulletin, 81,* 256-260.

Stewart, D. E., Cheung, A. M., Duff, S., Wong, F., McQuestion, M., Cheng, T., Purdy, L., & Bunston, T. (2000). Long-term breast cancer survivors: Confidentiality, disclosure, effects on work and insurance. *Psycho-Oncology, 10,* 259-263.

Tesauro, G. M., Rowland, J. H., & Lustig, C. (2002). Survivorship resources for post-treatment cancer survivors. *Cancer Practice, 10,* 277-283.

Thewes, B., Butow, P., Girgis, A., & Pendlebury, S. (2004). The psychosocial needs of breast cancer survivors: A qualitative study of the shared and unique needs of younger versus older survivors. *Psycho-Oncology, 13,* 177-189.

Van der Kam, W. J., Branger, P. J., van Bemmel, J. H., & Meyboom-de Jong, B. (1998). Communication between physicians and with patients suffering from breast cancer. *Family Practice, 15,* 415-419.

Weisman, A. D., & Hackett, T. P. (1961). Predilection to death. *Psychosomatic Medicine, 23,* 232-256.

CHAPTER 11

"So, When Are You Two Having a Baby?" Managing Information about Infertility within Social Networks

Keli Ryan Steuber

THE UNIVERSITY OF IOWA

Denise Haunani Solomon

PENNSYLVANIA STATE UNIVERSITY

In American society, there are two generally held assumptions: "that married couples should reproduce, and…that married couples should *want* to reproduce" (Miall, 1986, p. 268). Given these pronatalistic attitudes, many people expect to eventually become parents (Greil, 1991), which can make the diagnosis of infertility particularly devastating to a person's identity and family goals (Miall, 1986). Infertility touches the lives of 15% of couples in the United States (Chandra, Martinez, Mosher, Abma, & Jones, 2005), and many indicators suggest that the prevalence of reproductive disabilities will increase in the future. For example, sexually transmitted diseases that contribute to infertility are on the rise (Center for Disease Control and Prevention, 2007). In addition, demographic trends suggest that individuals are marrying later in life and, consequently, delaying childbearing (Amato, Booth, Johnson, & Rogers, 2007). Because there is a positive relationship between age and the risk of fertility problems, this demographic shift may contribute to an increased number of conception difficulties in the near future. A sizable body of research documents the challenges that couples face as they cope with difficulty conceiving (e.g., Chandra et al., 2005; Greil, 1991), including financial and medical decisions, threats to psychological well-being, and relationship strain. In fact, many infertile individuals nominate the disability as one of the greatest stressors they face in their marriage (Greil, 1991).

People often turn to their family and friends to help them cope with infertility, which can strain those individuals as well. One person's health condition can create considerable stress within social networks as the system copes with the diagnosis of an ailment, offers advice or information about a treatment plan, provides support, and lives with the personal implications of the illness or condition. When the health condition is infertility, a couple's friends and family are confronted with a great deal of uncertainty as well. Just as an individual copes with the possibility of never becoming a parent, family members face the prospect of missing out on having nieces, nephews, or grandchildren. Communication within the network may also be strained as members identify types of support that are and are not helpful and as they navigate privacy boundaries. The complexity of the communication issues experienced by infertile couples and their social networks makes this a prime topic for further study.

Whereas previous research provides insight into the marital implications of infertility (e.g., Steuber & Solomon, 2008), we know relatively little about the challenges couples experience as they interface with their social networks during this time. Thus, the goal of this chapter is to explore the ways families go through infertility together, by considering how a person's social network changes and is changed by infertility. To this end, we first describe infertility and stressful aspects of reproductive disabilities. Next, we discuss how social networks can contribute to personal and marital well-being. Then, we propose research questions directed toward uncovering the ways that individuals interface with their social network members during this time. To address our research questions, we report a content analysis of transcripts from in-depth interviews with infertile individuals. To conclude, we discuss directions for future research within the context of marriage and infertility.

Infertility

The diagnosis of infertility brings with it psychological distress, difficult treatment decisions, and chronic uncertainty surrounding the final outcome of parenthood (Greil, 1991). These issues contribute to heightened emotions within the marital unit, which can be catalysts for marital strain. The following sections review treatment decisions and psychological stress in relation to infertility, followed by the difficulties couples face within their marriage as they cope with this condition.

Treatment Stressors

Decades ago, infertility treatment largely consisted of non-invasive procedures such as charting menstrual cycles and home remedies; however, today's technological advancements make possible surrogate mothers, sperm donors, multiple births, and frozen embryos. With the variety of these assisted reproductive technologies (ART) available, 50—75% of infertile couples will seek some variation of medical assistance (Schmidt, 2006). Along with these advanced and intricate treatment options come complicated personal and health decisions.

Many individuals receive care from reproductive endocrinologists, specialists who are able to utilize a variety of assisted reproductive technologies to help couples achieve a successful pregnancy. ART procedures are time consuming, expensive, often not covered by insurance in the United States, and, depending on the age of the woman trying to conceive, have an approximately 25% success rate (Center for Disease Control and Prevention, 2007). As reported in Peterson, Gold, & Feingold (2007), even with a successful conception, these procedures often result in miscarriage, low birth rate, and preterm labor (see Shevell, Malone, Vidaver, Porter, Luthy, & Comstock, 2005). Thus, a variety of medical interventions can result in biological offspring, but usually not without serious financial, physical, and emotional implications for couples.

Psychological Stressors

In addition to the practical issues couples have to cope with, experiencing infertility can evoke considerable psychosocial distress. Research shows that women experiencing infertility often feel inferior to other women, feel socially isolated, and lack self-esteem (Wirtberg, Moller, Hogstrom, Tronstad, & Lalos, 2007). Infertile women also report depression, anxiety, anger, and feelings of guilt (Schmidt, 2006).

Daniluk (1997) asserted that women may contend with these emotions because they feel their inability to conceive directly and negatively reflects on their identity and self-image. This evidence highlights the threats to personal and emotional well-being infertile women experience.

Similar to women, men experiencing infertility identify shame, guilt, anger, isolation, loss, personal failure, and low self-esteem as some of the negative feelings they have (Wright, Duchesne, Sabourin, Bissonnette, Benoit, & Girard, 1991). Schmidt (2006) also found that men with a non-pregnant wife experience higher levels of depressive symptoms and lower levels of sexual and relational satisfaction than men with a pregnant wife. Likewise, Daniluk (1997) reported that infertile men attach more negative attributes to themselves, such as being useless or defective.

Marital Stressors

Being diagnosed with infertility is often a turning point in the life course of a marriage, which can prompt couples to seek counseling for numerous personal and relational issues (see Greil, Leitko, & Porter, 1988; Leiblum, 1997; Schneider & Forthofer, 2005). Prior research has shown that, depending on how a couple communicates about the situation, infertility can have both negative and positive effects on personal relationships (Pasch, Dunkel-Schetter, & Christensen, 2002). For example, stress from infertility is associated with lower quality of marriage (Abbey, Andrews, & Halman, 1994; Wright, Allard, Lecours, & Sabourin, 1989), and spouses may experience conflict about treatment options and costs (Epstein & Rosenberg, 1997). At the same time, surviving the experience of infertility sometimes forges a stronger relational bond between husband and wife (Steuber & Solomon, 2008).

In a study of online discussion boards and blogs, Steuber and Solomon (2008) found a range of themes present in relationships struggling with infertility. Feelings of relational invalidation were present during treatment, especially when partners prioritized treatment differently. Tensions also emerged when people blamed either themselves or their partner for the infertility; this theme was especially prominent with individuals who had been coping with infertility for an extended period of time. The goal of facilitating a successful pregnancy often becomes an obsession for one or both individuals in the partnership and the process of treatment (e.g., keeping medical appointments and performing prescribed sexual activities) overwhelmed some marriages. Many individuals also experienced frustration when their partners focused too much or too little on overcoming infertility. Finally, feelings of a stronger relational identity emerged as couples worked together towards their goal of overcoming their reproductive disability.

As this brief review suggests, the stressors that follow a diagnosis of infertility are substantial. In particular, partners must cope with choosing among, and affording, numerous and complex treatment options, they experience a great deal of psychological distress, and their marriage may be strained by the burden of treating or living with infertility. With this understanding of the infertility experience within marriage in place, our attention turns to how marital experiences can be shaped by other significant relational partners, namely close friends and family.

Social Networks and Well-Being

As noted by Felmlee "No couple is an island" (2001, p. 1283). In fact, couples are embedded within a social structure that has the potential to provide both positive and negative support throughout the lifespan. These structures, known as social networks, can alter an individual's role within a couple, affect how a couple interacts, and influence the decisions a couple makes (see Felmlee, 2001). Social networks are social structures comprised of the people individuals interact with on a regular basis. They often consist of family members, friends, and other people with whom an individual interacts with routinely. Regardless of role, those people closest to the individual often evoke the most influence on them (Kahn & Antonucci, 1980). This section documents the impact social network members can have on a person and a marriage.

A large body of evidence connects network interaction with well-being. The availability of network members, particularly friends, has been found to contribute to both marital satisfaction and personal well-being (Willits & Crider, 1986). Lewis and Spanier (1979) reported that a feeling of belonging contributes to higher self-concept, which is associated with marital quality. Other empirical evidence offers further support for the notion that people's perceptions of network support predicts a variety of relationship components, including stability, satisfaction, and commitment (Bryant & Conger, 1999; Felmlee, 2001).

Close friends outside the marriage may be especially beneficial to marriages. For example, Birditt and Antonucci (2007) found that people who report having a best friend and at least one other high-quality relationship (spouse or friendship) demonstrated the highest level of general well-being. Amato and colleagues (2007) examined the relationship between friendship and marital quality and found that people with a large number of friends reported being happier with their marriages, engaged in less conflict with spouses, perceived fewer problems with their spouses, and were less divorce prone than individuals reporting only a few friends.

Friends outside the marriage are most beneficial when they do not eclipse the marital relationship. For example, Lee (1988) reported that marital satisfaction in older couples was the greatest for those individuals who confided the most in their spouse, whereas those people who primarily revealed to someone other than their partner experienced below-average marital satisfaction. Similarly, Julien and Markman (1991) found that younger individuals who confided in their friends about marital problems reported more marital distress than those who revealed their concerns directly to their spouse.

Taken together, results suggest that individuals routinely share information related to their marriage with members of their social networks. When experiencing transitions or stressful times, individuals turn to their loved ones for support; however, they also have to balance their desire for support with their preferences for privacy. Information regulation seems especially relevant during transitions that are private in nature, much like the experience of infertility.

Revealing and Concealing Infertility

When coping with a health issue like infertility, people must make decisions about how much information to reveal about their personal and marital conditions. The amount of information shared likely varies from person to person, but the process of concealing and revealing information can be stressful for both the person coping with the condition and the family and friends who are attempting to make sense of it. The following paragraphs offer a brief review of the communication literature on information management and discuss the implications of this work within the infertility context. Finally, we consider how revealing and concealing information can have immediate and long-term relationship implications.

A primary reason to conceal information is to avoid adverse reactions (e.g., Afifi, Olson, & Armstrong, 2005; Cloven & Roloff, 1993). People have a natural tendency to defend themselves from aggressive responses (see Tesser, Martin, & Cornell, 1996), perhaps because it threatens identity, risks being evaluated negatively, or because this information can be used against them (Infante, Myers, & Buerkel, 1994; Straus & Sweet, 1992). Individuals not only retain information in an attempt to protect themselves from mild negative reactions such as rejection or ridicule (e.g., Cline & McKenzie, 2000; Harber & Pennebaker, 1992), but also to maintain the status quo of the relationship (Afifi & Schrodt, 2003; Afifi & Burgoon, 1998) and to protect themselves and others (Afifi & Guerrero, 2000).

If individuals choose to be extremely private about their infertility status, they may share their diagnosis and treatment decisions with just a few confidants. Other individuals may be initially more open with the details of their diagnosis and treatment, and then retroactively be more shielded with those individuals who did not respond supportively. Other people may simply avoid interacting with those people who they do not feel are privy to the details of their condition. With the variety of possible strategies for concealing information, we pose the following research question:

RQ1: How do individuals describe concealing infertility-related information?

Individuals make decisions about sharing information based on many considerations (Caughlin & Petronio, 2004; Petronio, 2000). A large portion of their decision is likely based on the specifics of their situation and personalities, but there are some universal trends that may inform their decisions. Specifically, individuals might be more likely to reveal private information to people of the same sex (Caughlin &

Petronio, 2004). In addition, culture can have considerable influence on decisions to reveal. If a person comes from a culture that has high expectations for parenthood, then it might be monumentally more difficult to reveal an infertility diagnosis than it would be for a person without those pressures. Another reason people may be proactive about sharing their information is if they think their secret will be revealed to people in other ways (Caughlin & Petronio, 2004; Petronio, 2002). In cases when families are open with information or friends are questioning unusual behaviors, some individuals may decide to reveal their diagnosis rather than have those individuals come to false conclusions on their own.

When individuals do decide to unveil information about their infertility status, those revelations can elicit a variety of responses. In general, supportive behaviors can be perceived as negative or positive. Negative interactions include behaviors that discourage the expression of feelings, invade privacy, and interfere in another person's affairs (Lincoln, 2000), but the construct is usually operationalized as "those actions by which a member of one's social network can cause distress (e.g., resentment, sadness, shame)" (Lincoln, 2000, p. 233).

Positive support, on the other hand, can come in the form of instrumental, emotional, esteem, or tangible support. With regard to infertility, it would be helpful to understand not only the frequencies of positive and negative support individuals feel they garner from their social network members, but also what type of behaviors are considered positive and negative in this particular context. Therefore, a second research question is offered:

RQ2: How do individuals perceive positive and negative support from their social networks?

Research suggests that stressful events can actually result in a loss of social support because the stressor can increase the cost for the social network, leading members to withdraw from that individual rather than provide constant or demanding support (Peronance, Boivin, Schmidt, 2007). Research also suggests that consistently unsuccessful treatments may act as a stressor and put increasing burden on social networks. These relational hindrances can gradually aggravate and breakdown a person's social network, which further isolates an individual when they most need support from their interpersonal relationships.

The challenge of infertility, and communication about it, can have long-term effects on relationships as well. The way individuals and their social network jointly react to a stressor can shape the trajectory of their future relationship. Some people experience a positive change in their relationships, perhaps due to the perception of positive support during their stressor. Other relationships may negatively suffer as a result of unsupportive behaviors displayed during infertility. Still, some friendships and family relationships might not necessarily experience a strong positive or negative change, but may decrease in intensity. Research suggests that infertile couples tend to withdraw temporarily from situations that remind them of their infertility status (e.g., niece or nephew's birthday parties, church gatherings; e.g., Greil, 1991) or avoid events that are likely to give away the fact they are receiving treatment (e.g., a woman might not go to happy hour with coworkers because she cannot drink alcohol while taking infertility medicine). Therefore, these communicative behaviors may have immediate or long-term consequences for social networks. With these thoughts in mind, we present the final research question:

RQ3: How does concealing or revealing infertility-related information influence social network relationships?

The research reviewed to this point suggests that individuals both impact and are impacted by their social networks and that the experience of a stressor can alter the dynamic of relationships. Knowing little about how individuals experience and cope with their social relationships during infertility, we set out to uncover the role information management plays within the social networks of people experiencing reproductive disabilities.

Method

To address our research goals, we turned to the transcripts from 17 in-depth interviews that we previously conducted with infertile individuals. These interviews were focused mostly on issues pertaining to marriage, treatments, and identity. Although communication and relationships with friends and family were not the explicit focus of the interviews, these issues emerged as a topic within the discussions. Thus, the interviews provide us with insight into how privacy management and social issues are a prominent component of the infertility experience.

Participants

Participants were 15 women and 3 men (*N* = 18) ranging in age from 26-44 years (*M* = 35.7, *SD* = 4.68). All participants identified as being infertile and were married (*M* = 9.4 years, *SD* = 5.77). Most participants were Caucasian (88.9%) and Christian (83.3%); those individuals who were not Christian (16.7%) reported no religious affiliation or Atheism. The participants' average annual income ranged from $50,000 - $62,500. Although 18 individuals were interviewed, there were technical difficulties with the audio recording of an interview with one female, resulting in only 17 interviews being analyzed.

Procedures

The study was announced on a faculty and staff Listserv at a large, eastern university in an email that is distributed weekly to graduate students, support staff, academic faculty, and administrators. Respondents were distributed across these groups and some were spouses or friends of people connected to the university. Once potential participants contacted the researchers and confirmed that they met the requirements of the study, a time was set to meet in a private location for the interview.

The interview schedule covered a variety of topics related to infertility, including self, relationship, and treatment questions. The interview began by prompting participants to share their infertility story, and then continued through a semi-structured interview format. Specifically, individuals were asked to talk about changes in their marital, social, and work routines, as well as any changes in their family goals as they coped with their reproductive disability. Issues pertaining to treatment, insurance, and financial constraints were also discussed. Finally, individuals were asked to reflect on any self or relational identity changes they may have experienced, as well as their future family plans. Interviews lasted approximately one hour, were conducted individually, and participants were compensated $30 for their time. Interviews were transcribed into 238 pages of single-spaced text with all identifying information removed.

Because the interviews addressed issues unrelated to interfacing with the social network, we employed a sieve coding scheme to identify portions of the transcripts relevant to our research questions. Specifically, independent coders identified participant speaking turns that pertained to communication with friends and families. Coders were instructed to read the interviews through twice, then go back and identify those speaking turns that addressed social network support or information management pertaining to individuals external to the marriage. Coders established acceptable reliability (α = .77) and then divided the remaining data equally with a 20% overlap to ensure they maintained reliability throughout the coding process. For those units coded by both assistants, speaking turns identified by either coder were retained (κ = .78), which yielded a total of 169 applicable speaking units (N = 169) for further analysis.[1]

Analysis

Independent coders were trained to evaluate the speaking units for the presence and absence of three topics: (a) references to *concealing* infertility-related information (n = 88; κ = .70), (b) references to *revealing* infertility-related information (n = 135; κ = .70), and (c) references to the *social implications* of revealing or concealing infertility-related information (n = 117; κ = .86). The categories were not mutually exclusive, and if a speaking turn did not fit into any of the above three categories, it was considered not applicable (n = 22). This stage was conducted to filter information into the three categories so that a content analysis could be completed within each category.

Once the information had been sifted into categories, attention was paid to the perceived valence of social network behaviors, as well as the general forms the behaviors took. We used the extant literature on information-management, in general (e.g., Caughlin & Petronio,

1 The process of establishing an acceptable initial Cohen's Kappa (> .70; Cohen, 1960), dividing the remaining data with 20% of units overlapping, and the calculation of a final reliability score was utilized throughout each stage of coding. The final Cohen's Kappa is reported for each stage.

2004; Lincoln, 2000), and infertility and privacy specifically (e.g., Demyttenaere, Nijs, Evers-Kiebooms, & Koninckx, 1991) as a framework for reading the discourse. Then, the first author read the relevant segments of the transcripts multiple times to identify those central concepts pertaining to each research question. As a final step, independent coders evaluated the presence of the categories of discourse in each segment of the transcripts.

Results

The following sections report our findings with respect to each research question. In each case, we focused on the subset of the discourse relevant to the research question. We first provide examples to illustrate how people discussed concealing information (RQ1), reactions to revealing information (RQ2), and relationship implications of their infertility experiences (RQ3). Then, we report content analyses that revealed the types of experiences described in each subset of the discourse.

Concealment

In an effort to answer RQ1, we focused on discourse that referenced concealing infertility-related information. In some cases, participants described a decision to conceal their condition from others right from the start of their diagnosis. Other times, the interviewees discussed limiting information sharing because of the way others responded to previous revelations. After sharing examples of this discourse, we report the results of the content analysis.

Many descriptions of concealing highlighted an inherent tension associated with communicating about infertility. For example, a 34-year old female graduate student perceived discomfort from her friends when she talked about infertility, which in turn caused her to limit the information she shared with them. Whereas her married friends were generally supportive of her pregnancy quest, her unmarried friends were more dismissive:

> My single friends, I just don't think they're in the same stage of their lives to understand the frustrations. So I think they just kind of dismiss it a lot. Yeah, so I don't really talk too much about it with them cause it's just, it's probably uncomfortable to them too.

Even people who did not report stress with their family or social network attempted to limit the information they shared with them. A 36-year old woman from another country, who is in the United States so her husband can pursue a graduate education, desperately wished that her family was around her to support her during her infertility struggles, especially when she experienced a miscarriage. Despite her desire for social support from her loved ones, she still filtered information to protect her mother, "With my mom I tell her a lot and then I don't cause she gets really sad about it. So she tends to get sadder than what I think the issue is to a point, and then I'm like 'Oh no! It *is* a big issue so she *should* be worried or sad or whatever!'" The reasoning behind why these two women limited their information was very different, but the underlying premise stemming from the speaking turns was that, at some point during conception difficulties, information to social networks is filtered.

Our reading of the discourse about concealing information revealed three recurring categories: (a) *complete concealment,* (b) *limited information sharing,* and (c) *limited contact with others*. Two independent coders then judged the presence or absence of each category in each of the 88 speaking turns that addressed concealing information. These categories were not mutually exclusive, and they accounted for 72% of the units.

Speaking units were coded as *complete concealment* when the infertile person talked about having kept his or her diagnosis secret from others, often from the initial diagnosis of reproductive difficulties. These comments usually indicate the infertile having one or two confidants outside the marriage, but the conception difficulties are kept secret from the general social network. For example, one woman explicitly stated:

> We have decided to keep it private. I, um, had told a very close friend of mine at the beginning of this and the only other person we told is my mother. Those are the only people we've told, as far as my co-workers, nobody knows.

A total of 26 of the 88 units (30%) referenced *complete concealment* (n = 26, $\kappa = .78$).

Statements coded as limiting information indicated that decisions had been made to start to filter the infertility-related information, usually because of past experiences. Some people described initially sharing their diagnosis and initial treatment details with their social network, but then eventually limiting the information they shared to avoid negative input, unsupportive reactions, or increased stress. Others just talked about only offering pieces of information as they became necessary. For example, one woman commented how it became tiresome to rehash the details of treatment, "We had friends after a test was done and you're just down and out. And they ask if everything's okay, and I don't feel like explaining everything I had." Coders identified 17 of the 88 units (19%) as those referencing *limited information* (κ = 1.0).

Units were identified as *limiting contact* when they referenced a decrease in opportunities for communication to avoid explaining a lack of children, discussing treatment decisions, or experiencing a lack of understanding. For example, some people described avoiding pregnant family or friends, people who were parents already, or people in their social network who make inquiries about their parenthood status. Other people just wanted to avoid being around their friends who were pregnant or already parents. One woman commented on the difficulty balancing her friendship with the emotional pain brought on by infertility, "These two friends that are pregnant... I'm very, very happy for them, but I'm not too excited to spend a whole lot of time with them." Rather than just limiting the information shared with others, limiting contact involved avoiding individuals to decrease the chance for uncomfortable or painful encounters. A total of 19 of the 88 units (22%; κ = .83) were identified as referencing *limited contact*.

Revelations

To address RQ2, we turned to discourse that referenced revealing infertility-related information. In some situations, individuals suggested that sharing their private information resulted in a positive reaction from their network members, whereas other cases highlighted the strain that surfaces when they feel their friends and family are overstepping their boundaries. We first share some examples from the discourse and then turn to findings from the content analysis.

Many individuals who shared some aspect of their condition spent time talking about behaviors they witnessed after they revealed their infertility status to their social networks. Some people noted the support they felt by their friends and families, whereas others were overbearing or insensitive. One 34-year old woman revealed how her sisters were a source of both support and annoyance during her infertility experience:

> You know it's funny because they all have kids, so, but they're supportive…There might be a sister or two that's like, "What are you doing? You're not getting any younger!" And I'm like "Leave me alone, I'm fine. Just leave me be." So that can be annoying.

Whereas some people felt annoyance or frustration, other individuals experienced hurt after a negative interaction. A 39-year old woman shared her trials with her husband's family, "We have issues with his family and they've pressured us in a lot of ways and they say very inappropriate things, which is very hard because we'll walk away from gatherings and I'll be crying in the car." Her 40-year old husband, in a separate interview, mirrored those feelings, "They don't know, certain words, sting or hurt someone who doesn't have children." Similarly, in a conversation with a close friend, a female graduate student also found herself surprised at the lack of sensitivity demonstrated when her friend talked about her own successful pregnancy. Although she did not state her hurt to her friend out loud, she admitted she was internally upset, "And I just was kind of like, really? You're going to tell me that (crying)?" There were a variety of responses individuals faced when they chose to share details of their infertility diagnosis and treatments, and people described spending a good deal of time processing the responses they received from their social networks.

Our review of the discourse referencing revealing infertility-related information suggested that people perceived their disclosure to be met with a variety of responses. In general, infertile individuals interpreted behavioral responses as either supportive and positive or damaging and negative. Accordingly, two independent coders were trained to assign the valence of responses to revelations as *positive* and *negative.* These codes, which were not mutually exclusive, applied to 62% of the units.

Positive responses consisted of those speaking turns that represented accommodation (e.g., working around the participant's treatment schedule or other cooperative behaviors), relating to the participant (e.g., showing sympathy or empathy), being a supportive confidant (e.g., offering instrumental or emotional support), and unspecified positive behaviors (e.g., the general understanding that the participant thought this person reacted in a constructive way by making ambiguous statements such as "She was great!"). One woman mentioned a specific encounter in which a new mother sensed that the infertile woman wanted to hold her infant:

> She knows what the situation is and she was probably aware that it was something I'd probably enjoy doing—caring for this child and nurturing it a little bit. So that to me was kind of wonderful and I was so glad I was able to do it, and…it was really sweet [of her].

Coders assigned 73 of the 135 units (54%) as positive reactions (κ = .77).

Negative responses took various forms, but they were universally experienced as unpleasant or upsetting. Specifically, negative responses consisted of people being nosy (e.g., asking frequent questions or making inquiries), being dismissive (e.g., acting in ways that do not validate a person's concerns or diminishes the severity of an issue), and offering unsolicited advice (e.g., offering comments or tips that are not requested by the infertile). An excerpt from a woman's interview highlights how unsolicited advice leaves her feeling frustrated, "You hear all the time, you know, just stop thinking about it and it'll happen. Like, if I hear that one more time I'm gonna...smack somebody!" Of the 135 speaking units, coders assigned 29 of them (22%) as negative (κ = .75).

Relational Implications

To address RQ3, we examined the discourse that suggested the experience of infertility may have impacted social network relationships in some way. In some cases, participants talked about how their relationships have gotten stronger due to the intimacy of sharing private details of their reproductive condition, or because of the support demonstrated by a friend or family member. Other times, the interviewees suggested that they stopped maintaining some relationships due to the strain induced by infertility. Finally, some individuals reported that their social networks took a negative turn since they started treating their infertility. After citing examples of this discourse, we report the results of the content analysis.

Many individuals mentioned a withdrawal from friends as they continued to struggle with reproduction issues, whereas others chose to socially isolate themselves as a way to limit negativity. One man mentioned the discomfort some friends, who had children, felt being around them:

> They're kind of uncomfortable around you. If they have a newborn and they know the situation you're coming from, they may steer away from you. And you can tell it's very hard for people...because people are very uncomfortable in this conversation, especially if they have children.

Similarly, another woman mentioned how she would avoid social situations she used to partake in, mostly because she was tired of having to explain her situation, "A lot of my friends still go out. They have relationships, they're hanging out, they're having parties. I'll go sometimes, but I steer more away from it because why go and say, I can't drink cause of this medicine." The same woman mentioned how her close friends would keep secrets about their own pregnancies from her out of fear of hurting her, "They don't want to tell me. They wait for a little while, they wait until there's a little bump and I'm like is there something you should be telling me (laughing)?" Although she found humor in the situation, she seemed torn between being grateful over the fact they were considerate enough to think of her feelings and feeling sadness that she could not completely share in their pregnancy joy. Once again, there was an array of examples pertaining to how information related to infertility influenced social partnerships.

The 117 units that referenced the ramifications of revealing or concealing infertility-related information on social relationships were coded based on the relational implications apparent: *positive relational perception*, a *lack of involvement*, and a *negative relational perception*. The three groups were not mutually exclusive, and they accounted for 76% of the total units.

Positive relational perceptions represented those units in which the participant explicitly or implicitly suggested a constructive or positive aspect of their relationship as a result of the social network member's response to the infertility. Specifically, this reaction could occur in the form of increased closeness or intimacy, satisfaction with the support provided, or a positive expectancy violation the participant had with the person's response to the information. One woman stated how pleased she was that her group of friends maintained their closeness despite their own successful pregnancies and her failed attempts at having a child, "We have a really nice bunch of friends…What I love is that they're really open, I would hate it if some of them would have talked about stuff with care cause I'm there. I mean it's going to hurt in some way, but I love that it's really open." Of the 117 units, 38 (32%) were coded as a *positive relational perception* (κ = .86).

Lack of involvement applied to those units suggesting that either the participant or the social network member adjusted their behavior in a way that decreased encounters. Reducing involvement was achieved by a decrease in frequency of interaction, a withdrawal from friends who do not understand their situation, or an avoidance of particular events (e.g., baby showers, church, family gatherings). In addition, this category referenced a particular relationship (e.g., avoiding that person specifically) and social behavior in general (e.g., avoiding social gatherings). Some individuals even noted that they just had different schedules than their friends with children, which resulted in them being unable to spend as much time together, "It changes your lifestyle and who you do things with. Because the friends we had…they had children, they have ball games, piano recitals. They're not as free, and we notice that."A total of 34 of the 117 units (29%) were coded as *lack of involvement* (κ = .90).

The *negative relationship perception* category encompassed the feeling that a social network member's reaction caused hostility, hurt, disappointment, frustration, or a general negativity in the relationship. Some participants explicitly stated their feelings of negativity or implicitly suggested it when talking about their feelings and the relationship. One woman felt strain with her sister because she grew tired of the constant badgering about treatment, "She's the one that's kind of like, she'll ask my mom a lot, is she doing anything, she's not sitting still, is she doing anything? And you know what, I'm tired of that." Of the 117 units, a total of 31 (27%; κ = .70) were considered *negative relational perceptions*.

Discussion

The goal of this study was to explore how the experience of infertility exists within a greater social context and to recognize that as spouses cope with this disability within their marriage, they also navigate through this stressor with their families in tow. A content analysis conducted on 17 in-depth interviews reported the frequency with which individuals reveal and conceal their infertility-related information to family and friends, as well as the way these information-management decisions influenced the trajectories of those relationships. To conclude this chapter, we review how individuals communicate with their social networks during reproductive difficulties, address the strengths and limitations of our findings, and suggest directions for future study.

Communicating with Social Networks During Infertility

Results from the content analysis (see table 11.1) suggest that individuals are selective with not only their infertility status, but also the details of their treatment plan. Of the 88 units tagged as referencing concealing their private infertility information to any degree, 30% of those units indicated that the participant was completely concealing that content with individuals within their social network. Although not as frequent, 19% of the units alluded to limiting information with network members and 22% purposely limited contact to avoid explaining their actions related to infertility. Although the reasoning behind these concealments were not always offered, these results suggest that people not only are consciously managing their infertility-related information differently with individual network members, but that, perhaps, they often readjust their approach with friends and families when they see how those individuals respond to the infertility information they share with them.

When participants chose to share aspects of their infertility story with their network members, they were confronted with varying forms of support. Fortunately, 54% percent of the 135 units relating to revealing infertility-information alluded to positive support responses from friends and family. Interestingly, whereas a smaller 29% referenced negative support responses, the participants seemed to remember the negative encounters in more colorful detail than those constructive responses. For example, when discussing the general support from social network members, many participants would offer simple and vague statements about positive support (e.g., "they're supportive"), but be able to dissect their negative encounters in more detail (e.g., "they say very inappropriate things…and I'll be crying in the car," "they don't know certain words hurt or sting,"). Whereas the percentage of units was smaller than the positive units, the examples and memories referencing those destructive encounters were given in greater emotional detail.

Table 11.1 Frequencies of Content Analysis Categories

	Units	Percentage	Kappa
Total Units	169		
Conceal	88	52%	.70
Reveal	135	80%	.70
Relational Implication	117	69%	.86
Conceal	88		
Complete Conceal	26	30%	.78
Limited Information	17	19%	1.00
Limited Contact	19	22%	.83
Reveal	135		
Positive	73	54%	.77
Negative	29	22%	.75
Relational Implications	117		
Positive Perceptions	38	32%	.86
Lack of Involvement	34	29%	.90
Negative Perception	31	27%	.70

Note. Categories are not mutually exclusive.

Finally, decisions to reveal or conceal important information from family and friends likely have repercussions on those relationships. The results from the relational implications content analysis suggest that individuals perceived varying changes in their partnerships as they coped with their reproductive disability. Specifically, of the 117 units in this category, 32% of them referenced a positive shift in network relationships. Participants referenced feelings of increased closeness or emotional bonding as their friends and family offered support and shared in their coping of infertility. Despite this positive representation, 29% of the units referenced relationships that dissipated in some capacity as a result of coping with infertility. Whether it was because the couple isolated themselves from difficult social situations or network members were uncomfortable with their own pregnancy success around their struggling friends, approximately one-third of the units alluded towards a distancing effect within some relationships. Even worse, a surprising 27% of the units hinted towards hostile or hurtful encounters that resulted in disappointing and negative changes in some of their relationships as a direct or indirect result of their infertility experience.

Our results suggest that people might not make one universal decision when it comes to managing their infertility-related information. Because revealing secrets or other forms of private information leaves people susceptible to scrutiny or judgment (Petronio, 1991, 2000, 2002), past experiences with social network members may influence if a person chooses to reveal or conceal details of their infertility. When it is anticipated that the confidant will be accepting, supportive, or open-minded about an issue, a person might be more willing to share information; however, if the other person is distrusted, an individual may be especially inclined to keep sensitive information private (Harber & Pennebaker, 1992; Pennebaker, 1990).

Our findings also suggest that there are factors beyond experiences with the social network member that might influence disclosures. In particular, the information management decisions of people experiencing reproductive difficulties might fluctuate based on their current approach to treatment—and the information they reveal may vary in levels of detail and accuracy. For instance, some couples may have shared all details of their experience the first year they coped with infertility; however, they may remain more discreet about their plans as they cope with chronic treatment failures. Another trend that emerged was that some couples even offer misguided information to social network members in an attempt to maintain their privacy or ward off unsolicited advice. These findings suggest that individuals may rely on a series of decisions and employ a repertoire of behaviors when they are regulating their infertility information.

Although we interviewed only individuals experiencing infertility, and not the social network members they described, the results we obtained hint at the ways that infertility pervades social systems. Participants in the study described changes in the communication behaviors their friends and family enacted in response to the infertile individual's experiences. Whereas some network members withheld information, perhaps about their own pregnancy, others were more forthcoming with advice or disclosures about their own experiences. These divergent reactions showcase how an infertile person's relationships with friends and families are likely to change due to the experience of infertility. From a dual perspective, family members have to discern which support tactics are perceived as most supportive by their infertile loved ones and the infertile couple has to negotiate the best way to manage their privacy while simultaneously seeking the support they might need to cope with their reproductive disability.

The insights offered by our results are tempered by unanswered questions. Notably, our interview script consisted largely of inquiries about marital communication issues, insurance problems, and medical procedures. Within the discussions of those topics, an overarching theme of information-management issues was unveiled. The idea that these communication aspects surfaced without prompting speaks to the prominent influence they evoke on the infertility experience. At the same time, the focus of the interviews on other topics limited our ability to gather specific details about the processes at work as individuals supervise the private aspects of infertility. Future studies should probe these issues further, and set out to apply theoretical frameworks to the exploration of these communication issues.

A second issue meriting further study concerns the coordination between spouses as they negotiate social network relationships together. This study, and a large majority of extant research, focuses on how individuals manage privacy. Future research studying information-management within the marital context should consider the processes at work as couples decide, together, how to supervise their private information. Understanding how couples negotiate the alignment of each of their individual privacy preferences into a set of rules with which both spouses are comfortable would extend our theoretical understanding of ownership and management of a marriage's private information.

Conclusion

Infertile couples cope with a plethora of personal and relational struggles surrounding their reproductive disability. The heart of this stressor exists within the marriage; however, individuals often rely on family and friends to help them cope with infertility. Similarly, the health condition of a loved one can exert considerable stress on social network members as they, too, struggle through diagnosing an ailment, deciding on treatments, offering support, and living with the issue. Specific to infertility, a couple's friends and family face the prospect of missing out on having nieces, nephews, or grandchildren. They also have to figure out the best way to support their infertile loved ones—a task that might need to be readdressed at multiple times throughout the experience.

This chapter took the first steps towards understanding how infertility does not merely impact the life of individuals diagnosed with the disability, but it also impacts the social network relationships in a way that can ignite short and long-term distress. Sharing this disability with loved ones forces individuals to make decisions about their privacy boundaries, and perhaps have to readjust them as the condition progresses. At the same time, how network members support their loved ones as they cope with infertility can greatly influence the trajectory of their relationships. Thus, health conditions like infertility are not experienced solely by the individuals and couples who are diagnosed with the ailments, but rather extend into the lives of those individuals who care most about them.

References

Abbey, A., Andrews, F. M., & Halman, J. L. (1994). Psychosocial predictors of life quality: How are they affected by infertility, gender, and parenthood. *Journal of Family Issues, 15,* 253-271.

Afifi, W. A., & Burgoon, J. K. (1998). "We never talk about that": A comparison of cross-sex friendships and dating relationships on uncertainty and topic avoidance. *Personal Relationships, 5,* 255-272.

Afifi, W. A. & Guerrero, L. K. (2000). Motivations underlying topic avoidance in close relationships. In S. Petronio (Ed.), *Balancing the secrets of private disclosures* (pp. 165-180). Mahwah, NJ: Lawrence Erlbaum Associates, Inc.

Afifi, T. D., Olson, L. N., & Armstrong, C. (2005). The chilling effect and family secrets. *Human Communication Research, 31,* 564-598.

Afifi, T. D., & Schrodt, P. (2003). Uncertainty and the avoidance of the state of one's family/relationships in stepfamilies, post-divorce single parent families, and first marriage families. *Human Communication Research, 29,* 516-533.

Amato, P.R., Booth, A., Johnson, D. R., & Rogers, S. J. (2007). *Alone together: How marriage in America is changing*. Cambridge, MA: Harvard University Press.

Birditt, K. S., & Antonucci, T. C. (2007). Relationship quality profiles and well-being among married adults. *Journal of Family Psychology, 21,* 595-604.

Bryant, C. M., & Conger, R. D. (1999). Marital success and domains of social support in long-term relationships: Does the influence of network members ever end? *Journal of Marriage and the Family, 61,* 437-450.

Caughlin, J. P., & Petronio, S. (2004). Privacy in families. In A. L. Vangelisti (Ed.), *Handbook of family communication* (pp. 379-412). Mahwah, NJ: Erlbaum.

Center for Disease Control and Prevention. (2007). 2004 Assisted Reproductive Technology Retrieved from http://www.cdc.gov/ART/.

Chandra, A., Martinez, G. M., Mosher, W. D., Abma, J. C., & Jones, J. (2005). Fertility, family planning, and reproductive health of U. S. women: Data from the 2002 National Survey of Family Growth. National Center for Health Statistics. *Vital and Health Statistics, 23,* 1-160.

Cline, R. J. & McKenzie, N. J. (2000). Dilemmas of disclosure in the age of HIV/AIDS: Balancing privacy and protection in the health care context. In S. Petronio (Ed.), *Balancing the secrets of private disclosures* (pp. 165-180). Mahwah, NJ: Lawrence Erlbaum Associates, Inc.

Cloven, D. H., & Roloff, M. E. (1993). The chilling effect of aggressive potential on the expression of complaints in intimate relationships. *Communication Monographs, 60,* 198-219.

Cohen, J. (1960). A coefficient of agreement for nominal scales. *Educational and Psychological Measurement*, 37-46.

Daniluk, J. C. (1997). Gender and infertility. In S. Leiblum (Ed.), *Infertility: Psychological Issues and Counseling Strategies* (pp. 103-125). New York: John Wiley & Sons.

Demyttenaere, K., Nijs, P., Evers-Kiebooms, G., & Koninckx, P. R. (1991). Coping, ineffectiveness of coping and the psychoendocrinological stress responses during in-vitro fertilization. *Journal of Psychosomatic Research, 35,* 231-243.

Epstein, Y. M., & Rosenberg, H. S. (1997). He does, she doesn't; she does, he doesn't: Couple conflicts about infertility. In S. R. Leiblum (Ed.), *Infertility: Psychological issues and counseling strategies* (pp. 129-148). Oxford, England: John Wiley & Sons.

Felmlee, D. H. (2001). No couple is an island: A social network perspective on dyadic stability. *Social Forces, 79,* 1259-1287.

Greil, A. (1991). *Not yet pregnant: Infertile couples in contemporary America.* New Brunswick, NJ: Rutgers University Press.

Greil, A. L., Leitko, T. A., & Porter, K. L. (1988). Infertility: His and hers. *Gender and Society, 2(2),* 172-199.

Harber, K. D., & Pennebaker, J. W. (1992). Overcoming traumatic memories. In S. A. Christianson (Ed.), *The handbook of emotion and memory* (pp. 359-387). Hillsdale, NJ: Erlbaum.

Infante, D. A., Myers, S. A., & Buerkel, R. A., (1994). Argument and verbal aggression in constructive and destructive family and organizational disagreements. *Western Journal of Communication, 58,* 73-93.

Julien, D. & Markman, H. (1991). Social support and social networks as determinants of individual and marital outcomes. *Journal of Social and Personal Relationships, 8,* 549-568.

Kahn, R. L., & Antonucci, T. C. (1980). Convoys over the life course: Attachments, roles, and social support. In P. B. Baltes and O. G. Brim, (Eds), *Life-span development and behavior* (pp. 81-102). Academic Press: New York.

Lee, G. R. (1988). Marital satisfaction in later life: The effects of nonmarital roles. *Journal of Marriage and the Family, 50,* 775-783.

Leiblum, S. R. (1997). Love, sex, and infertility: The impact of infertility on couples. In S. R. Leiblum (Ed.), *Infertility: Psychological issues and counseling strategies* (pp. 149-166). Oxford: John Wiley & Sons.

Lewis, R. A., & Spanier, G. B. (1979). Theorizing about the quality and stability of marriage. In W. R. Burr, R. Hill, F. I. Nye, & I. L. Reiss (Eds.), *Contemporary theories about the family* (pp. 268-294). New York: Free Press.

Lincoln, K. D., (2000). Social support, negative social interactions, and psychological well-being. *Social Service Review, 74,* 231-252.

Miall, C. E. (1986). Perceptions of informal sanctioning and the stigma of involuntary childlessness. *Deviant Behavior, 6,* 383.

Pasch, L. A., Dunkel-Schetter, C., & Christensen, A. (2002). Differences between husbands' and wives' approach to infertility affect marital communication and adjustment. *Fertility and Sterility, 77,* 1241-1247.

Pennebaker, J. W. (1990). *Opening up: The healing powers of confiding in others.* New York: Morrow.

Peronace, L. A., Boivin, J., & Schmidt, L. (2007). Patterns of suffering and social interaction in infertile men: 12 months after unsuccessful treatment. *Journal of Psychosomatic Obstetrics & Gynecology, 28,* 105-114.

Peterson, B. D., Gold, L., & Feingold, T. (2007). The experience and influence of infertility: Considerations for couple counselors. *The Family Journal, 15,* 251—257.

Petronio, S. (1991). Communication boundary management: A theoretical model of managing disclosure of private information between marital couples. *Communication Theory, 1,* 311-335.

Petronio, S. (2000). The boundaries of privacy: Praxis of everyday life. In S. Petronio (Ed.), *Balancing the secrets of private disclosures* (pp. 37-49). Mahwah, NJ: Lawrence Erlbaum Associates, Inc.

Petronio, S. (2002). *Boundaries of privacy: Dialectics of disclosure.* Albany, NY: SUNY Press.

Schmidt, L. (2006). *Infertility and assisted reproduction in Denmark.* Copenhagen: University of Copenhagen.

Schneider, M. G., & Forthofer, M. S. (2005). Associations of psychosocial factors with the stress of infertility treatment. *Health and Social Work, 30(3),* 183-191.

Shevell, T., Malone, F. D., Vidaver, J., Porter, F., Luthy, D. A., & Comstock, C. H. (2005). Assisted reproductive technology and pregnancy outcome. *Obstetrics & Gynecology, 106,* 1039-1045.

Steuber, K. R., & Solomon, D. H. (2008). Relational uncertainty, partner interference, and infertility: A qualitative study of discourse within online forums. *Journal of Social and Personal Relationships, 25,* 831-855.

Straus, M. A., & Sweet, S. (1992). Verbal/symbolic aggression in couples: Incidence rates and relationships to personal characteristics. *Journal of Marriage and the Family, 54,* 346-357.

Tesser, A., Martin, L., & Cornell, D. (1996). On the substitutability of self-protective mechanisms. In P. M. Gollwitzer & J. A. Bargh (Eds.), *The psychology of action: Linking motivation and cognition to behavior* (pp. 48-68). New York: Guilford.

Willits, F., & Crider, D. (1986). *Well-being at midlife.* (Agricultural Experiment Station Bulletin 863). University Park, PA: Pennsylvania State University.

Wirtberg, I., Moller, A., Hogstrom, L., Tronstad, S. E., & Lalos, A. (2007). Life 20 years after unsuccessful infertility treatment. *Human Reproduction, 22,* 598-604.

Wright, J., Allard, M., Lecours, A., & Sabourin, S. (1989). Psychosocial distress and infertility: A review of controlled research. *International Journal of Fertility, 34,* 126-142.

Wright, J., Duchesne, C., Sabourin, S., Bissonnette, F., Benoit, J., & Girard, Y. (1991). Psychological distress and infertility: Men and women respond differently. *Fertility and Sterility, 55,* 100-108.

CHAPTER 12

Caring for the Family: Teaching Systems and Cycles in a Family Medicine Residency Program

Elissa Foster, Ph.D.

MEDICAL EDUCATOR

Joanne Cohen-Katz, Ph.D.

FAMILY SYSTEMS ASSOCIATE

DEPARTMENT OF FAMILY MEDICINE
LEHIGH VALLEY HEALTH NETWORK

The role of communication within the family system is integral to understanding the meaning of and formulating a response to any health crisis for both the individual and the family member. By extension, an equally important constituent of the system of care is the communication among the patient, family members, and health care provider or providers. As provider patient communication becomes ever more compromised by the complexity and expense of health care in the United States, it is vital to examine ways in which providers and consumers of health care are working to overcome these challenges and forge positive relationships. Just as a systems perspective is integral to any understanding of families, developments in medical education at the local and national levels have recognized that physicians operate within a system of care that encompasses the patient, family members, and other health care professionals.

Our chapter approaches the topic of families and health transitions from the perspective of the family physician and, specifically, describes current approaches to professional training through the family medicine residency. As inherently interdisciplinary and generalist traditions, communication studies and family medicine are kindred spirits—both span scientific and humanistic paradigms, both are situated within hierarchies that privilege "hard science" specialties, and both embrace as the focus of their efforts the diversity and complexity of human experience and relationships. Our chapter, coauthored by a communication scholar and a clinical psychologist, is also inherently interdisciplinary and draws from both fields of research as we present a representative case of how family medicine physicians are trained to care for families. The case we describe is the Family Medicine Residency Program at Lehigh Valley Health Network (LVHN); specifically, the philosophies, tools, and particular learning experiences of the family systems curriculum. For health care professionals, this chapter will outline fundamental theory as well as useful practices for working with families. For patients and family members, having a clearer understanding of the dynamics that affect a meeting with a health care provider, as well as the goals of an effective family meeting, can inform and potentially improve communication among family members, whether or not the physician is present. For scholars of health and family communication, this account of a residency program that sees family relationships as integral to the healer's work may be revelatory and should inspire confidence in the potential of the two disciplines—medicine and communication—to inform one another more fully.

Situating Family Medicine and the Family Systems Approach

The family systems perspective stands in direct contrast—and perhaps opposition—to the individualism that characterizes Western culture generally and, specifically, the disciplines of psychology and medicine (Morris, 1998; Seale, 1998). Within the communication studies tradition, relational theory (Bochner, 1978, 1984; Millar & Rogers, 1976; Rogers & Escudero, 2004) emphasizes what goes on *between* people as they communicate in relationship rather than what goes on *within* them. Family communication scholarship emerged as a subdiscipline within communication studies by building on the understanding of communication as relational and by incorporating theoretical frameworks that would address the interactional complexity of the family group. Drawing on general systems theory (Sieburg, 1985), structural family therapy (Lannamann, 1989; Minuchin, 1974; Minuchin & Fishman, 1981), and the work of Bateson (1972) and the Palo Alto group (Watzlawick, Beavin, & Jackson, 1967), family communication scholars have generated a body of research that establishes interaction, ritual, and story as primarily constitutive of family life (e.g., Bavelas, 1984; Baxter & Clark, 1996; Bochner, 1981, 1989; Jorgenson, 1989; Jorgenson & Bochner, 2004; Koenig Kellas, 2006; McNamee, 1989).

Parallel developments occurred within psychology, as the individualist model of therapy made space for a systemic, family-oriented approach, in which all symptoms were assumed to occur within the context of the family, and therapy was likewise conducted with all or at least some of the family members present in the interaction (Ackerman, 1966; Bowen, 1978; Haley, 1963; Minuchin, 1974; Satir, 1967). Within systems approaches to therapy, even when only one person is present in the room, all problems are conceptualized as reflecting systemic problems. To take a classic example, the "acting out child" reflects difficulties the family is experiencing in negotiating their way—perhaps reflecting a distant marriage, a parent with an alcohol abuse problem, or a child with a severe illness who has derailed the family. There has been great variability in the degree to which systemic approaches have been adapted in behavioral health treatment settings and, recently, systemic approaches to therapy have attempted to more fully integrate biologic and genetic factors that influence individuals' difficulties. Nevertheless, systemic and relational theory has dramatically reshaped thinking and practice in the treatment of behavioral health issues.

Despite the ubiquitous image of the white-coated family physician making house calls, which dates back to the 19th century, *family medicine* as a distinct specialty emerged relatively recently, partly as a by-product of the counter-culture of the 1960s (Stephens, 1979), emphasizing a "low-technology, whole-person, whole-family approach" (Candib, 1995, p. xv). Two features that distinguish family medicine from other primary care specialties[1] are (a) its emphasis on the life-

1 The other primary care specialties are (a) internal medicine, which focuses on the medical care of adults; (b) obstetrics/gynecology, which focuses on women's medical services including prenatal, delivery, and postnatal care; and (c) pediatrics, which focuses on care of infants and children.

span of the patient (i.e., "from womb to tomb") and (b) the identification of the family, rather than the individual, as the context of care. Although variation exists in the extent to which an individual physician incorporates a family approach into her or his practice (Dougherty & Baird, 1986), a rich tradition has developed that integrates the insights from family therapy into the medical care of the family. Key theorists of the family systems approach to practice include Susan McDaniel and her colleagues (McDaniel, Campbell, Hepworth, & Lorenz, 2005; McDaniel, Campbell, & Seaburn, 1990), William Dougherty and Macaran Baird (1983; 1987), Lucy Candib (1985; 1995), Jeri Hepworth (McDaniel et al., 2005; McDaniel, Hepworth, & Dougherty, 1992), and Susan Thrower (Thrower, Bruce, & Walton, 1982), to name just a few. In the early 1980s, these and other scholar-practitioners formed a group called the Family in Family Medicine Group in order to share resources and developments in the field and to advance family systems practice within various residency programs across the country. Interestingly, after 28 years, this group held its last conference in 2008. Opinions differ as to the meaning of the demise of this conference; it may reflect that the ideas developed by these pioneers have become so mainstream that they no longer need their own conference, or it may indicate that family systems thinking has receded in its influence. Additionally, it is likely to be related to the fact that many attendees have become involved in the work of a relatively new organization that reflects a growing national interest in collaborative health care: the Collaborative Family Healthcare Association, formed in 1995.

The mission of the Collaborative Family Healthcare Association is to promote a comprehensive and cost-effective model of healthcare delivery that integrates mind and body, individual and family, patients, providers, and communities. The first two goals are: (a) to develop the knowledge base of collaborative family healthcare, and (b) to present and advocate for the collaborative family healthcare perspective locally, nationally, and internationally (Collaborative Family Healthcare Association, 2008). This movement towards establishing family-oriented behavioral health within medical settings would appear to hold great promise for delivering health care services that are family friendly and that integrate the rich tradition of theory and practice that grew out of the family therapy field and the work begun by the Family in Family Medicine group. Thus, within family medicine, many programs now implement curricula that support physicians' capacity to perceive their patients as embedded in a network of relationships and an ongoing family story that is integrally related to their patients' health and wellness.

The Case of LVHN Family Medicine Residency

The family medicine residency at LVHN was founded in 1995 with the understanding that the family, rather than the individual, is the relevant focus of care for primary practice. As a consequence of that commitment, the residency program established family systems as a foundational aspect of its curriculum, hiring second author Joanne Cohen-Katz as a Family Systems Associate, charging her with the development of the family systems curriculum. An important feature of the residency was that, unlike the majority of residency programs, the curriculum was longitudinal rather than divided into blocks. In contrast to a required sequence of continuous rotations (weeks or months long) of various inpatient specialties—such as surgery, critical care, obstetrics and gynecology, pediatrics, neonatal critical care, radiology—the residents spend the majority of their time in the outpatient setting with time to pursue focused training in shorter periods (days or half-days) during the week. Although the family medicine Residency Review Committee requires a number of rotation experiences, especially in the internship year (Accreditation Council for Graduate Medical Education, 2001), the longitudinal residency model allows for more frequent integration of key aspects of the curriculum—such as family systems and behavioral medicine—into the residents' training. In addition, the longitudinal integration is a more effective way for the family systems perspective to permeate the culture of the residency rather than approaching it as an add-on experience (Cohen-Katz, Miller, & Borkan, 2003).

Although a number of other family medicine residency programs employ both a longitudinal curriculum and integrated family systems training, a unique aspect of the LVHN program is that it is very explicit about the tools considered central to the craft of family medicine. These tools provide the intellectual, theoretical, and philosophical underpinnings of family practice. Three of these incorporate family systems thinking: (a) the relationship-centered clinical method (Tresolini & the Pew Fetzer Task Force, 1994), the ecological-transactional-system method (Miller, 1999), and the clinical hand (Miller, 2004). The fourth core clinical tool is the family development spiral, which we describe in more detail in the next section. Four large posters representing these tools hang in the conference room of the health center where many of our residents see patients, underscoring the centrality of family systems work in all medical care.

The family systems curriculum includes (a) extensive training in family assessment and history taking, (b) a modified version of the family life-cycle that we call the family development spiral, described below, (c) how to conduct family meetings, with an emphasis on the hospital setting, and (d) experience with family-oriented, collaborative, behavioral healthcare in the outpatient setting. The sections that follow describe this curriculum, how the various elements fit within the overall philosophy and approach of the residency program, and how the experiences in this residency program can inform family and health communication more generally.

Integrating Family Systems into the Residency

Within the three-year family medicine residency, there are several learning environments in which the family systems curriculum is taught and practiced. At the beginning of the residency, the interns participate in what is called Foundations Month, an orientation program that introduces key family medicine tools in addition to preparing the interns for inpatient and outpatient practice. Currently, the residents spend three to five half-day sessions during Foundations Month learning how to construct a genogram (see description below), complete family circle activities (Thrower, Bruce, & Walton, 1982), and break bad news; additionally, residents obtain some preliminary information about family meetings and are introduced to the family development spiral, a reformulation of the family life-cycle model (Carter & McGoldrick, 1980, 1988, 1999).

The second context of family systems education is what our residency calls learning labs—half-day sessions that primarily involve faculty-led, didactic and experiential workshops covering core content of the residency. Family systems is one of several curricular portfolios around which the content of the learning labs is currently organized.

The third context for teaching and learning the family systems curriculum is the Behavioral Medicine Clinic (BMC, formerly called Co-therapy), in which residents spend one half-day per week for their second and third years working with behavioral medicine faculty and providing family systems oriented therapy sessions to patients and families from their own clinical practices, explicitly using a family systems approach to care. Residents attend the clinic with a group of their peers. BMC adapts a classic teaching tool of family therapy training so that, with patients' consent, the residents who are not providing counseling during a given hour are able to view the session from another room on closed-circuit video. During this time, residents may discuss what they are seeing with another faculty member. At times, the group that is viewing the case has functioned as a supervisory team, providing the therapist and resident in the room with feedback and suggestions for intervention with the family. The BMC models an integrative approach to care by including psychology, social work and psychiatry faculty; therefore, patients are viewed simultaneously from the biologic lens and the systemic lens.

A fourth teaching and learning context is the delivery of care in the inpatient and outpatient settings, where residents work under the supervision of a family medicine attending physician (inpatient) or preceptor (outpatient), who may ask them to describe cases or apply family systems thinking to their management of a particular patient's condition. They are also asked to conduct family meetings regularly and to have at least one of these meetings observed per year by a faculty member trained in family systems health.

In the sections that follow, we describe three of the specific tools in more detail: (a) genograms, (b) the family meeting, and (c) the family development spiral. We explain how the tools are taught and assessed by faculty members in the four settings mentioned above: (a) Foundations Month, (b) learning labs, (c) BMC, and (d) clinical care, both inpatient and outpatient. We also address why the family systems perspective is helpful and necessary when it comes to health transitions in the family, as well as some of the challenges that we face when integrating family systems tools and perspectives into the delivery of medical care.

Genograms

A genogram (McGoldrick, Gerson, & Shellenberger, 1999) is a type of family tree diagram that is designed to summarize emotional and relational history in addition to basic familial relationships. Thus, the genogram includes symbols for relationship dynamics (e.g., estrangement, enmeshment, hostility, violence, close friendship, neglect, love, and many others) in addition to medical history including serious illness, death, miscarriage, adoption, and so on. One of the core ideas of the tool is that in order to look at a patient a practitioner must look at what is probably the most important context of that patient's life, the family, as the primary mechanism through which cultural practices and beliefs around health and illness are taught. The genogram is a tool that helps the therapist or physician generate a map for understanding the family context.

During Foundations Month, the residents are taught how to complete a genogram as a way of conceptualizing cases. The session always starts out with a number of medical cases, and the family genogram is written up on the whiteboard. Joanne regularly presents a case in which she was the consulting therapist many years ago, which involves an obese three-year-old whose mother brings her to the family physician. Typically, when presented with this case, a resident will ask, "Well, what's going on in the immediate family, with the mother? Is she overweight? How does the family eat?" This question comes from a basic understanding of the role of families in the health of a child. The residents may ask about grandparents; however, they generally won't ask more probing questions, such as these: Where is the mother in her own family life-cycle? Where is she geographically in relation to her own family of origin? Who are all the grandparent figures? What are their belief systems? As the story of the case unfolds, it is clear that the child's obesity only can be understood by finding out that this very young mother is thousands of miles away from home and that her mother-in-law rules the roost and is integrally involved in food preparation and providing the young child with treats.

Another case that often surprises the residents is that of a 67-year-old man with chest pain, who has been admitted for 24-hour observation in the hospital several times and has been ruled out for any cardiac problems. Filling in the genogram tells the story; he recently retired and witnessed the chronic illness and death of three parents and parents-in-law, all in one year. The genogram also helps to add to the potential solutions; for example, one of the core interventions in this case was in getting this man to be more involved in his grandson's school.

These cases reinforce the rationale for why health care practitioners need to know the family system of the patient and how the genogram can be the tool for understanding it. The idea is that the picture is worth a thousand words; the picture, the genogram, is a way to conceptualize and to understand the patient and the family.

To further enrich the physician's understanding of families and systems, during Foundations Month all residents are asked to have another resident or faculty member take their own genogram, looking at specific issues such as the role of illness in their own family of origin, the way in which their family might have influenced their choice of medicine as a career, and likely clinical strengths or "allergies" (challenges) that arise from their own experience in their families of origin. We also speculate about how different family experiences might directly impact some of the cases we have discussed. So, for example, when talking about the case of the young mother who is geographically far from her own mother and has an overweight child we ask how a resident who is a new mom herself and far from her own family might react to this case. How about a resident who had an obese family member or struggles with eating issues himself? How about a very athletic resident who is single and very happy to be away from home? These discussions deepen the residents' understanding of the power of the family system, their own as well as their patients'.

In addition to Foundations Month and Learning Labs, residents have opportunities to present family genograms during an activity called Continuity Case Conference, in which second- and third-year residents present hour-long analyses of patients with whom they have experienced a long-term practitioner-patient relationship. Cases presented during BMC also, ideally, start with the presentation of the patient's genogram. The BMC is both psychiatrically focused and systemic, providing opportunities to develop an intake process that incorporates elements of both, including the genogram and a description of where the family is in the family development spiral, so that they can be incorporated into the patient's medical record. In addition, there are opportunities for residents to generate and present genograms when precepting in the outpatient clinic and when presenting on rounds in the hospital.

Consistently integrating the genogram into patient care forces the physician to think systemically. To illustrate this point, during one of the residents' learning labs, Joanne shows the film *What's Eating Gilbert Grape?*(Hallström & Hedges, 1993) and asks the residents to draw the genogram of the family. In that movie, the father committed suicide 17 years prior and the autistic son is just turning 18, while the mother is agoraphobic and obese and has not left the house since her husband's death. Looking at the genogram, which includes the dates when significant family events occurred, raises an interesting question: Did the father committing suicide have anything to do with giving birth to a son who was so impaired and having to deal with a disabled child? As a teaching resource, this film also provides rich illustrations of the roles that family members adopt in a family system—another core feature of family systems theory. For example, the central character in this film (Gilbert Grape) becomes a caretaker to both his autistic younger brother and his disabled mother, with all the incumbent challenges. Exploring Gilbert's storyline leads into a rich discussion of the impact of mental and physical illness on the family system. Physicians may believe they consider the family, but without the genogram they think in terms of the individual *having* a family versus *being embedded within* the family—a distinction that has significant implications for health care.

In the early years of the LVHN family medicine residency, presenting genograms was standard practice for both case presentations in what was then called Co-therapy (now BMC) and also for Continuity Case Conference. As Joanne puts it, "You had to put a genogram up before you saw a case. You couldn't just *talk* about a family; you had to put the genogram up on the board." One of the reasons for genograms becoming less common in the presentation of cases is the arrival of the electronic medical record (EMR). Whereas patients once had paper charts in which hand-drawn genograms and family circles could reside comfortably, the EMR is relatively inflexible in the kinds of documents that it will accommodate. The physician no longer sits with a paper and pencil, but with a laptop, which means that to complete a genogram the physician must put down the laptop and draw the genogram and have somebody else scan it in to the EMR. Although these are only a few extra steps, they are sufficiently time consuming to prevent the genogram from being completed or incorporated into the patient's medical record. However, the commitment to this particular tool is strong enough to warrant renewed effort within the residency to both require the presentation of genograms more consistently during patient care and educational activities and to find an efficient way to include a genogram in the EMR.

The Family Meeting

A significant feature of the longitudinal family systems curriculum is the form and practice of conducting a family meeting. Although there are a number of different models for conducting a family meeting, common functions are found in a given meeting structure (see table 12.1). The meeting generally includes tasks of preparation prior to the meeting; greeting and connecting with the family when they arrive; collaboratively setting an agenda for the meeting; sharing thoughts, feelings, goals, concerns, questions and needs; establishing and agreeing to a plan; and post-meeting tasks of review and documentation. Although the meeting format and functions are fairly self-evident, residents face a challenge in the competent execution of the family meeting in practice.

The most common context for a family meeting is in the inpatient setting, because a crisis is often associated with an acute onset of a condition or exacerbation of an existing condition that indicates a change in the health of the patient. Not coincidentally, at these times multiple family members likely are involved, with multiple perspectives on what needs to be done, especially in cases where the patient is no longer able to speak. The philosophy of the family meeting is for the physician to serve as a facilitator who is able to validate the feelings and needs of multiple family members, assisting them to clarify their needs while maintaining a clear view of the patient's best interests. Although the inpatient setting is the most common context for a family meeting, there may be occasions for family meetings in the outpatient setting, whether planned and initiated by the physician or patient or impromptu when the patient and family are present during an office visit.

Common scenarios for family meetings include giving the family bad news about their loved one's prognosis, which is often most challenging when the family was expecting a very different outcome. Another common scenario is a conflict among family members about how to handle end-of-life treatment decisions. Most residents have stories to tell about a family member who flies in from another part of the country and challenges the care that their mother or father is receiving. Yet another common scenario is one in which the family insists the patient needs hospitalization, when the family itself is struggling with issues around chronic caregiving and burnout. These types of cases are predicted and discussed in learning labs that address how to deliver bad news to a family, how to negotiate around end-of-life treatment decisions, and how to help families that are struggling with caregiving issues. Family systems therapy training provides skills of conflict management and communicating and managing a family meeting, which are extremely helpful tools to the resident in resolving these cases.

For any resident who spends any length of time caring for patients in the hospital, the family meeting is impossible to avoid; however, the extent to which residents are able to be observed and provided with feedback varies greatly. In the early years of the program, Joanne was able to go to the hospital to supervise the family meetings, but the logistics of providing that support have proven challenging, mostly because there is rarely an opportunity to know in advance when the family will arrive at the hospital. Despite the occasional unpredictability of the hospital family meeting, Joanne notes that residents are often willing to partner with her or an attending physician to prepare for the meeting, often with a genogram, in order to make the best plan for facilitating the meeting. The most significant

Table 12.1 Common Tasks Associated With a Family Meeting

Stage	Tasks
Stage One (Premeeting) Setting the Stage: Reading Oneself for the Meeting	Reviewing the genogram Developing hypotheses about the family situation and needs Preparing self to be fully present for the family
Stage Two Joining With the Family: Greeting and Building Rapport With Family Members	Greeting and thanking the family for coming Orienting the family to the room and the building Talking with each member about who they are and relationship to the patient
Stage Three Agenda Setting: Determining the Goals of the Meeting	Hearing from everyone Noting any conflicting goals Balancing and prioritizing multiple agendas
Stage Four Discussing	Soliciting each person's view of the problem Recognizing and acknowledging emotions Negotiating multiple points of view Dealing with strongly conflicting points of view, by "converting positions into interests" Avoiding taking sides and triangulation Encouraging questions from the patient and family members Providing education as needed Addressing people who monopolize the conversation Avoiding advice giving too early in the family meeting
Stage Five Brainstorming Resources: Identifying family, medical, community, and spiritual resources	Helping the family come up with multiple options Focusing on solutions that address multiple interests
Stage Six Developing a Plan	Summarizing options Emphasizing common ground Developing "next steps" for everyone Keeping options open for future discussion Referring to a therapist if it seems helpful Checking for understanding before adjourning
Stage Seven (Post-Meeting) Debriefing	Revising the genogram Revising the hypotheses Documenting the meeting

Note: Adapted from *Family-oriented primary care* (2nd Ed.) by S. H. McDaniel, T. L. Campbell, J. Hepworth, & A. Lorenz, 2005, p. 89. Copyright 2005 by Springer-Verlag.

aspect of this particular tool, from a communication perspective, is that it provides a framework within which the physician is able to improvise, focusing on the essential functions of the communicative event while remaining open and fully present to the patient and members of the family.

A core strength of the family systems perspective and the family meeting is that they debunk the myth of the individual that permeates our systems of care whether psychiatric, psychological, or medical. A corollary of this myth is that individuals are fully autonomous and can best make their health care decisions in the context of a rational discussion with one other person. Indeed, this is often more comfortable for the provider, because it is generally much more comfortable to have a discussion with one person than to have several people in the room interacting with each other, which can be complex, complicated, and daunting (Levine & Zuckerman, 1999). Nevertheless, the learning experiences we provide to our residents reinforce the message to them that they are always stepping into a family system when they step into a room with a patient.

At times, the implication of the family system is impossible to ignore, even when the physician would prefer to do so. Such times might include when there is a health transition such as a new diagnosis, a terminal diagnosis, an accident, or a life transition, such as a pregnancy or birth, a change in sexual function, a divorce, or a death. In these cases, the family becomes integral to the meaning of the experience and the approach to the care of the patient. In the case of a terminal illness, the physician can expect to start getting phone calls from "all over the genogram." If the physician had no relationship with the family before, and no training to help them work with all of the relational complexities, she or he would become overwhelmed very quickly.

Family Development Spiral

The family development spiral is our attempt to articulate a model of family development that acknowledges the importance of developmental phases and transitions in the life of a family. It is drawn from the family life-cycle model developed by Betty Carter and Monica McGoldrick (1980; 1988), and the family life spiral developed by Lee Combrinck-Graham (1985, cited by McDaniel et al., 2005, p. 32). Like relational developmental models (e.g., Knapp & Vangelisti, 2000) that have been critiqued for valorizing a heteronormative view of the family (Elia, 2003; Foster, 2008), the family life-cycle model has been similarly criticized for its normative, generalizing impact. For example, Candib (1995, pp. 38-39) took one version of the family life-cycle stages and pointed out that it was a particularly gendered view, devoid of cultural context, and conservative to the extent that it assumed a nuclear vision of the family to which few would belong these days. In their later articulations of this model, Carter and McGoldrick (1988) acknowledged the variety of ways that culture and nonnuclear family models influence the way families negotiate the life-cycle. Combrinck-Graham's family life spiral names ubiquitous stages and notes the spiraling cycle that occurs in family development. We have found it helpful to develop a model that integrates the best of these two models and adds other pieces. Like Combrinck-Graham's model, ours uses a spiral to depict ubiquitous family stages of development (birth, raising children, aging, death), and also explicitly acknowledges some of the many variants that different families and cultures experience in negotiating these stages, such as re-evaluating one's sexual orientation, alternatives to traditional childbearing and childrearing, and so on (see Figure 12.1.). Like the family life-cycle model, we delineate the developmental tasks of each of these stages.

The family development spiral introduced in this chapter was developed by Will Miller and Joanne Cohen-Katz specifically for the family medicine residency at LVHN. In contrast to other, more linear descriptions of the family's development, this model emphasizes transitions of shifting roles for different members of the family, adding and losing generations, forming new family units, and changing existing ones. One implication of this model is that everyone can find themselves reflected in the model, regardless of whether they are coupled or not, bearing children or not, heterosexual or homosexual, or in a single- or multiple-generation family. The model reminds physicians that even if the family they are working with does not look like a "typical" family, family stories of coming together and coming apart accompany many of the health transitions they see in the office and the hospital.

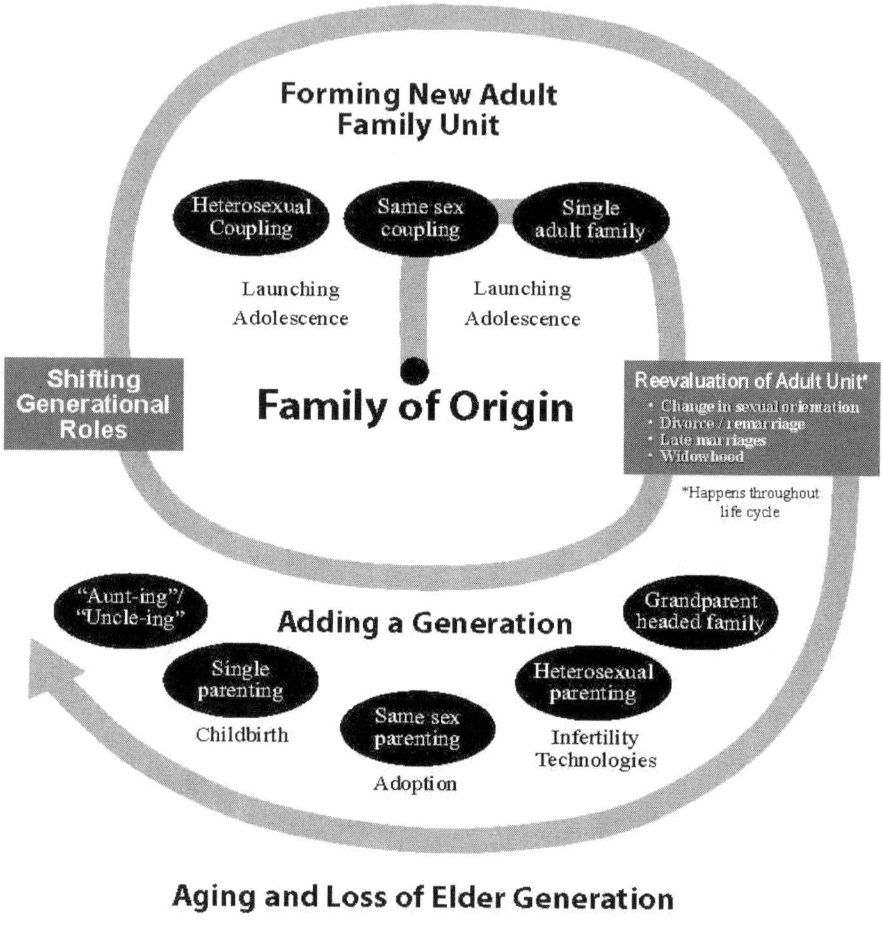

Figure 12.1 The Family Development Spiral © 2010 by William L. Miller, MD, & Joanne L. Cohen-Katz, PhD

In addition to the spiral, the model includes a table that indicates the developmental tasks for the family at a particular stage of development; many of these tasks are drawn directly from the work of Carter and McGoldrick (1980; 1988); others are based on our own work. The ideas that life-cycle transitions are stress points that can produce symptoms, particularly when combined with understanding family developmental tasks, are powerful concepts that inform residents' practice with families. Therefore, in our model we included and expanded upon the family life-cycle model's articulation of developmental tasks; for the developmental stages we added, such as changing one's sexual orientation, we have developed our own list of potential developmental tasks.

For example, our formulation of the tasks of the family for shifting generational roles at midlife, adapted directly from the work of Carter and McGoldrick, include (a) renegotiation of adult unit without parenting as primary task, (b) development of adult-to-adult relationships between grown children and their parents, (c) making decisions about and facing retirement, (d) realignment of relationships to include children's in-laws and their own children, and (e) dealing with disabilities and death of the eldest generation.

Our formulation of the tasks of re-evaluating and changing one's sexual orientation include (a) coming out to oneself, (b) coming out to family, (c) coming out to work community and friends, (d) becoming ready to couple as a gay person, (e) becoming ready to formally commit to a relationship, (f) dealing with homophobia (family, public, societal), (g) grieving loss of fantasy of heterosexual family life for couple and extended family, and (h) learning as a family how to include same-sex couple into larger family rituals and events.

The strength of the spiral and the developmental tasks is that it gives physicians another approach and helps them to conceptualize the symptoms they see during the office visit as potential reflections of developmental transitions with which the family is struggling. This insight then can be applied by the residents in their everyday practice. In our residency, the family development spiral tool is introduced in Foundations Month and revisited in family systems learning labs, Continuity Case Conference, and BMC.

In one half-day of BMC, Joanne saw three patients with a resident, all three of whom were greatly informed by the use of the family development spiral. One case involved a young working mother who had been referred for symptoms of depression: irritability, tearfulness, and negative feelings about herself. Although one legitimate way to integrate the biologic and family systems models with this patient might be to normalize her difficulties as a new mother (*individual* life-cycle transition) and to provide her with an antidepressant, what proved even more useful in this case was to see the underlying *family* transition at the root of her presentation. Her husband kept telling her to "get it together" and be less stressed. Underlying this pressure was their transition to parenthood and the belief that the couple had been lost. The more the husband missed her, the more he told her to "just relax," and the more she felt inadequate. Working with this family from this perspective allowed for more effective treatment; helping the couple to reconnect was more powerful than treating the mother individually and identifying her as the one with the problem.

The second patient was a man in his mid-50s who was also struggling with family developmental issues. His children were now launched, and he and his wife had witnessed a traumatic injury and subsequent rehabilitation in their younger son in recent years. The impact of the son's illness on our patient was devastating, but more debilitating was the recent distance in his marriage, exacerbated further by his wife's drinking. An immediate exploration of this case might point to a "classic midlife crisis"; however, taking some additional time in collaborative care to flesh out the genogram provided for a new set of possibilities for the family physician. Facilitating conversations between this man and his wife, particularly around the developmental crisis represented by their child's illness, added to the perspective and options for sense-making by the physician and collaborator.

The third case was a classic story of a teenager presenting to the clinic with his mother, where the biologic lens was pervasive in the family's explanation of the teen's behavioral problems. Specifically, the family perceived Ritalin to be the cure for the behavioral issues, but much more work needed to be done within the family system to fully address these issues. Thus, the challenge for the physician and family was to reframe the problem as concerning family relationships in addition to brain function. In this case, enhancing the family's ability to navigate a divorce and adjust to living as a single-parent family (all part of the family development spiral) was integral to resolving this case.

In all three of these cases, the family developmental spiral helped the treatment team understand the major contributing factors creating symptoms, and provided solutions that would not otherwise have been apparent. Best of all, the family development spiral pointed toward treatment approaches that used relationships within the patient's own life as a source of healing.

Family Systems and Health Transitions

From the beginning, a fundamental philosophy of family medicine was for physicians to enact long-term relationships with their patients. In that context, it is possible to imagine a physician saying to a family member,

> I've treated four generations of this family, we go way, way, back—you and I both know how helpful it was when your Grandma died—and we all share these stories together and these experiences; at the very least we share this trust. So now I'm telling you I really think it's time for you to think about your mom getting some assisted living because her health is failing.

Such a conversation comes from a very different place than the physician who "thinks that my mother is just an invalid and wants me to send her away to an institution." In this age of managed care and transcontinental families, it may not be possible to enact a four-generational relationship with a given family; however, by keeping the family system in mind, the physician is far more likely to ask the right questions, to remain open to multiple needs within the family, and to honor family relationships towards the best outcome for the patient.

An additional dynamic to keep in mind when taking a family systems approach is the effect of centripetal and centrifugal forces (Baxter & Montgomery, 1996) as the system encounters a crisis. The family dynamic can become more centripetal around an illness or a death in the family, which means they want to be involved in each other's decisions. A myth related to the individualism of the US culture is that people make decisions by themselves when they are in health transitions; however, patients commonly will say, "I want to do whatever my husband, the doctor, thinks is right," or "I have some ideas, but I want everyone in the family to be comfortable." Patients might even say,

> It's more important to me that my kids are getting along right now and I have a peaceful death than it is that you give me a particular medicine or put me in a particular setting. We just need to come up with a plan that

> people are comfortable with and I don't make that decision in a vacuum. I want to find out what other people in the family think about it.

Although the physician may feel frustrated when a patient says, "I want what my husband wants" or "I want what my wife wants," a family systems approach requires the physician to acknowledge the value of the relationship and put it on an equal or higher footing with the ideals of individualized patient care.

After making a health transition—into wellness or chronic illness—or a life transition (e.g., childbirth), patients will enter a maintenance phase. In this phase, family relationships remain present but are acknowledged less than during times of transition. Some cases in which a physician might be slow to acknowledge the implications of the family system include smoking cessation; the impact of others smoking in the home is one dimension of the system, but smokers also may be using tobacco to set boundaries or establish identity within the family. Similarly, diet and exercise are related not only to the roles within the family—including responsibilities for shopping, cooking, working outside the home, caring for children—but also to beliefs about food and caregiving, hospitality, nurturance, and so on. Thus, with an adult who is not obviously in a life-cycle transition, the physician may not think to consider the embeddedness of the patient within the family.

It is also important to consider the relevant family development stage of the patient alongside the potential life transition and health transition. For example, from a family systems perspective, there is a difference between diagnosing an 8-year-old with diabetes and diagnosing a 17-year-old with diabetes. The 17-year-old is in a centrifugal phase where they are ready to be launched from the family and yet they are being diagnosed with an illness that will pull him or her back into their family for support. In some situations stages of the life-cycle and the health transition are completely at odds; the developmental cycle of the family may involve relaxing the bonds tying a person to family (e.g., when a child gets married), yet the diagnosis will tend to pull that family member back forming even tighter bonds. In our example above, the young adult son who had suffered a traumatic injury was 22, a time when he quite naturally would have been leaving home and moving toward more independence. Thus, the stress of the health transition may be compounded by the stress of the family life-cycle transition.

The illness transition also may be a time where the family pathology becomes clearer, sometimes more exacerbated, to the point where the family will fracture around the health transition. In this case, the dynamic is centrifugal instead of centripetal, and the instinct will be towards distance rather than closeness. This outcome is particularly likely if there are significant, negative, and unresolved issues within the family at the time when the crisis occurs. A common indicator of this outcome could be when a family member declares, "The way they treated my mother at the end-of-life I'll never talk to my [sibling] again." Whatever dynamic prevails at the time of the crisis will become more highlighted and more accentuated, and the wise physician will not avoid the family during those times.

Although we have outlined a comprehensive approach to family systems within residency training and family practice, this approach does face numerous challenges in our current health care system. In our own program, the BMC brings together family therapeutic techniques and philosophies with psychiatry and some individual models of care. As a result, there is a certain tension between viewing the illness as integral to and an extension of family relationships and viewing it as the province of the individual. Because the medical hierarchy already privileges an individualistic and biomedical model, the family systems curriculum may lose some of its impact by using psychiatrists who are not family systems trained. Similarly, when the residents become trained to give medication, the family therapy approach may become less attractive, which is, of course, a tension that exists in the larger context of medicine. Although systems approaches have permeated the way we think about health in different pockets of the health care system, we still have a largely reductionistic, individually focused medical culture. It is simply cheaper and easier to prescribe a pill, especially when pressured by an insurance company or a patient or family member to "fix the problem, quickly!" Nevertheless, we feel that when we model collaboration and integration in our BMC, the patient gets the best care and the physician gets the best training.

Over the past several years, one phenomenon that promises to enable a more robust family systems approach in primary care practices is the growing prevalence of behavioral health practitioners in medical settings, some of whom have had exposure to family systems thinking and therapy. Our own work in the BMC models this type of work, although the presence of the resident physician as a co-therapist is likely to be very limited in actual primary care once physicians are no longer in training.

To take an example from Joanne's work in primary care, a faculty physician referred a woman to her who was newly married and having problems with eating behaviors. The physician, who was male, had a good relationship with both the patient and her husband, so he was able to serve as a co-therapist in several marital therapy sessions that helped this family. Although many therapists have been working in this way in primary care for years, they remain a relatively small subculture. The flowering of the Collaborative Family Healthcare Association and the growing number of therapists in primary care settings may predict a greater number of physicians integrating family systems ideas and practice into their work with families experiencing health transitions.

For family and health communication researchers, this chapter's overview of family systems residency training highlights something of our absence from developments within medical education. At the same time, it is clear that we share many of the foundational concepts and theories that inform this training. Likewise, there is much research from communication that could support the family perspective in medical practice. For example, the theme of "transitions" that unites the chapters of this edited collection has been articulated clearly in research around relational dialectics (Baxter & Harper, 1998; Baxter & Montgomery, 1996; Conville, 1991; Conville, 1998; Rawlins, 1992; Yerby, 1995), particularly in the notion of centripetal and centrifugal—or coming-together and coming-apart—dynamics. Just as an individualistic perspective continues to serve as the default mode of most medical encounters, so too does a curative mindset. Familiarity with relational dialectics could complement existing systems thinking in the clinical context by emphasizing change and its associated tensions as a feature of relationships to be *negotiated* through communication rather than *mitigated* through treatment. Much may be gained on both sides if communication scholars recognize the efforts of family practitioners to address the needs of families, frame our communication research in ways that will positively impact clinical practice, and support the notion that practitioners and families alike must traverse health transitions in partnership.

References

Accreditation Council for Graduate Medical Education (2001). *Program requirements for residency education in family medicine, Effective July 1, 2001.* Available from the ACGME website http://www.acgme.org/acWebsite/downloads/RRC_progReq/120pr701.pdf.

Accreditation Council for Graduate Medical Education. (2009). *Outcome Project: Enhancing residency education through outcomes assessment.* Available from http://www.acgme.org/outcome

Ackerman, N. (1966). *Treating the troubled family.* New York: Basic Books.

Bateson, G. (1972). *Steps to an ecology of mind.* New York: Ballantine.

Bavelas, J. B. (1984). On "naturalistic" family research. *Family Process, 23,* 337-341.

Baxter, L. A., & Clark, C. L. (1996). Perceptions of family communication patterns and the enactment of family rituals. *Western Journal of Communication, 60,* 254-268.

Baxter, L. A., & Harper, A. M. (1998). The role of rituals in the management of the dialectical tensions of "old" and "new" in blended families. *Communication Studies, 49,* 101-120.

Baxter, L. A., & Montgomery, B. M. (1996). *Relating: Dialogues and dialectics.* New York: Guilford Press.

Bochner, A. P. (1978). On taking ourselves seriously: An analysis of some persistent problems and promising directions in interpersonal research. *Human Communication Research, 4,* 179-191.

Bochner, A. P. (1981). Forming warm ideas. In C. Wickler-Mott & J. H. Weakland (Eds.), *Rigor and imagination: Essays from the legacy of Gregory Bateson* (pp. 65-81). New York: Praeger.

Bochner, A. P. (1984). The functions of communication in interpersonal bonding. In C. Arnold & J. Bowers (Eds.), *The handbook of rhetoric and communication* (pp. 544-621). Needham Heights, MA: Allyn & Bacon.

Bochner, A. P. (Ed.) (1989). Applying communication theory to family process [Special issue]. *Journal of Applied Communication Research, 17,* 1-2.

Bowen, M. (1978). *Family therapy in clinical practice.* New York: Jason Aronson.

Candib, L. M. (1985). The family approach at each moment. *Family Medicine, 17*(5), 201-208.

Candib, L. M. (1995). *Medicine and the family: A feminist perspective.* New York: Basic Books.

Carter, B., & McGoldrick, M. (Eds.) (1980). *The family lifecycle: A framework for family therapy.* New York: Gardner Press.

Carter, B., & McGoldrick, M. (Eds.) (1988). *The changing family lifecycle: A framework for family therapy.* New York: Gardner Press.

Carter, B., & McGoldrick, M. (Eds.) (1999). *The expanded family lifecycle: Individual, family and social perspectives* (3rd ed.). Needham Heights, MA: Allyn & Bacon.

Cohen-Katz, J. L., Miller, W. L., & Borkan, J. M. (2003). Building a culture of resident well-being: Creating self-reflection, community, and positive identity in family practice residency education. *Families, Systems, & Health, 21*(3), 293-304.

Collaborative Family Healthcare Association. (2008). *Mission Statement.* Available from http://www.cfha.net/pages/Mission-Statement.

Conville, R. L. (1991). *Relational transitions.* Westport, CT: Praeger.

Conville, R. L. (1998). Telling stories: Dialectics of relational transition. In B. M. Montgomery & L. A. Baxter (Eds.), *Dialectical approaches to studying personal relationships* (pp. 17-40). Mahwah, NJ: Erlbaum.

Dougherty, W. J., & Baird, M. A. (1983). *Family therapy and family medicine: Toward the primary care of families.* New York: Guilford Press.

Dougherty, W. J., & Baird, M. A. (1986). Developmental levels of physician involvement with families. *Family Medicine, 18,* 153-156.

Dougherty, W. J., & Baird, M. A. (Eds.) (1987). *Family-centered medical care: A clinical casebook.* New York: Guilford Press.

Elia, J. (2003). Queering relationships: Toward a paradigmatic shift. *Journal of Homosexuality, 45,* 61-86.

Foster, E. (2008). Commitment, communication, and contending with heteronormativity: An invitation to greater reflexivity in interpersonal research. *Southern Communication Journal, 73,* 84-101.

Haley, J. (1963). *Strategies of psychotherapy.* New York: Grune & Stratton.

Hallström, L. (Director), & Hedges, P. (Writer). (1993). *What's eating Gilbert Grape?* [Motion picture]. United States: Paramount Pictures.

Jorgenson, J. (1989). Where is the "family" in family communication? Exploring families' self-definitions. *Journal of Applied Communication Research, 17,* 27-41.

Jorgenson, J., & Bochner, A. P. (2004). Imagining families through stories and rituals. In A. Vangelisti (Ed.), *Handbook of family communication* (pp. 513-538). Mahwah, NJ: Erlbaum.

Knapp, M. L., & Vangelisti, A. L. (2000). *Interpersonal communication and human relationships* (4th ed.). Needham Heights, MA: Allyn & Bacon.

Koenig Kellas, J. (2006). Finding meaning in difficult family experiences: Sense-making and interaction processes during joint family storytelling. *Journal of Family Communication, 6,* 49-76.

Lannamann, M. (1989). Communication theory applied to relational change: A case study in Milan systemic family therapy. *Journal of Applied Communication Research, 17,* 71-91.

Levine, C., & Zuckerman, C. (1999). The trouble with families: Toward an ethic of accommodation.. *Annals of Internal Medicine, 130*(2), 148-152.

McDaniel, S. H., Campbell, T. L., Hepworth, J., & Lorenz, A. (2005) *Family-oriented primary care* (2nd Ed.). New York: Springer-Verlag.

McDaniel, S. H., Campbell, T. L., & Seaburn, D. (1990) *Family-oriented primary care: A manual for medical providers.* New York: Springer-Verlag.

McDaniel, S. H., Hepworth, J., & Dougherty, W. (1992). *Medical family therapy: A biopsychosocial approach to families with health problems.* New York: Basic Books.

McGoldrick, M., Gerson, R., & Shellenberger, S. (1999). *Genograms: Assessment and intervention* (2nd ed.). New York: Norton.

McNamee, S. (1989). Creating new narratives in family therapy: An application of social constructionism. *Journal of Applied Communication Research, 17,* 92-112.

Millar, F. E., & Rogers, L. E. (1976). A relational approach to interpersonal communication. In G. R. Miller (Ed.), *Explorations in interpersonal communication* (pp. 87-104). Beverly Hills, CA: Sage.

Miller, W. L. (2004). The clinical hand: A curricular map for relationship-centered care. *Family Medicine, 36*(5), 330-335.

Miller, W. L. (1999). The ecological-transactional systemic map of primary care. In B. Crabtree & W. Miller (Eds.), *Doing qualitative research* (p. xii). Thousand Oaks, CA: Sage Publications.

Minuchin, S. (1974). *Families and family therapy.* Cambridge, MA: Harvard University Press.

Minuchin, S., & Fishman, C. H. (1981). *Family therapy techniques.* Cambridge, MA: Harvard University Press.

Morris, D. (1998). *Illness and culture in the postmodern age.* Berkeley: University of California.

Rawlins, W. K. (1992). *Friendship matters: Relational dialectics and the life course.* New York: Aldine DeGruyter.

Rogers, L. E., & Escudero, V. (Eds.) (2004). *Relational communication: An interactional perspective to the study of process and form.* Mahwah, NJ: Erlbaum.

Satir, V. (1967). *Conjoint family therapy.* Palo Alto, CA: Science and Behavior Books.

Seale, C. (1998). *Constructing death: The sociology of dying and bereavement.* Cambridge, England: Cambridge University.

Sieburg, E. (1985). *Family communication: An integrated systems approach.* New York: Gardener Press.

Stephens, G. G. (1979). Family medicine as counter-culture. *Family Medicine Teacher, 11*(5), 14-18.

Thrower, S. M., Bruce, W. E., & Walton, R. F. (1982). The family circle method for integrating family systems concepts in family medicine. *Journal of Family Practice, 15,* 451-457.

Tresolini, C. P., & the Pew Fetzer Task Force (1994). *Health professions education and relationship centered care.* San Francisco, CA: Pew Health Professions Commission.

Watzlawick, P., Beavin, J., & Jackson, D. D. (1967). *Pragmatics of human communication.* New York: Norton.

Yerby, J. (1995). Family systems theory reconsidered: Integrating social construction theory and dialectical process. *Communication Theory, 5,* 339-365.

PART 5

End-of-Life Transitions

CHAPTER 13

Transitioning from Independence to Dependence: Family Relational Adaptation to Alzheimer's Disease

Thomas J. Hipper

BLOOMBERG SCHOOL OF PUBLIC HEALTH, JOHNS HOPKINS UNIVERSITY

Danielle Catona and Jon F. Nussbaum

THE PENNSYLVANIA STATE UNIVERSITY

> *"I was devastated, frightened, and upset. But I knew that our family would make the best of it. I knew my grandmother was in good hands, and that I would be a big part of [taking care of her]." —Grandchild*[1]

In caring for an older adult with Alzheimer's Disease (AD), family caregivers demonstrate remarkable strength and courage when attempting to physically and emotionally care for a loved one. While there is an ample amount of academic and popular literature addressing the care of individuals with AD, there has been less attention paid to explaining how the caregiving process impacts the entire family system. In this chapter we will review what is known about the profound effects of AD on families. In this review we seek to highlight the impact of AD on primary caregivers and secondary caregivers while acknowledging how environmental factors affect how families manage care during this health transition. We conclude the chapter by discussing implications for future research and argue that the

1 Brief interviews were conducted with former Alzheimer's caregivers in order to provide unique insight into how the disease truly impacts the entire family system.

"ripple effect" of caregiving, in which the entire family system is affected by the monumental caring effort, deserves more attention.

Alzheimer's Disease

AD is a progressive disorder characterized by the insidious onset of cognitive difficulties, ranging from minor confusion in its early stages toward severe dementia in its later stages, and ultimately leading to death (Harwood, 2007). It is the most common form of dementia (it is estimated to account for over half of all dementia cases) and currently affects over 4 million people in the United States (Liu & Gallagher-Thompson, 2009). Named after Dr. Alois Alzheimer, a German physician who lived during the early 1900s and studied changes in the brain tissue of mentally ill patients, AD is characterized by abnormal clumps (amyloid plaques) and tangled bundles of fibers (neurofibrillary tangles) composed of misplaced proteins in the brain (Kemper, Anagnopoulos, Lyons, & Heberlein, 1994). Though the causes are still unclear, it is believed that the disease is caused by a combination of genetic and environmental risk factors including diet, exercise, and mental activity throughout the lifespan. In fact, AD can only be definitely determined after death following an examination of the brain (Harwood). In addition to being difficult to diagnose, the diagnosis is likely to be made in the context of pre-existing health problems. As a result of the fact that physiological problems and disease states accumulate in late life, co-morbidity has become known as the "ultimate geriatric syndrome" (Stephens & Franks, 2009; Yancik et al., 2007).

The risk for the disease increases with age, though in extremely rare cases, it can be found in younger individuals. AD is found most frequently in older adults over the age of 85 (Wright, Sparks, & O'Hair, 2008). While only about 3% of 65-75-year-olds suffer from the disease, prevalence of AD increases dramatically beyond the age of 65, with up to 50% of people over the age of 85 currently suffering from the disease (Baltes, 1997; Harwood, 2007; U.S. Department of Health and Human Services, 2005). The life expectancy for an individual diagnosed with AD is variable, ranging from 5 to 20 years with an average survival rate of 8.5 years from initial diagnosis (Kemper et al., 1994). The degenerative nature of the disease makes living with or caring for someone with AD an incredibly difficult experience.

Alzheimer's Disease in an Aging Society

With advances in medical care and increased life expectancy, individuals are advancing into later years in life. As a result, our society is experiencing an epidemiological shift in which individuals are becoming increasingly susceptible to chronic physical and mental health problems (Stephens & Franks, 2009). By 2050, the total population over age 65 within the U.S. is expected to double, while the number of people older than 85 is expected to triple (U.S. Census Bureau, 2000). As the Baby Boomer generation ages, an unprecedented increase in the rates of AD is expected. Despite the fact that Baby Boomers have, on average, higher levels of education, which is a protective factor against AD, the number of AD cases is expected to increase to between 11 and 16 million by the year 2050 (Hebert, Scherr, Bienias, Bennett, & Evans, 2003; Mortimer & Graves, 1993). In fact, some have likened the expected prevalence rates of AD to an epidemic tantamount to the AIDS crisis (Flint, Query & Parrish, 2005). As the prevalence of AD increases, so, too, does the likelihood that individuals will need assistance performing daily activities and that they will be cared for by one or more of their family members (Schulz & Martire, 2004; Stephens & Franks).

Caregiving for Family Members with Alzheimer's Disease

Although the primary objective of this chapter is to move beyond individual caregiver stress and, instead, focus on the entire family system, it is important to note that a considerable amount of research has examined individual primary caregivers in the context of AD. Development of dementia is associated with nearly twice the likelihood of dependency onset, significantly increasing the need for family caregivers (Wolff, Boult, Boyd, & Anderson, 2005). The primary responsibility of caregiving often falls to one family member, referred to as the primary caregiver, and does so in a fairly predictable way (Aneshensel, Pearlin, Mullan, Zarit, & Whitlatch, 1995). The spouse of the ill person is the most likely to assume the role of primary caregiver, followed by adult children, and then siblings (Bourgeois, Schulz, & Burgio, 1996; Davey, 2000). The likelihood of assuming the role of adult-child caregiver is highly gendered, as daughters are three times more likely than sons to assume the role of primary caregiver (Stephens &

Franks, 2009). Moreover, as the severity of the illness for the care receiver increases, daughters are even more likely to assume the role of primary caregiver (Stone & Kemper, 1990).

> *"The lack of privacy was also difficult for me. I don't need a lot of alone time, but everybody needs some. It was almost impossible to find a time that I could spend by myself." —adult daughter caregiver*

The debilitating nature of AD, coupled with the many difficulties of caring for a patient with Alzheimer's, can cause both patients and caregivers to suffer (Orange, 2001). Primary caregivers of family members with AD experience an incredible burden including high levels of psychological, emotional, social, financial, and physical stress (Hummert & Nussbaum, 2001; Kramer, 1997). The frequency of caregiving burdens has led some to define family caregivers as "hidden patients" (Gilliland & Bush, 2001). Caregiving has been found to be positively associated with depression (Adams, 2007; Cohen & Eisdorfer, 1988; Haley, 1997), and depression associated with AD caregiving has often been studied within the marital context (Choi & Marks, 2006). Most caregiver spouses indicated a decline in marital quality and disruptions in the marital relationship that lead to feelings of sorrow, guilt, anger, resentment, and even hostility (Knop, Bergman-Evans, & Wharton, 1998; Robinson, 1990; Wright, 1993). Pecchioni, Wright, & Nussbaum (2005) explain that, "As caregivers, marital partners may have to spend an enormous amount of time meeting the physical needs of a parent, and most people do not have the experience, skills, or training that are necessary to handle the responsibility of caregiving" (p. 84).

Congruent with the notion that caring for a loved one with AD induces significant stress, non-dementia caregivers were found to have significantly lower levels of stress than AD caregivers (Bertrand, Fredman, & Saczynski, 2006). In fact, dementia caregivers were commonly found to commit 40 or more hours per week of additional time than non-dementia caregivers, or the equivalent of a full-time job (Liu & Gallagher-Thompson, 2009). Compounding this problem, the Family Caregiver Alliance (2009) notes that more than one-third of caregivers suffer from poor health themselves while trying to provide care for others.

The stage of the disease plays a significant role in the responsibilities and stress of the primary caregiver (Pfeiffer, 1999). Earlier stages of AD include symptoms such as mild confusion and memory problems, and communication impairments including a failure to take part in family conversations or an inability to sustain conversations (Harwood, 2007; Wright, et al., 2008). However, as the disease progresses, symptoms worsen and people often become more dependent on caregivers, increasing the magnitude of caregiving difficulties. At later stages of the disease, patients are unable to manage activities of daily living (ADL), including getting out of bed, getting dressed, incontinence, bathing, and feeding. Primary caregivers are also likely to assist with instrumental activities of daily living (IADL), including medication management, transportation, shopping, house work, preparing meals, and managing finances (Wolff et al., 2005). The functional limitations experienced by Alzheimer's patients lead to an increased functional dependency on caregivers, increasing the responsibilities and, in many cases, the stress of family caregivers (Harwood; Stephens & Franks, 2009).

> *Although I knew Mom was having trouble with remembering things, when I finally convinced her to go to the neurologist and was told she had Alzheimer's, I was devastated and worried... I was so afraid she would not remember her family and that broke my heart. —Adult-child (Daughter)*

It is important, however, to note that, in addition to the negative effects of caregiving, primary caregivers have also reported a number of positive aspects associated with caring for a family member with AD (Beach, 1997). Many adult-caregivers find that their parent-care responsibilities are quite rewarding. In fact, women were more likely to report the rewards of providing parent care than they were to report stressors (Stephens & Franks, 2009). While the positive effects of providing care to family members with AD are important and must be considered, the tremendous burden placed on family caregivers, coupled with the expected increase in AD prevalence, means that other family members will play a significant role in the caregiving duties. In the remainder of this chapter we focus on this comparatively understudied area of family caregiving, explicating what we currently know and what deserves greater attention if we hope to improve the ability of families to care for their loved ones and cope with this terrible disease.

The Ripple Effect

We contend that it is important to view Alzheimer's as a family problem rather than solely the problem of the afflicted individual or his/her primary caregiver. When a family member becomes seriously ill, the entire family system is often affected and adjustments are necessary for effective family functioning and in maintaining family relationships (Segrin & Flora, 2005). This effect of Alzheimer's disease on the entire family system is what we refer to as *the ripple effect*. Data from national surveys indicate that 38% of caregivers are spouses, compared to 31% who are daughters or daughters-in-law, and 11% who are sons. The remaining 20% of caregivers consist of siblings, grandchildren, other relatives, and non-kin (Wolff & Kasper, 2006).

> *"Mom lived with me so I was the primary caregiver. Thankfully my immediate family was willing to do all they could to help Mom and I. We worked together keeping her active and keeping her company. My family (husband, 2 young adult children) gave me full support, letting me vent, laugh, cry, and helped me to take time for myself." —Adult-child (Daughter)*

Regardless of the family role of the caregiver, studies find there are consequences of providing long-term care for a loved one suffering from dementia (e.g., Gaugler, Mendiondo, Smith, & Schmitt, 2003). Moving beyond an examination of the effects of caregiving on an individual caregiver, this next section explores consequences of care for the marital relationship, adult children, grandchildren, and siblings. In addition, we review what we currently know about family decision making and social support networks with respect to caregiving.

Caregiving Networks

According to family systems theory, all family members are interdependent (Boss, 1987; Whitchurch & Constantine, 1993). The actions of one member affect all other members of the family and the family unit as a whole. For example, when one member becomes a caregiver for an Alzheimer's patient, the family dynamic is dramatically altered (Brody, 1989). Depending on the stage of life of the family caregiver, various relationships are affected in different ways. Spousal caregivers experience changes in the marital relationship. Adult-children caregivers experience changes in their multiple roles as an adult-child, spouse, parent, and employee (Goode, 1960). Grandchildren caregivers experience changes in the parent-child, sibling, and grandparent-grandchild relationship (Beach, 1994, 1997).

While family systems theory provides an important framework for understanding the systemic nature of families, it does not address an important assumption that is present in much of the caregiving research. Much of the current research literature uses the term "primary caregiver" to refer to the individual (usually the spouse or daughter) who assumes caregiving responsibilities. In this case then, "secondary caregivers" would be described as other family members or friends who provide assistance both to the primary caregiver and the impaired adult (Stephens & Franks, 2009). However, we argue that it is helpful to view the process of family caregiving as comprised of caregiving teams or *caregiving networks*, in which multiple caregivers share authority and responsibility and, ideally, "perceive themselves to be organized in a clear and integrated manner" (Brewer, 2002; Keith, 1995, p. 184). The following describes what we know about caregiving for different players in the caregiving network.

Adult Child

> *"Our family pulled together tightly. The kids took Mom on outings and kept her company. My daughter was home during the day and made lunch and snacks for her. My son took time off from school to be with Mom when she was hospitalized. He was with her all day and kept her spirits high. My husband would cook for her, help me get her to doctor appointments and spar verbally with her, which she loved. They had a particularly strong relationship for mother and son-in-law." —adult daughter caregiver*

Several major trends have altered the nature of family environments including: increased longevity of older adults, the changing role of women in our society, the time of marriage, the time of childbirth, more adult children choosing to live at home during college years, and more adult children returning home after divorce (Brody, 1981; Lindgren & Decker, 1996; Treas, 1979). As a result, middle-aged adults may find themselves "sandwiched" between caregiving for their elderly parent and parenting their adolescent children (Williams & Nussbaum, 2001).

"Sandwich generation caregivers" is a term for individuals who care for an older family member while also caring for a child under 18 years old living at home (Tebes & Irish, 2000). These individuals are typically between 45 and 65 years old, and are faced with the challenge of finding time, energy, and resources to balance the needs of aging parents, with the needs of dependent children, and responsibilities associated with work (Lindgren & Decker, 1996).

Several studies have focused on the parent-adult child relationship and the subsequent effects on the adult child's relationship with his/her children. Hamill's (1994) study reported relationship strain between the adult child caregiver and parent negatively influenced communication with the caregiver's own children. Similarly, more psychological stress was reported between parents and children in elderly caregiving families (Malone-Beach, DeGenova, & Otani, 1998; Pruchno, Peters, & Burant, 1996). Caregiver stress associated with elder parent care was also expressed physically. Stolley and Szinovacz (1997) found that caregiving mothers were more likely than non-caregiving mothers to use physical force and spank their children.

Grandchild

Beach (1994) indicated children's relationships with their parents, siblings, and grandparents are both negatively and positively affected when their parent became a caregiver. Specifically, these children expressed frustration with vying for attention from the primary caregiver and confronting the Alzheimer's-afflicted grandparent's violent behavior. Children also mentioned growing closer to the caregiver and spending more time with siblings during the period of providing care for a grandparent.

Many studies have supported both negative and positive caregiving consequences. Creasey and Jarvis (1989) found that mothers' caregiver burden negatively affected children's relationships with their fathers and Alzheimer's-afflicted grandparents, and similar studies suggest an explanation for this occurrence. Brody's (1989) study reported resentment of mother's caregiving burdens and tension between grandparents and grandchildren. Some granddaughters were upset with the amount of bickering between their grandmother and mother, while others resented that the burden reduced the time their mother spent with them. Similarly, in a study by Szinovacz (2003) children expressed resentment of their parent paying more attention to and spending more time with their Alzheimer's-afflicted grandparent than with them. Children also reported parents taking out caregiving stress on them, becoming stricter, and imposing more rules. These negative consequences resulted in an increase in the number of arguments among parents and children (Szinovacz).

In a follow-up study, Beach (1997) further examined positive caregiving consequences. Children attributed sibling and parent bonding to the caregiving predicament. For example, caregiving tasks for a relative with Alzheimer's disease increased the number of opportunities for sibling interactions. Older siblings (living away from home) acknowledged younger siblings' caregiving responsibilities and therefore visited more regularly. Children often assisted mothers with caregiving responsibilities. Mothers' positive reinforcement and verbal praise for these efforts resulted in children feeling valued. Discussions about the serious aspects of caregiving, which included the care recipients' health condition and care plan, reinforced the children feeling valued and fostered a greater sense of intimacy between mothers and children. A greater sense of closeness was described as a result of children listening about mothers' caregiving stress and helping them work through emotional outbursts. Observing the physical and emotional toll of caregiving led to children's greater appreciation and respect for their caregiving mother.

> *"My entire family helped out in my grandmother's care. My parents were her primary caregivers but my brother and I helped out when we could. I saw my role as to try and continue to treat her as the same grandmother as I always knew even though there was always this sense of changing. I have very vivid memories of helping her do things that she had always done on her own."* —*Grandchild*

Similarly, Szinovacz (2003) found children showed empathy and respect for the parent who was the primary caregiver. Joint involvement in the caregiving experience strengthened the relationship between the child and the caregiving parent. Stronger relational ties were also reported as a result of the caregiving parent asking the child for assistance and openly discussing the care recipient's needs. Care recipients prompted parent-child interactions by sharing stories about the caregiving parents' youth. This allowed parents and children to learn more about each other while sharing similar experiences about growing up. In another example, Fruhauf, Jarrott, and Allen (2006) found that grandchildren caregivers reported filial obligation and preparing for future caregiving responsibilities as reasons for assisting with the caregiving process.

Sibling

> *"I have two sisters. My younger sister dropped out after we decided to move Mother here. During the 7 years Mother lived here, both in my guest house and in nursing care, she visited her twice. Even then, one of those times [my older sister] and I basically forced her to come. She has chosen to live her life according to different values than those held by the rest of the family, so our relationship has never been really close. However she was close to Mother, and rather dependent on Mother as well. I can't explain why she chose to close Mother out for the last 7 years of her life.*
>
> *I have a much closer relationship to [my older siste] than I had before. There is 9 years difference in our ages, and we had not lived in the same city as adults in 25 years. So I was given the opportunity to get to know her in a whole new way. Not only that, but I enormously appreciated her sacrificial giving up of her own life to move here to help with Mother's care. I could not have done what I did without her." —Adult-Child (Daughter)*

Sibling relationships are potentially the longest-enduring family relationships of all (Bedford, 1995). The National Survey of Families and Households reported that individuals usually consider siblings potential sources of support even if they do not actually help each other very often. This is especially true of older adult siblings (White, 2001; White & Riedmann, 1992). Similar studies reported that siblings are considered potential sources of instrumental and emotional support for the 80 percent of individuals age 65 and over who have at least one living sibling (Avioli, 1989; Connidis, 1989, 1994). Connidis (1994) found one-fifth to one-third of older adults would turn to a sibling for longer-term help when ill, and one-fifth to one-quarter would live with a sibling if needed. Due to the equal distribution of power and generational solidarity that characterizes sibling relationships, siblings are especially suited to provide emotional support. Being from the same generation increases the ability to empathize with similar others and reflect on the importance of shared experiences (Cumming & Schneider, 1961). Based on the various types of support provided by siblings, it is not surprising that they serve a protective role against the risk of nursing home admission. Freedman (1996) found having at least one sibling reduced an older person's chances of admission by about one-fourth. While, in many caregiving cases, siblings have been found to provide support and care for one another; in other cases, differences of opinion among siblings may generate considerable conflict (Pecchioni et al., 2005). Despite the significant potential role that siblings can play within the family caregiving system, they remain largely understudied in this context.

Family Unit as a Whole

Caregiving for Alzheimer's patients affects the dynamics of the family unit as a whole. When a diagnosis of a chronic illness like AD occurs, family anxiety is typically quite high, which may negatively affect the well-being of all members of the family, with subsequent consequences rippling throughout the family system (Leske & Jiricka, 1998: Pecchioni, Thompson, & Anderson, 2006). Strains experienced by caregivers have repercussions for other family members "as the balance of roles and responsibilities changes and shifts occur in the family homeostasis," (Brody, 1981, p. 472). In a study by Szinovacz (2003), negative family dynamics included an increase in the number of family tensions and a decrease in the number of family activities. Specifically, family members mentioned heightened conflict between parents, arguments directed against the care recipient, and significant decrease or altogether elimination of "normal" family discourse. Research implies that most families eventually adapt to care predicaments, sometimes furthered by outside support and counseling (Szinovacz). Some family members even express closer family bonding as a result of coping with the Alzheimer's-afflicted patients' aberrant behaviors (Beach, 1997). In Beach's studies, family bonding was facilitated primarily by the use of humor as a coping mechanism (Beach, 1994, 1997).

These findings suggest that caregiving does, indeed, have a ripple effect on the entire family. In fact, a study by Fisher and Lieberman (1996) found that family environment, when operationalized as organization, conflict avoidance, and avoidance of guilt reduction, is more strongly associated with the well-being of Alzheimer's caregivers than the actual severity of the disorder. Indeed, the manner in which the entire family system interacts can play a vital role in either keeping caregivers from becoming overburdened, or contributing to their burden (Segrin & Flora, 2005). As Pecchioni et al., (2006) pointed out:

> Having a seriously ill family member alters the ways in which family members interact with each other and the responsibilities each person takes on in the family system. Not only must families adjust to their new situation, but they must also make sense of what is happening to the sick person and to the family unit, especially if the illness is terminal. (p. 458)

Families often restructure their lives in order to provide care for their ill family member. This period of reorganization includes the process of making difficult decisions.

Family Decision Making

Bethea (2002) pointed out that "the decision of moving an older adult parent into the home is much more than knowing how to set-up the guest bedroom, fill prescriptions, or cook a meal" (p. 122). Despite the large numbers of older adults requiring familial caregiving, we know little about how families make decisions related to care (Whitlatch, 2008). When decisions are made concerning family members with AD, stakeholders of the decision include the care receiver and other family members who provide varying degrees of care. In making these decisions, balance is sought between the needs of the care receiver and the abilities of the family network to provide care, and rarely is this an easy process (Feinberg, Newman, Gray, & Kolb, 2004; Pecchioni, 2001; Wackerbarth, 1999). The most difficult decisions revolve around providing care, including deciding between in-home and nursing home care, and deciding who will assist with the caregiving. For example, we do know that family responsibility and societal expectations can make caregivers feel guilty about using support services, and that many caregivers will even put themselves at risk to avoiding sending their loved one to a nursing home (Wackerbarth).

> *"We followed our usual procedure and called a family confab. We chose to hold this meeting in my home because it was centrally located. After much discussion, it was decided that Mother would move to live here, that [my older sister] would also move here, and that Mother would live with [my older sister] after she had gotten settled in. We used a white board and brainstormed ideas for possible solutions, then prioritized and eliminated. Everyone was pleased with our ultimate decision except Mother, who still thought she could live by herself." —Adult-child (Daughter)*

Even when agreement is reached and "optimal" choices are made, families still experience grief due to a lack of guidance in the decision-making process. Tension among family members as a result of differing opinions contributes to the stress of caregiving and indecision. Often those family members farther from the primary caregiver do not realize the full extent of the situation, may feel left out, or may be suggesting decisions based on different information (Wackerbarth, 1999). More information is needed to understand how members of the family caregiving system make important decisions about care provision and roles so that the entire family can work cohesively to provide care for their loved ones. Social support networks have the potential to play an integral role in the ability of families to provide care.

Social Support Networks

Considering our discussion thus far, it is clear that there can be significant stress associated with caring for an individual with Alzheimer's. Yet, there are also processes that serve to buffer this stress. It is well established that social support can act as a buffer for stress, and studies have shown that increased social support leads to better well-being and a lower risk of depression for caregivers (Atienza, Collins, & King, 2001; Cohen & Wills, 1985). Social support received in the context of family networks has been found to result in positive effects, benefits, and rewards for both the care recipient and provider

(Bearon, 2004; Donelan et al., 2002; Kramer, 1997). Communication is a vital conduit for the provision of support, and family communication has been shown to influence both patient and family adaptation to illness (Ell, 1996). However, it is important to consider both the ways in which individuals have trouble obtaining support from their network and the consequences of non-support.

Alzheimer's caregivers often have difficulty obtaining social support from both family and outside sources. Evidence suggests that family members repeatedly express a need for more information from health professionals, but experience difficulty in obtaining this information (Ell, 1996). Family members also report receiving inadequate or misguided support from family and friends, including a lack of information and assistance, and few opportunities to express distress. Poor flow of information in families also may result in less satisfactory reallocation of roles, more role conflict and role strain, less family cohesion and greater family conflict (Ell).

Perhaps the most alarming concern is that, as a result of the demanding process of caring for a family member with AD, one risks reducing one's access to the very social networks that he or she needs to rely on during this period (Schulz & Martire, 2004). Spending tremendous amounts of time and energy with the patient can cause distance between caregivers and their network, making it less likely that the caregivers will receive the support they need. Family caregivers have shown reluctance to request assistance until their needs become severe, and by then it may be more difficult to obtain that support (Ell, 1996). In addition, the mere perception that social support has been lost can result in similar psychological consequences for the caregiver as those associated with actually losing the support (Cohen & Wills, 1985). As a result, when considering caregiving from a family perspective, it is vital to acknowledge the positive potential of social support networks, while also considering the common ways in which they become inaccessible to family caregivers.

Environmental Factors

While the focus of this chapter is on family and relational dynamics, it is important to consider that the caregiving process does not occur in a vacuum; but rather, the process is subjected to and impacted by a number of macro-level environmental factors. Two of the relevant environmental factors, long-term health care and institutional care, are outlined briefly below.

Long-term care policy. The Alzheimer's Association (2006) revealed that, "Alzheimer's disease is the most expensive uninsured illness older Americans are likely to face" (p. 12). This emphasizes the need for improved medical, long-term, and social care for individuals with Alzheimer's or related dementias (ADRDs) (Chodosh et al., 2007; Schubert et al., 2006; Sloan, Trogdon, Curtis, & Schulman, 2004; Warchol, 2004). Many factors influence the current health care received by individuals with ADRDs including policy issues, medical reimbursement systems, and nursing home care (Brauner, Muir, & Sachs, 2000; Luchins & Hanrahan, 1993; Newcomer, Fox, & Harrington, 2001; Sloan et al.).

Two publicly funded programs that provide health assistance for older adults include Medicare and Medicaid. Medicare is a health insurance program under the Social Security administration and Health and Human Services that provides reimbursement to physicians and hospitals for medical treatment of adults who are over the age of 65. Medicaid is an income needs based public policy program for the poor (Whitlatch & Feinberg, 2007). Eligibility for older adults includes being a United States citizen or legal immigrant over the age of 65 who is poor or has become poor due to long-term care spending. In 2005, Medicare costs for individuals with ADRDs were $91 billion. Medicaid costs for nursing home care were $21 billion (Alzheimer's Association, 2007).

Despite good intentions, these programs have many limitations. For example, the majority of long-term care and drug costs for individuals with ADRDs are not covered by Medicare (Alzheimer's Association, 2001). Utilization of assessment criteria such as activities of daily living (ADLs), behavioral issues, and mini-mental status cutoff points decreases the numbers of individuals with ADRDs who are eligible for publicly funded long-term care benefits (Fox, Maslow, & Zhang, 1999). As a result, families have to pay for much of Alzheimer's-afflicted individuals' care costs (Alzheimer's Association). This is especially alarming considering that restricted health care access and unmet care-recipient needs have been shown to be predictive of earlier nursing home placement or even mortality (Gaugler, Kane, Kane, & Newcomer, 2005).

Programs such as the National Family Caregiver Support Program (NFCSP) provide funding to support caregivers of older relatives (Whitlatch & Feinberg, 2007). While such funding is needed and helpful, many states still receive such modest funding that the overall impact is minimal. In addition, awareness of the availability of programs like NFCSP is quite low. There are several policies currently under review that would serve to improve the health care and address unmet needs of individuals with ADRDs including the Geriatric Assessment and Chronic Care Coordination Act of 2007, Alzheimer's Treatment and Caregiver Support Act of 2007, and Nurse Faculty and Physical Therapist Education Act of 2007 (Murray, & Boyd, 2009). However, it remains to be seen if these policies, if instituted, would have similar budgetary concerns as programs like the NFCSP.

> *"Our role was just to go visit, seemingly more for our benefit than hers because she no longer remembered who we were." —Grandchild*

Institutions. When families are no longer able to care for their Alzheimer's-afflicted relative they may opt for formal care. Common formal care options include nursing homes (NHs) and assisted living facilities (ALFs). NHs are defined as facilities that have three or more beds and routinely provide nursing care services (Gabrel, 2000). Transitioning to the around-the-clock care setting includes relinquishing decisions such as when to eat, bathe, and sleep (Abrams & Beers, 1995). Nursing home caregivers contribute to feelings of powerlessness (Ryan, Giles, Bartolucci, & Henwood, 1986). Caregiver interaction with residents is often controlling (Lanceley, 1985), task-oriented (Grainger, 1995; Lubinski, 1995; Williams, Ilten, & Bower, 2005), and patronizing (Ashburn & Gordon, 1981; Ryan, Hummert, & Boich, 1995). Such interactions contribute to learned helplessness (Rodin & Langer, 1980), reinforce dependency (Baltes & Wahl, 1996), and negatively affect older adult self-concept and future interpersonal interactions (Ryan et al., 1986). The SUPPORT study revealed NH resident dissatisfaction. Findings indicated 30% of older adults preferred death to permanent NH placement (Matimore et al., 1997).

ALFs are possible alternatives to NHs. These facilities differ in their levels of service and privacy, and offer qualities somewhere between the privacy and family caregiving experienced by older people living in their homes and nursing homes (Mitchell and Kemp, 2000). The goal of ALFs is to enable residents to maintain independence by promoting autonomy, dignity, and personal choice (National Center for Assisted Living, 2001). The success of ALFs in achieving these goals and overcoming the problems encountered in traditional NHs remains unknown.

Implications for Future Research

In light of demographic trends, the difficulty of providing care for an individual with Alzheimer's, and the strong evidence that suggests that multiple family members can and should be part of the caregiving process, we suggest that future research continue to examine caregiving from a family systems perspective. Care in this context is no longer the work of one "primary caregiver." Instead it involves several people being able to contribute in a variety of ways. In addition to future research, interventions must also take this into account. Whitlatch and Feinberg (2007) found that the best interventions are targeted to the caregiver's needs and stressors and are structured in a manner that is receptive to the caregiver. This includes taking into account the relationship to the person with AD, the stage of disease, and the setting in which care is taking place.

While we concur with these recommendations, we also suggest that these interventions take all family members into account, not just the patient and primary caregiver. By taking into account this key component, we can strengthen interventions that have already been found to reduce the stress of both caregivers and other family members who are less active in providing care (Amirkhanyan & Wolf, 2006; Mitrani et al., 2006) We are not alone in these recommendations, as Brewer (2002) suggested that macro-level policies should focus on caregiving systems rather than focusing exclusively on either primary caregivers or care recipients.

A greater focus on communication, from both an interpersonal and message strategy perspective, is needed in this area as well. While significant attention has been paid to communication deficits resulting from AD (Harwood, 2007), and to communication strategies between caregivers and care receivers (Small & Guttman, 2002), more attention should be paid to understanding effective communication strategies between multiple caregivers within the family network. A better understanding of how families can effectively communicate caregiving concerns and strategies will help families deal with the difficult decisions associated with caregiving as well as ensure that all members of the family get the most out of the entire family support network.

From a message strategy perspective, more effort needs to be placed on encouraging men to take a more active role in the caregiving process. Lawrence, Goodnow, Woods, and Karantzas (2002) suggest that effectively framing recommended action can help to increase male involvement. They posit that messages are likely to be more effective if they involve tasks that are seen as able to be done by either sons or daughters rather than those that are typically seen by the group as being tightly tied to gender. The purpose of doing this is not to make blanket assumptions about what men and women should (or are willing) to do, but to tailor messages in such a way that men perceive the departure from the norm of doing very little as realistic and doable. While this is but one suggestion, the authors agree that greater involvement of men, and all family members for that matter, is vitally important to ensuring that caregivers and care receivers alike can make the best of this terrible and increasingly prevalent disease.

> *"The whole process brought our family closer at a time when we needed each other. Doing the right thing by caring for our mom was a great life lesson for our children. Her being with us made our family closer." —Son-in-law*

References

Abrams, W., & Beers, M., et al. (Eds.). (1995). *The Merck Manual of Geriatrics*. Whitehouse Station, NJ: Merck Research Laboratories.

Adams, K. B. (2007). Specific effects of caring for a spouse with dementia: Differences in depressive symptoms between caregiver and non-caregiver spouses. *International Psychogeriatrics, 20* (3), 508-520.

Alzheimer's Association. (2001). Medicare and Medicaid costs for people with Alzheimer's disease. Retrieved June 1, 2009, from www.alz.org

Alzheimer's Association. (2006). 2006 national public policy program to conquer Alzheimer's disease. Retrieved June 1, 2009, from www.alz.org

Alzheimer's Association. (2007). Alzheimer's disease facts and figures. Retrieved June 1, 2009, from www.alz.org

Amirkhanyan, A. A., & Wolf, D. A. (2006). Parent care and the stress process: Findings from panel data. *The Journals of Gerontology; Series A; Biological Sciences and Medical Sciences, 61*, 248–255.

Aneshensel, C. S., Pearlin, L. I., Mullan, J. T., Zarit, S. H., & Whitlatch, C. J. (1995). *Profiles in caregiving: The unexpected career*. San Diego, CA: Academic Press.

Ashburn, G., & Gordon, A. (1981). Features of a simplified register in speech to elderly conversationalists. *International Journal of Psycholinguistics, 23*, 7-31.

Atienza, A. A., Collins, R., & King, A. C. (2001). The mediating effects of situational control on social support and mood following a stressor: a prospective study of dementia caregivers in their natural environments. *The Journals of Gerontology; Series A; Biological Sciences and Medical Sciences, 56*, 129-139.

Avioli, P. (1989). The social support functions of siblings in later life. *American Behavioral Scientist, 33*, 45-57.

Baltes, M. M., & Wahl, H. W. (1996). Patterns of communication in old age: The dependence-support and independence-ignore script. *Health Communication, 8*(3), 217–231.

Baltes, P. B. (1997). On the incomplete architecture of human ontogeny: Selection, optimization, and compensation as foundation of developmental theory. *American Psychologist, 52*, 366-380.

Beach, D. L. (1994). Family care of Alzheimer victims. An analysis of the adolescent experience. *American Journal of Alzheimer's Disease and Related Disorders, 9*, 12–19.

Beach, D. L. (1997). Family caregiving: The positive impact on adolescent relationships. *The Gerontologist, 37*, 233–238.

Bearon, L. (2004). *The burden and blessings of family caregiving*. North Carolina Cooperative Extension Service.

Bedford, V. H. (1995). Sibling relationships in middle and old age. In R. Blieszner & V. H. Bedford (Eds.), *Handbook of aging and the family* (pp. 201-222). Westport, CT: Greenwood.

Bertrand, R. M., Fredman, L., & Saczynski, J. (2006). Are all caregivers created equal? Stress in caregivers to adults with and without dementia. *Journal of Aging and Health, 18*(4), 534-552.

Bethea, L. S. (2002). The impact of an adult parent on communicative satisfaction and dyadic adjustment in the long-term marital relationship: Adult-children and spouses' retrospective accounts. *Journal of Applied Communication Research, 30*, 107–125.

Boss, P. (1987). Family stress. In M. B. Sussman, & S. K. Steinmetz (Eds.), *Handbook of marriage and the family* (pp. 695–724). New York: Plenum.

Bourgeois, M. S., Schulz, R., & Burgio, L. (1996). Interventions for caregivers of patients with Alzheimer's disease: A review and analysis of content, process, and outcomes. *International Journal of Aging and Human Development, 43*, 35-92

Brauner, D. J., Muir, J. C., & Sachs, G. A. (2000). Treating non dementia illnesses in patients with dementia. *Journal of the American Medical Academy, 283*(24), 3230-3235.

Brewer, L. (2002). Families that care: A qualitative study of families engaged in the provision of elder care. *Journal of Gerontological Social Work, 39*(3), 41-56

Brody, E. M. (1989). The family at risk. In E. Light, & B. D. Lebowitz (Eds.), *Alzheimer's disease treatment and family stress: Directions for research* (pp. 2–49). Rockeville, MD: National Institute of Mental Health.

Brody, E. M. (1981). Women in the middle and family help to older people. *The Gerontologist*, 21, 471-480.

Chodosh, J., Mittman, B. S., Connor, K. I., Vassar, S. D., Lee, M. L., DeMonte, R. W. (2007). Caring for patients with dementia: How good is the quality of care? Results from three health systems. *Journal of the American Geriatrics Society, 55*, 1260-1268.

Choi, H., & Marks, N. F. (2006). Transition to caregiving, marital disagreement, and psychological well-being: A prospective U.S. National Study. *Journal of Family Issues, 27*, 1701-1723.

Cohen, D., & Eisdorfer, C. (1988). Depression in family members caring for a relative with Alzheimer's disease. *Journal of the American Geriatrics Society, 36*(10), 885-889.

Cohen, S., & Wills, T. A. (1985). Stress, social support, and the buffering hypothesis. *Psychological Bulletin, 98*, 310-357.

Connidis, I. A. (1989). *Family ties and aging*. Toronto: Butterworths.

Connidis, I. A. (1994). Sibling support in older age. *Journal of Gerontology, 49*(6), 309-317.

Creasey, G. L., & Jarvis, P. A. (1989). Grandparents with Alzheimer's disease: Effect of parental burden on grandchildren. *Family Therapy, 16*, 79–85.

Cumming, E., & Schneider, D. M. (1961). Sibling solidarity: A property of American kinship. *American Anthropologist, 63*(3), 498-507.

Davey, A. (2000). Aging and adaptation: How families cope. In P. C. McKenry & S. J. Price (Eds.), *Families and change: Coping with stressful events and transitions* (2nd ed., pp. 94-119). Thousand Oaks, CA: Sage.

Donelan, K., Hill, C. A., Hoffman, C., Scoles, K., Feldman, P. H., Levine, C., & Gould, D. (2002). Challenged to care: Informal caregivers in a changing health system. *Health Affairs, 21*, 222-231.

Ell, K. (1996). Social networks, social support and coping with serious illness: The family connection. *Social Science and Medicine, 42*, 173-183.

Family Caregiver Alliance (2009). *2009 National policy statement*. San Francisco, CA.

Feinberg, L. F., Newman, S. L., Gray, L., & Kolb, K. N. (2004). *The state of the states in family caregiver support: A 50 state study*. San Francisco, CA: Family Caregiver Alliance.

Fisher, L., & Lieberman, M. A. (1996). The effects of family context on adult offspring of patients with Alzheimer's disease: A longitudinal study. *Journal of Family Psychology, 10*, 180-191.

Fitting, M., Rabins, P., Lucas, M. J., & Eastham, J. (1986). Caregivers for dementia patients: A comparison of husbands and wives. *The Gerontologist, 26*, 248-252.

Flint, L. J., Query, J. L., & Parrish, A. (2005). Negotiating communication obstacles while experiencing Alzheimer's disease: The case of one family. For E. B. Ray (Ed.), *Case studies in health communication* (2nd ed.). Mahwah, NJ: Erlbaum.

Fox, P., Maslow, K., & Zhang, X. (1999). Long-term care eligibility criteria for people with Alzheimer's disease. *Health Care Financing Review, 20*(4), 67-84.

Freedman, V. (1996). Family structure and the risk of nursing home admission. *Journal of Gerontology, 51*(2), 261-269.

Fruhauf, C. A., Jarrott, S. E., & Allen, K. A. (2006). Grandchildren's perceptions of caring for grandparents. *Journal of Family Issues, 27*, 887-911.

Gabrel, C. S. (2000). *Characteristics of elderly nursing home current residents and discharges: Data From the 1997 National Nursing Home Survey, Advance Data From Vital and Health Statistics, No. 312*. Hyattsville, MD: National Center for Health Statistics.

Gaugler, J. E., Kane, R. L., Kane, R. A., & Newcomer, R. (2005). Unmet care needs and key outcomes in dementia. *Journal of the American Geriatrics Society, 53*, 2098-2105.

Gaugler, J. E., Mendiondo, M., Smith, C. D., & Schmitt, F. A. (2003). Secondary dementia caregiving and its consequences. *American Journal of Alzheimer's Disease and Other Dementia, 18*, 300-308.

Gilliland, M. P., & Bush, H. A. (2001). Social support for family caregivers: Toward a situation-specific theory. *The Journal of Theory Construction & Testing, 5*, 53-62.

Goode, W. J., (1960). A theory of role strain. *American Sociological Review, 25*, 483-496.

Grainger, K. (1995). Communication and the institutionalized elder. In J. F. Nussbaum & J. Coupland (Eds.), *Handbook of Communication and Aging Research* (pp. 417–436). Mahwah, New Jersey: Lawrence Erlbaum Associates.

Haley, W. E. (1997). The family caregiver's role in Alzheimer's disease. *Neurology, 48*, 25–29.

Hamill, S. B. (1994). Parent–adolescent communication in sandwich generation families. *Journal of Adolescent Research, 9*, 458–482.

Harwood, J. (2007). *Understanding communication and aging: Developing knowledge and awareness*. Los Angeles, CA: Sage.

Hebert, L. E., Scherr, P. A., Bienias, J. L., Bennett, D. A., & Evans, D. A. (2003). Alzheimer disease in the US population: Prevalence estimates using the 2000 Census. *Archives of Neurology, 60*(8), 1119-1122.

Hummert, M. L., & Nussbaum, J. F. (2001). *Aging, communication, and health: Linking research and practice for successful aging*. Mahwah, NJ: Lawrence Erlbaum Associates.

Keith, C. (1995). Family caregiving systems: Models, resources, and values. *Journal of Marriage and the Family, 57*, 179-189.

Kemper, S., Anagnopoulos, C., Lyons, K., & Heberlein, W. (1994). Speech accommodations to dementia. *Journal of Gerontology, 49*, 223-229.

Knop, D. S., Bergman-Evans, B., & Wharton, B. (1998). In sickness and in health: An exploration of the perceived quality of the marital relationship, coping, and depression in caregivers of spouses with Alzheimer's disease. *Journal of Psychosocial Nursing & Mental Health Services, 36*(1), 16-21.

Kramer, B. J. (1997). Gain in the caregiving experience: Where are we? What next? *The Gerontologist, 37*, 218-232.

Lanceley, A. (1985). Use of controlling language in the rehabilitation of the elderly. *Journal of Advanced Nursing, 10*, 125–135.

Lawrence, J. A., Goodnow, J. J., Woods, K., & Karantzas, G. (2002). Distributions of caregiving tasks among family members: The place of gender and availability. *Journal of Family Psychology, 16*, 493–509.

Leske, J. S., & Jiricka, M. K. (1998). Impact of family demands and family strengths and capabilities on family well-being and adaptation after critical injury. *American Journal of Critical Care, 7*, 383-392.

Lindgren, H. G., & Decker, H. (1996). The sandwich generation: A cluttered nest. *Adulthood and Aging*. Retrieved May 28, 2009, from http://ianrpubls.unl.edu/familuy/g1117.htm

Liu, W., & Gallagher-Thompson, D. (2009). Impact of dementia caregiving: Risks, strains, and growth. In S. H. Qualls, & S. H. Zarit (Eds.), *Aging families and caregiving* (pp. 85-112). Hoboken, NJ: John Wiley & Sons, Inc.

Lubinski, R. (1995). State-of-the-art perspectives on communication in nursing homes. *Topics in Language Disorders, 15*(2), 1–19.

Luchins, D. J., & Hanrahan, P. (1993). What is appropriate health care for end stage dementia? *Journal of the American Geriatrics Society, 41*, 25-30.

Malone-Beach, E. E., DeGenova, M., & Otani, H. (1998). Conflict, well-being, and depression: Young adults in intergenerational caregiving and noncaregiving families. *Korean Journal of Research in Gerontology, 7*, 5-16.

Matimore, T., Wenger, N., Cesbiens, N., Teno, J., Hamel, J., & Liu, M. (1997). Surrogate and physician understanding of patients' preferences for living permanently in a nursing home. *Journal of the American Geriatrics Society, 45*, 818–824.

Mitchell, J. M., & Kemp, B. J. (2000). Quality of life in assisted living homes: A multidimensional analysis. *The Journals of Gerontology; Series A; Biological Sciences and Medical Sciences, 55*(2), 117-127.

Mitrani, V. B., Lewis, J. E., Feaster, D. J., Czaja, S. J., Eisdorfer, C., & Schulz, R. (2006). The role of family functioning in the stress process of dementia caregivers: A structural family framework. *The Gerontologist, 46,* 97-105.

Mortimer J. A., & Graves, A. B. (1993). Education and other socioeconomic determinants of dementia and Alzheimer's disease. Neurology, *43,* 39-44.

Murray, L. M., & Boyd, S. (2009). Protecting personhood and achieving quality of life for older adults with dementia in the U.S. health care system. *Journal of Aging Health, 21,* 350-374.

National Center for Assisted Living. (2001). Assisted living: Independence, choice, and dignity, from http://www.ncal.org/about/alicd.pdf

Newcomer, R. J., Fox, P. J., & Harrington, C. A. (2001). Health and long-term care for people with Alzheimer's disease and related dementias: Policy research issues. *Aging and Mental Health, 5,* 124-137.

Orange, J. B. (2001). Family caregivers, communication, and Alzheimer's disease. In: M. L. Hummert, & J. F. Nussbaum (Eds.), *Aging, communication, and health: Linking research and practice to successful aging* (pp. 225-248). Mahwah, NJ: Lawrence Erlbaum Associates.

Pecchioni, L. L. (2001). Implicit decision-making in family caregiving. *Journal of Social and Personal Relationships, 18,* 219–237.

Pecchioni, L. L., Thompson, T. L., & Anderson, D. J. (2006). Interrelations between family communication and health communication. In: L. H. Turner & R. West, (Eds.), *The family communication sourcebook* (pp. 447–468). Thousand Oaks, CA: Sage.

Pecchioni, L. L., Wright, K. B., & Nussbaum, J. F. (2005). *Life-span communication.* Mahwah, NJ: Lawrence Erlbaum Associates Publishing.

Pfeiffer, E. (1999). Stages of caregiving. *American Journal of Alzheimer's Disease, 14,* 125–127.

Pruchno, R. A., Peters, N. D., & Burant, C. J. (1996). Child life events, parent–child disagreements, and parent well-being: Model development and testing. In C. D. Ryff, & M. M. Seltzer (Eds.), The parental experience in midlife (pp. 561–606). Chicago: University of Chicago Press.

Robinson, K. M. (1990). Predictors of burden among wife caregivers. *Scholarly Inquiry for Nursing practice: An International Journal,* 4(3), 189-202.

Rodin, J., & Langer, E. J. (1980). Aging labels: The decline of control and the fall of self-esteem. *Journal of Social Issues, 36,* 12–29.

Ryan, E. B., Giles, H., Bartolucci, G., & Henwood, K. (1986). Psycholinguistic and social psychological components of communication by and with the elderly. *Language & Communication, 6,* 1-24.

Ryan, E. B., Hummert, M., & Boich, L. (1995). Communication predicaments of aging: Patronizing behavior toward older adults. *Journal of Language and Social Psychology, 14,* 144-166.

Schubert, C. C., Boustani, M., Callahan, C. M., Perkins, A. J., Carney, C. P., Fox, C. (2006). Comorbidity profile of dementia patients in primary care: Are they sicker? *Journal of the American Geriatrics Society, 54,* 104-109.

Schulz, R., & Martire, L. M. (2004). Family caregiving of persons with dementia: Prevalence, health effects, and support strategies. *American Journal of Geriatric Psychiatry, 12*(3), 240-249.

Segrin, C., & Flora, J. (2005). *Family communication.* Mahwah, NJ: Lawrence Erlbaum Associates Publishing.

Sloan, F. A., Trogdon, J. G., Curtis, L. H., & Schulman, K. A. (2004). The effect of dementia on outcomes and process of care for Medicare beneficiaries admitted with acute myocardial infarction. *Journal of the American Geriatrics Society, 52,* 173-181.

Small, J. A., & Gutman, G. (2002). Recommended and reported use of communication strategies in Alzheimer caregiving. *Alzheimer Disease and Associated Disorders, 16*(4), 270-278.

Stephens, M., & Franks, M. M. (2009). All in the family: Providing care to chronically ill and disabled older adults. In S. H. Qualls, & S. H. Zarit (Eds.), *Aging families and caregiving* (pp. 61-83). Hoboken, NJ: John Wiley & Sons, Inc.

Stolley, K. S., & Szinovacz, M. (1997). Caregiving responsibilities and child spanking. *Journal of Family Violence, 12,* 99–112.

Stone, R. I., & Kemper, P. (1990). Spouses and children of disabled elders: How large a constituency for long-term care reform? *Milbank Quarterly, 67,* 485-506.

Szinovacz, M. (2003). Caring for a demented relative at home: Effects on parent–adolescent relationships and family dynamics. *Journal of Aging Studies, 17,* 445-472.

Tebes, J. K., & Irish, J. T. (2000). Promoting resilience among children of sandwiched generation caregiving women through caregiver mutual help. *Journal of Prevention and Intervention in the Community, 20,* 139-158.

Treas, J. (1979). Intergenerational families and social change. In P.K. Ragan (Ed.), *Aging parents* (pp.58-65). Los Angeles: University of Southern California Press.

U.S. Census Bureau. (2000). *The elderly population.* Retrieved June 6, 2009, from http://www.census.gov/population/www/pop-profile/elderpop.html

U.S. Department of Health and Human Services: National Institutes of Health and National Institute on Aging. (2005). *Progress report on Alzheimer's disease 2004-2005* (NIH Publication Number: 05-5724).

Wackerbarth, S. (1999). Modeling a dynamic decision process: Supporting the decisions of carers of family members with dementia. *Qualitative Health Research, 9*(3), 294–318.

Warchol, K. (2004). An interdisciplinary dementia program model for long-term care. *Topics in Geriatric Rehabilitation, 20*(1), 59-71.

Whitchurch, G. G., & Constantine, L. L. (1993). Systems theory. In P. G. Boss, W. J. Doherty, R. LaRossa, W. R. Schumm, & S. K. Steinmetz (Eds.), *Sourcebook of family theories and methods* (pp. 325–352). New York: Plenum.

White, L. K. (2001). Sibling relationships over the life course: A panel analysis. *Journal of Marriage and Family, 63,* 555-568.

White, L. K., & Riedmann, A. (1992). Ties among adult siblings. *Social Forces, 71,* 85-102.

Whitlatch, C. J. (2008). Informal caregivers: Communication and decision making. *American Journal of Nursing, 108*(9), 73-79.

Williams, A., & Nussbaum, J. F. (2001). *Intergenerational communication across the life span.* Mahwah, NJ: Lawrence Erlbaum Associates Publishing.

Williams, K., Ilten, T., & Bower, H. (2005). Meeting communication needs: Topics of talk in the nursing home. *Journal of Psychosocial Nursing and Mental Health Services, 43,* 38–45.

Wolff, J. L., Boult, C., Boyd, C., & Anderson, G. (2005). Newly reported chronic conditions and onset of functional dependency. *Journal of the American Geriatrics Society, 53*(5), 851-855.

Wolff, J. L., & Kasper, J. D. (2006). Caregivers of frail elders: Updating a national profile. *The Gerontologist, 46,* 344-356.

Wright, L. K. (Ed.). (1993). *Alzheimer's disease and marriage: An intimate account.* Newbury Park, CA: Sage Publications.

Wright, K. B., Sparks, L., & O'Hair, H. D. (2008). *Health communication in the 21st century.* Oxford, UK: Blackwell.

Yancik, R., Ershler, W., Satariano, W., Hazzard, W., Cohen, H. J., & Ferrucci, L. (2007). Report of the National Institute on Aging task force on comorbidity. *The Journals of Gerontology; Series A; Biological Sciences and Medical Sciences, 62,* 275–280.

CHAPTER 14

Dancing with the Spirit: Communicating Family Norms for Positive End-of-Life Transitions

Margaret Jane Pitts

OLD DOMINION UNIVERSITY

> *The creative possibility embedded in the experience of mortal time is facing the fact of the limitation of all human existence, which people are inclined to avoid, explicitly and deeply. This, in turn, carries the blessing of the opportunity to consider one's life, make amends where possible, and say what is in one's heart to family, friends, and associates—to finish one's life with a deliberateness and a measure of closure denied to those whose lives end unexpectedly.* (McQuellon & Cowan, 2000, p. 318)

At the center of the sunflower is Gigi. Her daughters, siblings, grandchildren, and friends are the petals arranged in a circle representing life and connection with Spirit. The sunflower represents the unbroken circle of living and dying. It is also the symbol for Gigi's spiritualist camp in the sanctuary of the Arizona desert. Over the last few years Gigi has been planning her departure from this world and transition into the next life. She has organized all of her important documents, ranging from property deeds to almost 80 years of photographs. Although Gigi does not have an acute illness, she has been diagnosed with a chronic disease affecting her heart and lungs. Her body is slowly dying while her spirit is still growing. Because of this, she has become a familiar personality at the hospital and emergency clinic. Family members are accustomed to late night calls or electronic messages updating them on her health status. Through hugs, tears, greetings, and farewells her family holds her hand and tries to honor, celebrate, and make sense of her end-of-life transition. For Gigi's family, news of her impending death is met with both sadness and a tingling sense of adventure. For them, when a family member dies, this represents an opportunity for rebirth and reunion with a spiritual source.

Over time, Gigi's family has co-constructed positive expectations about dying by openly communicating with one another about death, using metaphorical language that serves to connect dying with living, and accepting family members' spiritual experiences. By examining the communication practices of this family, I believe much can be learned about communicatively creating a *good death* for family members. Thus, the purpose of this case study is to examine how one family—Gigi's family—co-constructs positive end-of-life experiences and communicates positive expectations about death with all family members intergenerationally. Through the writing of this chapter, I seek to honor and maximize this family's authority over their belief system, while at the same time providing insight into their communication practices. This case study describes one family's experience and has the potential to increase understanding of how families might construct the end-of-life transition as a natural, positive event.

End-of-Life Experiences and Expectations

As recently as the late 19th and early 20th centuries, death and dying were an accepted part of living and of family relationships in the West. Of course, in the 21st century, people are still dying. The difference is that individuals don't talk about it. In fact, many people have distanced themselves from almost all aspects of the dying process (Keeley & Yingling, 2007). And, in the US in particular, people are generally averse to the thought of death (Gelfand, Raspa, Briller, & Myers Schim, 2005), often expressing fear, anxiety, and feelings of disgust or morbidity at the mere mention of it. In part, this is the result of medical and technological "advancements" (Nuland, 1993). The life expectancy continues to creep upward as physicians and scientists are capable of sustaining life in a body—keeping death at a distance by prolonging life. With new medical developments, physicians are able to do more for their dying patients than before through palliative care, symptom management, and sustaining life. Unfortunately, this often results in the medicalization of death, distancing physicians (and others) from the more human elements of medicine and dying (Mitchell, 1997). Contemporary living also distances many people in the West from the process of living and dying. Birth and death most often happen in a sterile, depersonalized environment outside the family home. The elderly and people with terminal illnesses are frequently treated in hospitals, hospices, or other institutions. The body of a loved one is no longer housed in the family parlor for survivors to mourn, but rests instead in a funeral parlor, morgue, or mortuary until it is eventually buried or cremated—all processes undertaken by someone outside of the family (Lynch, 1997). The point is, as a culture, we have constructed a phenomenon wherein death and dying are happening at the outskirts of living and not as part of the process. There is a cultural tendency to forget that while we are *all* on our individual path toward dying. We are *all* also living (Foster, 2007).

Meaningful Scripts, Roles, and Conversations at the End-of-Life

Dying is a multidimensional and deeply personal experience (Emanuel & Emanuel, 1998). The search for meaning in that process differs from person to person (Leichtentritt & Rettig, 2001), "and these meanings have serious impact on how each person communicates with others as they deal with it together" (McQuellon & Cowan, 2000, p. 312). Indeed, just as every life is experienced uniquely, so is every death. The individual physical, psychological, social, and spiritual manners of dying ensure that. Nuland (1993) writes, "Every man will yield up the ghost in a manner that the heavens have never known before: every woman will go her final way in her own way" (p. 3). Each death, then, is "an occasion" that should be witnessed and honored (Foster, 2007). It is important, as Foster notes, "to transition from a generalized cultural understanding of death to an understanding based on the uniqueness of the individual patients and families" (p. 38). Moreover, it is not just the individual who is dying that experiences death uniquely, but also her/his social network. Dying is both an individual and a collective experience (Gelfand et al., 2005).

When death is not addressed as part of life in families, it becomes a challenge to find meaning in death and dying later in life. Having been largely sheltered from the dying process, people approaching the end-of-life have to make sense of their own life and death without the benefit of cultural norms for positive end-of-life experiences. Mitchell (1997), for example, argues that a good death needs to include open discussion about dying. Today, however, people do not understand the importance of talking about death: "When most people die in hospitals or nursing homes, this understanding and the ability to talk about death have been largely forgotten" (Mitchell, p. 92). The result is that there are few cultural *scripts* for dying well. Thus, as a person approaches the end-of-life it can seem as though s/he is on the first ever "quest for a good death."

Finding meaning in end-of-life transitions is also complicated because people are uncertain how to play the *role* of a dying person (Emanuel, Bennett, & Richardson, 2007). Because individuals are so often removed from the dying process (both psychologically and physically) when they are presented with end-of-life scenarios they often experience anxiety and uncertainty. Uncertainty about the role of the dying person makes positive end-of-life experiences and expectations difficult to imagine and enact. In fact, Foster (2007) argues that end-of-life communication seems so "foreign" that it can be understood through Gudykunst and Kim's (1997) concept of stranger and Berger and Calabrese's (1975) concept of uncertainty,

> The absence of a familiar social script for conversations about death and the high degree of uncertainty related to dying can cause us to treat even a close friend or relative who is dying as if he or she is a stranger. (p. 92)

A greater awareness of the dying person's role for all involved increases the likelihood of finding meaning in and achieving a good death (Emanuel et al., 2007). In particular, developing an understanding that the dying role has three interrelated domains that must be attended to—practical, personal, and relational—helps the dying person and her/his family adjust to all of their important new roles (Emanuel et al.). Specifically, attending to practical tasks of the dying role include logistical aspects of planning and preparing for the end-of-life. The personal dimension of the dying role focuses on achieving closure, forgiveness, and personal growth. Attending to the relational dimension of the dying role encompasses being able to maintain important relationships such as mother or husband, achieving a sense that one has contributed to a legacy, and/or passing on symbolic possessions (Emanuel et al.). According to Costello (2006), "acknowledgment of the social life of the dying and the creation of an open climate about disclosure" is important for individuals to collaborate with loved ones in creating a script for a "good death" (p. 595). Just as people model other life roles (being a father or being a wife) after influential family members, it is also possible to create positive dying roles through open communication. Keeley and Yingling (2007) aptly ask, "if the death process is unseen, if there are no examples to demonstrate how to act when a loved one is dying, then how is the Living one to know what to say or what to do" (p. 4)?

People nearing the end-of-life have an opportunity to build a "bridge of empathy" (McQuellon & Cowan, 2000, p. 315) between the living and dying and a spiritual bridge between two worlds for the dying person through communication. Research on final conversations with loved ones demonstrates the importance of confirming and celebrating relationships during the transition (Keeley, 2007). Final conversations are important for the living and the dying because they create opportunities to communicate at the time of transition often leading to relational growth, identity development, and helping both parties to prepare for the transition (Keeley). Keeley and colleagues' work (Keeley; Keeley & Kellas, 2005; Keeley & Yingling, 2007) make evident the importance of communicating during the end-of-life transition. They identify five key messages shared in final conversations: messages about love, identity, spirituality, relational maintenance through everyday talk, and addressing difficult relationship issues.

A Lifespan Approach to Death and Dying: Narratives and Rituals of Death and Dying

Final conversations and open communication about the dying process is important as family members age, but a sole focus on communication at the end-of-life neglects the significance of talking about and understanding death throughout all stages of the lifespan. After all, death is a life course phenomenon (Gelfand et al., 2005; Nussbaum, Pecchioni, Robinson, & Thompson, 2000). Often the first, and sometimes only, experiences with death are family experiences. Thus, family death narratives and rituals throughout family life shape one's expectations about and experiences with death (Book, 1996).

Family death narratives and end-of-life narratives are important ways for dying people (and their families) to make sense of their life, narrate their legacy, and provide a family script for dying (Leichtentritt & Rettig, 2001). End-of-life narratives empower those who are dying by allowing them to construct a good life and a good death, thereby offering a sense of control and accomplishment (Leichtentritt & Rettig). Once the end-of-life narrative is finalized, people often feel a sense of completion and accept the transition into death (Emanuel et al., 2007). Personal storytelling also contributes to overall positivity and resilience in later life by allowing elders to reflect on the past, share their experiences in the present, and contemplate the future (Nakashima & Canda, 2005). In turn, personal storytelling across the lifespan about living, dying, and end-of-life experiences benefits the family by creating family death narratives and rituals. Death narratives play an important role in helping the family adjust to the transition and develop expectations for a positive end-of-life experience. Moreover, sharing the story of final conversations with loved ones and stories about experiences with death can also help families heal and make sense of end-of-life transitions (Keeley, 2007; Keeley & Kellas, 2005; Keeley & Yingling, 1997; Sedney, Baker, & Gross, 1994).

In addition to the important role that narratives play in constructing death in families, many family rituals, and even children's "make believe" games, prepare individuals for the death rituals they will later encounter (Kastenbaum, 2004). Children sometimes feign their own deaths to "test" their parents' bonds of love. Some parents might pray with their children for protection while they sleep. Kastenbaum suggests that

> the shape of our lives cannot be fully known until the entire journey has run its course—assuming we share the tenets of a traditional belief system. This system also gives us shelter along the way: *the intergenerational flow of stories and memories, the symbols, the daily practices and the grand rituals*, all working hard to hold back the anxieties, the doubts, and of course the irrational forces that seize and destroy our finest achievements, even our most innocent or gifted comrades [at death] (p. 23, emphasis added).

Embedded in the "intergenerational flow of stories and memories, the symbols, the daily practices and the grand rituals" (Kastenbaum, 2004, p. 23) within families are the bits of information that can be used to make sense out of death and dying. Thus, family death narratives, or lack thereof, contribute to the overall performance of living and dying. Likewise, Coffman and Coffman (1995-96) suggest it might be beneficial for people who are not dying to engage in behavioral rehearsals of the dying process—to construct and enact a good death. Like practicing married-life or parenting, practicing dying or imagining the death of a loved one might help ease death-related anxiety and create the stage for positive dying experiences. Although research about death-education (e.g., college courses on death and dying) suggests it does little to assuage death-related anxiety, what it might do is open the doors for more discussions about fears and expectations about the dying process earlier in life (Servaty & Hayslip, 1996-97).

The Importance of Studying Positive End-of-Life Experiences and Expectations

People nearing or perceiving the end-of-life often focus their attentions on finding meaning in living/dying and on maximizing emotional meaning to optimize psychological well-being (e.g., Carstensens' [1992] socioemotional selectivity theory). People who are dying often exclude all but their closest family and friends from their final transition—an opportunity, argue Keeley and Yingling (2007), for the living and the dying to turn toward each other at death (Keeley, 2007; McQuellon, & Cowan, 2000) and co-construct a meaningful transition. It is important to attend to the role of narrative and story telling in finding meaning in end-of-life transitions and sharing those experiences and expectations intergenerationally.

This brief review of literature brings to light the difficulties with and the importance of creating positive end-of-life experiences. Communication is central to this process. Although all families have the opportunity to plan for, to anticipate, and to experience this transition, few families participate in a lifespan approach toward creating, or even talking about, positive end-of-life expectations. In this regard, Gigi's family is unique in that they have communicated positive expectations about death and dying across three generations. There is much to be learned from Gigi's case about the ways everyday talk about death and dying influence final life transitions. The remainder of this chapter will describe a naturalistic case study (Stake, 1998) I conducted to obtain an in-depth understanding of how Gigi's family creates norms for achieving the good death and to identify what can be learned from their experiences.

Method

The central questions that drove the study of Gigi's family were *1) how do Gigi's family members communicatively establish norms for positive end-of-life experiences,* and *2) how do Gigi's family members co-construct positive expectations about end-of-life transitions?*

A case study methodology is uniquely suited to answer "how" questions, particularly "when the focus is on a contemporary phenomenon within some real-life context" (Yin, 2003, p. 1). Although dying is not a distinctively "contemporary phenomenon," the fact that as a culture the U.S. has pushed dying to the outskirts of living, and very few families generate plans for end-of-life transitions before they are faced with that reality, means that dying is quite often experienced as a contemporary issue situated in the very immediate real life context. Case studies are inquiries that offer the investigator insight into a specific phenomenon through intensive investigation of an event, an individual, or a social unit—in this case a family (Reinard, 2008). As in Gigi's case, the phenomenon under study is unique and holds potential to generate in-depth knowledge of a particular topic, especially one that has not received much research attention. A case study approach places emphasis on the *case* itself (i.e., a family that has positively framed the dying experience) and not variables. As Stake (1998) notes, "the purpose of case study is not to represent the world, but to represent the case" (p. 104). Finally, case studies are the quintessential modes of inquiry for capturing the complexity of a single case or social phenomenon (Stake, 1995), "allow[ing] investigators to retain the holistic and meaningful characteristics of real-life events—such as individual life-cycles" (Yin, p. 2).

Case studies are differentiated by their purpose (Stake 1995, 1998). A researcher conducting an *intrinsic* case study is most interested in the particularities of a specific case for the sake of better understanding that case. A researcher engaging in an *instrumental* case study is most concerned with investigating a specific case to provide insight into a wider cultural phenomenon. Finally, a researcher initiating a *collective* case study is less interested in the specific case per se than s/he is in examining and comparing multiple cases in an effort to better understand, and perhaps theorize about, a phenomenon, population, or general condition. Stake acknowledges that although it might be possible to distinguish types of case studies in this manner, it is rare that any case study should fit neatly in a single category. My primary purpose in conducting this case study was instrumental—a focus on the *issue* in the case (Stake). I sought to highlight the ways in which family norms are communicated across the lifespan and contribute to positive expectations about and experiences with death. However, Gigi's case is so compelling that it also tugs me toward the intrinsic nature of this investigation—a focus on the case itself (Stake). Thus, the purposes driving this case study were two-fold. First, I sought to use this case to advance understanding of the role of communication across the lifespan in developing positive end-of-life experiences. Second, I sought to bring attention to and honor the unique details of this case because the case itself is important.

Learning about Gigi's Family

This case study begins in a multigenerational family in which Gigi, the oldest living member of her family, is making plans for her transition into death. Although I have known Gigi for 14 years, and was introduced to her unique perspectives on death in our first meeting, this case study offered my first opportunity to sit down with Gigi and her family members to discuss her own passing. This report is the result of one year's study with this family and draws on multiple methods of data collection from several family members. Data triangulation enabled me to verify if what I was observing and reporting carried the same meaning under different circumstances (Stake, 1995). In-depth narrative interviews provided the foundation for this investigation. Family and life narratives served as important sense-making processes, particularly as this family was transitioning. My observations of the daily interactions and discussions among family members that occurred outside of the interview context (i.e., preparing dinner, driving in a car) were also important to the development of this case. In addition to interviews and observations, documents such as photographs, home videos, books, letters, and e-mail also informed this study. Documents not only offered additional insight into the family context, but also served as a stimulus for rich family narratives. Finally, this report draws from not only many day-to-day interactions with the family, but also my invited participation in family celebrations and holidays, including a large family reunion that spanned multiple generations and layers of extended relatives. Over the course of one year, I spoke to and observed interactions with numerous family members, nine of whom were key participants and informants in this investigation, including Gigi, her husband, her sister, her four daughters, and two of her nine grandsons (see Gigi's Family, Table 14.1). All participants have been assigned pseudonyms.

Table 14.1 Gigi's Family

Name	Relationship
Gigi	Grandmother—Matriarch
Pappy	Gigi's husband of 55 years
Auntie Dianne	Gigi's sister
Becky	Gigi's first (oldest) daughter
Meredith	Gigi's second daughter
Tabitha (Beth)	Gigi's third daughter
Jennifer (Jenny)	Gigi's fourth (youngest) daughter
Ethan	Gigi's grandson (Meredith's son)
Daniel	Gigi's grandson (Meredith's son)

Lessons Learned: Making Sense of End-of-Life Transitions

The research questions that frame this analysis are designed to capture the *perceptions* of end-of-life experiences and the *process* of communicating those expectations across generations. The process of communicating those perceptions is intimately linked with the unique features of this family. An understanding of how this family co-constructs positive end-of-life experiences; therefore, necessarily begins with a description of the family.

An Introduction to Gigi

Gigi Balin is quite a presence—she is big in everyway. Over time, her family teases, Gigi's body has grown larger and larger to accommodate for her loving, and perhaps eccentric, spirit. Described by her family as *the queen bee,* Gigi has a kind of commanding manner in any social scene that enables her to hold court among even the most able of socialites. She is often found at the center of a room, her children, friends, and grandchildren surrounding her like petals of a flower. Gigi is regarded by everyone as "the glue holding the family together." As the oldest member of her family, Gigi plays a significant role in shaping the "Balin family line." She is matriarch to her blood family as well as to many who have followed her spiritual guidance over the years. When her father insisted that if she wished to join a church she must first read the Bible in its entirety he set her on a unique path of enlightenment. Encouraged to find her personal spiritual path by her parents (albeit indirectly), she has since set the pace as spiritual leader for her family, encouraging them to find their own spiritual path. Until very recently, Gigi lived at and directed a spiritualist camp built on an energy vortex in western Arizona. Although she never received formal religious schooling, having turned away from organized religions, Gigi recalls having a connection with the God-energy as a young child. Recent health complications and family concerns resulted in Gigi and Pappy's (her husband of over 50 years) relocation to Sterling Lifescapes, a retirement center, in Phoenix. No longer an active member of her spiritualist camp, she has bestowed upon herself "Ministry of Music" of Sterling Lifescapes.

On the 20th day of November, 2000, Gigi, a true Scorpio, will celebrate her 78th birthday. The past 15 birthdays represent significant milestones for Gigi who did not expect to live beyond 63—the age that her own mother died. From all accounts, Gigi's mother, Nonny, was the life of a party. Late in life Nonny moved to Arizona to check into an alcoholism rehabilitation center. Gigi, who always played the mothering role in her relationship with Nonny, packed up her husband and four daughters, moved to Arizona, and began once more to care for her mother. The pain Gigi describes of grief and loss following her mother's death was insufferable. When Gigi witnessed the fear and anger that later accompanied her father's death, she embraced her spiritualist connections and sought greater meaning in the life/death cycle. Over the years she has taught her daughters and grandchildren to recognize and embrace their part in the encompassing God-energy. She teaches that everyone is part of a loving God-energy—"in life as it is in death, on Earth as it is in Heaven" (FN_3[1]). Dying, she says, is just the transition between this world and the spirit world—"like walking through a door" (FN_3).

Gigi's Teachings—Perceptions about and Principles Guiding Life

Gigi's spiritual beliefs guide both life on this "planet" and the transcendence to the "other side." What is remarkable about Gigi's family is the frequency and consistency with which each member articulates their beliefs about life and death. These beliefs are reminiscent of a range of theological sources, many stemming from biblical stories, but also including Navajo creationist ideas, Buddhism, Judaism, and specific readings in *A Course in Miracles, The Tapes of Abraham, The Secret, The Prayer of Jabez, Mary Summer Rain's Guide to Dream Symbols,* and *Past Lives, Future Healings* introduced to Gigi by her daughters. Although Gigi's family doesn't make a point of identifying individual beliefs, it is possible to organize these ideas into a set of principles that guide life/living and death/dying in the Balin family. These principles inform family experiences and expectations about the end-of-life.

Principle one: All things have life and are part of Spirit. This principle provides the context for understanding transcendence into the next life. The family believes that humans are energy temporarily encased in the vehicle that is your body ("like your Ford" [Gigi_1_15]). Humans are all connected to and through *Spirit.* Spirit is the embodiment of love and is called by many names, including God and Father. According to Gigi, the energy that humans identify as "Self" exists before birth and continues to exist after a body dies. She and

1 Excepts from field notes are denoted by FN followed by the page number (e.g., FN_3). Excerpts from interviews are denoted by the interviewee's name followed by the interview number if relevant (Gigi_1_39) and ending with the page number. In the case of single interviews, the excerpt is denoted by interviewees name followed by page number (e.g., Jenny_7).

Auntie Dianne warn, however that one must learn to disconnect from "Self" in order to transcend fear and pain. Gigi also explains that energy has different vibration levels. Most humans are only capable of perceiving a finite range of vibrations. Others are more sensitive to and open-minded about recognizing other vibrations. Those people, like Gigi, experience a deeper connection with the Spirit energy and may be able to harness it in order to communicate with people on *the spirit side* (those who have "passed over" before us).

Principle two: We can communicate in spirit with the other side. A person who accepts the Balin belief that people are all part of the same energy source interacting on different vibration levels is then able to recognize the "thin veil of reality" (Gigi_2_7) that separates physical lives from spiritual lives. The only thing separating what people perceive to be real on this planet from an infinite possibility of other realities is the limitation imposed upon us by our human form. Gigi teaches that the thin veil of reality can be transcended if one is open-minded in order to communicate in spirit with the other side. Gigi also believes that there is a host of spiritual guides conspiring to help people achieve their greatest potential. However, God requires that one must ask for guidance:

> All you have to do is talk—I used to tell my kids (pause) (laughs) Becky, Meredith, when they were little, (pause) I said, "God's phone number is the Lord's Prayer. Just say that, and it's his private line, nobody can hook into it." (pause) And Meredith was always seeing (pause) spirits (chuckles). And she's four and a half years younger than Becky, you know? (pause) So they slept together (laughs) in the same room, you know, and they had their beds in there. (pause) And Meredith was always wakin' Becky up, telling her to say the Lord's Prayer because (laughs) she couldn't remember it. (laughs) And she was always seeing (pause) somebody in the room. (Gigi_1_16)

Gigi's daughters and grandchildren acknowledge that they were taught to ask for and receive guidance from the angels and animal spirits that surround them, yet work on a different level of vibrations. "You can have a visitation [from angels] and they look and feel just as real as any other physical [being] (pause). They can just come and go. So when you get to that point (pause) there's (pause) you know, there would be no more fear" (Gigi_2_8).

Principle three: We construct our own experiences in this life. Gigi's family believes in a sort of energy reincarnation—that people cycle through this universe eternally, but with different purposes. Each time a person comes into this planet it is to learn about or experience something specific. Gigi's family refers to this life as a schoolhouse for learning with a sandbox for everyone to play in. People return to this form of life for new experiences. Some experiences are painful (abuse, illness) and others are joyful. In this sense, each person is responsible for the life s/he constructs. People choose when to come into this life, who their parents will be, and also what struggles and successes they will endure. Aunt Dianne offers an example referencing her relationship with her own family,

> I know that this isn't just some random thing that these kids are in my family. And that no matter what they think, I know that at some point, we were there together before [this life] and we're all going to be cycling through eternity forever. (Dianne_29)

The idea is that upon entering life on this planet, people experience a state of amnesia, forgetting all they learned in past lives—"Because if you remember who you are, you can learn nothing here" (Gigi_1_13). The conviction that people construct their experiences in this lifetime also reveals the belief that people have some control over end-of-life experiences.

Principle four: Dying is like being born on the other side. Through communication Gigi's family creates an intricate system of spiritual beliefs that result in the understanding that dying can be a positive experience as the spirit prepares to say "goodbye" to this world and "hello" to the next as it returns to the Source. The physical separation hurts until one realizes that the energy, the love-force, is still there, is real, and is perceivable. Dying, says Gigi, is no different than walking into another room. Meredith describes it like walking into a kitchen where all your elders are sitting, drinking coffee, playing cards, laughing, and waiting for you. Not as if you had been gone a long time, but as if you simply stepped outside for a smoke. Gigi describes the dying process much like conception and birth. Individuals are offered time to prepare for their grand entrance/exit in the womb or upon experiencing near-death awareness. It is understood that during these times people are able to experience and communicate with both worlds to prepare for arrival. When people die, she explains, it is just like when they are born. It's never easy. Giving birth isn't *easy*. Even if there is a C-section, the mother has to recover. Yet, the baby is received with love through the pain. In death, the deceased is received with love on the other side and there is joy at the spiritual reunion. Gigi imagines that birth into this life world is equally painful for the spirit side who must bid farewell as the spirit takes human form. Sharing stories and experiences with birth and death helps to prepare the whole family for these life-course transitions. Gelfand et al. (2005) argue for the importance and instinctive nature of storytelling from birth to death. Comparing death narratives to birth, they write:

> Birth, too, is a narrative. When we are born, we enter the world of story-making, as natural for us as breathing. We are born into a story that our parents and families have already begun inventing about us: where we fit into their lives, where we will live, who will take care of us, what dreams parents and families have about our future. (p. 5)

The Intergenerational Transmission of End-of-Life Expectations

The Balin family borders on Olson's Chaotically Enmeshed and Flexibly Enmeshed families (Olson, Sprenkle, & Russell, 1979). They are deeply connected; "stuck way close together" admits Becky (Becky_4). They experience a deep spiritual connection with each other and stay in each others' lives across distances. The younger two daughters live in Colorado, working together to maintain what is left of the original Balin homestead. The elder two daughters continue to make their homes in Arizona. They also work together. Mother, daughters, and sisters remain connected through daily phone calls, e-mail, and video conferencing on personal computers. Their enmeshed lives enhance their ability to develop, communicate, and practice family norms not only among each other, but also with their own children. Gigi is said to have "set the pace for the family by questioning life, seeking answers, and looking within the self" (Meredith_15). One of Gigi's later-life goals has been to "set the example for the girls" (Gigi_1_3). She wants them to learn from her experiences with healing, health complications, relocations, and maintaining a connection with Spirit. "Learn from this!" (Gigi_1_2) she implores her daughters when addressing her health complications.

Gigi's family has several patterns for communicating end-of-life experiences and expectations. First and foremost, open and expressive communication is encouraged. Thus, directly communicating about death and dying is one manner in which the Balin's share expectations about transitioning into death. However, two other less direct means also serve to communicate positive expectations or enhance understanding—sharing spiritual experiences and using metaphors.

Open communication about death and dying. The Balin family agrees open communication about the end-of-life is important, but not easy. At times "you have to just push through it with tears" (Becky_38). "It" refers to the many discussions and decision-making sessions that mark end-of-life transitions. Gigi's daughters and grandchildren emphasize the necessity to talk and listen to the elders. The elders have insight that only they can share concerning The Depression, starting a business, or healing. Even in the final moments of life, there is awe and wonder in the last words shared by a dying person. "It's so cool…to relive a person's life with them, especially when they flash back, all the way back, across their life" (Jenny_9). For Gigi, openly communicating about death and dying is the most important factor in constructing a successful end-of-life transition for all parties. Gigi argues that this is something she learned after experiencing her own parents' deaths. Recalling the fear in her father's eyes as he lay dying in hospice, she explained,

> I went in hospice (pause) with my dad, (pause) and I could see (pause) it was just like that (pause) a cross between fear (pause) and anger. (pause) with—with dying. . . You can see it (pause). And—and I says to him, "Daddy, do you need to talk," "Yeah, I need to talk." Well, they keep 'em drugged in hospice [and he was unable to]. (Gigi_1_26)

Since then, Gigi has made it her "platform" to sit down and talk to her children about "what death is, what we call death, because there is no death" (Gigi_1_48). People are more alive, Gigi believes, on the other side than they are here, because on the other side the spirit has access to a fuller range of vibrations and is not constricted by the human form. Over time, talking openly, "like you and I are talking about these things," becomes natural. "It's just as simple as talkin' about givin' birth" (Gigi_1_52).

> Oh! (mimicking) "So and so's gonna give birth? We're gonna have a new baby! We're all gonna celebrate. The hospital, it's so fun to go in there. And they announce, "welcome to the wooorld," and they play Rock-a-Bye Baby, and everybody celebrates. *They should be doing it, just the opposite* (Gigi_1_26).

Gigi believes it is important for her to teach her children and grandchildren to communicate openly with each other and to ask for guidance from the spirit side. "I taught my kids by *allowing* them (to find their own paths) and not by *forcing* them into a set of beliefs" (Gigi_1_22).

> My kids weren't raised in a church where everything was a mystery and there was some God sittin' on a cloud somewhere. They were raised talking to "Father" all the time. If I'd fall down and get a skinned knee I'd ask God "why—what'd I do?" And that's all it is, that's the whole secret to everything, quit making a mystery out of it. Keep it simple, stupid! (Gigi_1_53)

Meredith adds weight to this claim by explaining that whereas other families might have a more traditional understanding of a higher power God or Jehovah,

> Our family, on the other hand, is a little bit more alternative. Where we never went to church, but we always believed in the power of God which is the power of love to us. Gigi was the matriarch, and she was really kooky and would get into that weird stuff, but taught us all about the Bible, [and] other aspects of knowing within yourself, and listening to find your guidance, and follow your guidance, and learn how to hear God's voice and not listen to other people (Meredith_4).

Open communication helps family members prepare for their roles across the lifespan. It's like evolution, Meredith explains, when one starts to weaken, the other ones start getting stronger. And hopefully the elders have gleaned knowledge from the experiences of growing up and have passed that knowledge on to the youngsters who start stepping up to become the elders.

Relating spiritual experiences. Gigi and the Balin sisters spend a significant amount of their everyday talk with each other sharing spiritual insights and experiences. E-mailing inspirational messages, telling and interpreting dreams, and relating other spiritual experiences (visits from family members who have passed over, strange occurrences, accurate predictions) comprise much of their discussions. Their spiritual connectedness centers on acceptance and sharing of spiritual and cosmic experiences. For instance, Gigi's family accepts that astral travel is possible in dreams. A person can leave his or her body and travel and visit in spirit form while sleeping because the mind releases tight binds of logic and rules. According to Gigi, dreams and astral travel also provide a practice realm for transitioning into death:

> You're out preparing every night when you're asleep to come in and get another body and move into another cycle to finish your work. So uh—if you just get the understanding that life is *eternal*, there is no end and there is no death. (Gigi_1_13)

Dreams are also a natural channel for communication between the spirit and the human world. Each member of the Balin family interviewed has had significant conversations with deceased relatives in their dreams. "I mean I've experienced my grandparents coming in my dreams loud and clear and they're all dead, you know. And it's like—I'm like going, 'Welll hi!!! How are you!' and it's just a really nice visit" (Meredith_26). The Balin family believes that loved ones come through in dreams because it is easier to accept their presence than if a person receives a physical visitation. When a family member experiences a dream or visitation, she shares it with others. Sharing these experiences strengthens the inherent value of those experiences and belief in the truth that comes from them. The excerpt below from Gigi and also shared by Meredith and Jenny offers a good example:

> I didn't get to tell you what happened to Jenny. Night before last, I think it was. She called me and, you know, my dad, they called Gramps—and Brad was born on Gramps' birthday. And she's had so much trouble with Brad. You-know? Okay, so the other night, she's in this real deep dream. And while she's in this dream, Beth is yelling at her in the dream, 'Jenny, you're wanted on the phone.' And she says again, 'Jenny! Gramps is on the phone!'

> And Jenny says, 'okay,' she goes and picks up the phone, and she's talking to Gramps on the phone and he's—all he talks to her about, the whole time is about Brad. So when she woke up she says, 'Oh mom, you cannot believe the experience I had,' you know, and I said, (laughs) 'yeah. I could believe it.' But he's saying, she says, 'You know, I can't tell you word for word what he said, but we had this intense conversation.' But she says, 'I woke up knowing Brad's gonna be okay, everything is going to be okay.' Isn't that a neat experience? (Gigi_1_16)

This example highlights three points. First, Jenny's disclosure of this dream to her mother and all three sisters demonstrates the importance of the dream and importance of sharing that experience with the rest of the family. Second, her dream is immediately accepted as significant and meaningful by other family members (i.e., her experience is "believed"). Third, these types of dreams bring about a sense of peace and familial and spiritual connection.

In addition to sharing spiritual experiences with each other, the Balin daughters seek spiritual guidance from the same external sources. For example, all four of the Balin daughters have been taking the "Course," shorthand for *A Course in Miracles*, a sort of spiritual guide for manifesting miracles in life through the love and acceptance of God. The Course is accompanied by a workbook and exercises that are designed to help the reader master metaphysical principles of thought and behavior. Work schedules and life events often interrupt a continuous devotion to the Course, but it nonetheless informs their life practices. The daughters often draw on readings from the Course, or other sources, in conversations, especially those involving difficult decisions, challenging situations, or unclear paths. In seeking guidance for how to manage their parents' transition, the daughters turn to the Course and share their new insights with Gigi as she continues to expand her spiritual knowledge. Familiarity with principles of the Course gives the daughters a spiritual grounding for conversations about living, dying, and preparing for the transition. In perhaps overly simple terms, The Course teaches students to manifest miracles by accepting that the peace of God lies within two principles: Nothing real can be threatened and nothing unreal exists. In light of end-of-life transitions, the Course also teaches, "Miracles enable you to heal the sick and raise the dead because you made sickness and death yourself, and can therefore abolish both" (Course in Miracles, 2008).

Knowledge gained from the readings of various spiritual texts and discussions of those texts helps to ensure that family members share the same expectations about death and dying.

Creating shared family metaphors. The Balin family also co-constructs and communicates their expectations about living and dying through the frequent use of metaphor. Metaphors are interesting carriers of family and cultural norms as they are situated in the lay-language and everyday life experience of the speakers. Recurrent metaphors give insight into what themes are important in the lives of family members and identify features of a shared belief system. In a rudimentary way, metaphors allow family members to simplify an abstract concept (like death) into something that is familiar and concrete (like giving birth). In her research, Foster (2007) points to the frequency with which people who write about health and illness evoke metaphors of geography, travel, or quests. Families talking about the death of a loved one often employ life, living, growth, and change metaphors (FitzSimmons, 1994-95). It is not surprising, then, that the Balin family creates their own metaphorical language to talk about the process of dying and death. Discussions among the Balin family that center on living and dying reveal several metaphors. The following passage is a typical explanation of birth and death (metaphors are italicized):

> Because that poor baby's comin' in here *to go to school* and go through all these trials and tribulations. (pause) And *death is graduation day,* and it's *no different than walkin' from here into the other room.* (pause) *And then there's a (pause) biiig party waitin' for ya.* (pause) All your loved ones are there, your *teachers, guides,* "Hooorah (pause) you made it! (pause) *You're home,* welcome home!" (Gigi_1_26)

Several metaphors are pervasive throughout their discourse. Only the most salient ones are offered here as examples, but they speak to the richness of this mode of transferring a familial belief system.

School metaphors and metaphors about having spiritual guides and teachers is common in their discourse. School metaphors describe a sense of *purpose* for living and dying. Humans can achieve different "levels" in life, a metaphor for reaching different levels of spiritual awareness. "Graduation day" arrives when we have fulfilled our purposes and we return to spirit side (death). Jenny provides evidence of how such beliefs are transferred and manifested, "[In my life] all I see [are] lessons. And, my mom's always told me 'life is a big schoolhouse and you're learning it from the minute you come in to the minute you go out'" (Jenny_29). School metaphors are also evoked to explain that life is really just a forum for practicing what is done on spirit side. In the following passage Gigi explains that there is nothing to fear in death, because "as it is here on Earth, so it is in Heaven":

> What do you do on Earth? You go to school. You pick your electives. Whatdo you do in heaven? You do the same thing. (pause) It's a reflection (pause) of the same thing. (pause) Why would God have you do something that's foreign to ya? Why would this [physical life] be natural and that [spiritual life] be foreign? (pause) Common sense, right? (Gigi_1_32)

Gigi also explains that people are not sent to go to school on Earth alone, they have guides or babysitters:

> You're a baby creator. (pause) You're little baby gods and goddesses down here going to school, but *Heeeee* [God] (pause) sends you to boarding school with a team of baby-sitters, and believe me, you've got baby-sitters. (Gigi_1_15)

The preceding example not only emphasizes the purpose of life (learning at boarding school), but also draws upon a sense of creation, kinship, and connection familiar to the women in the Balin family who have all had children. "Women are nurturers" (Gigi_1_12), Gigi declares as a scientific fact. Other metaphors that emphasize connection instruct that "you're not dangling out here by yourself" (Gigi_1_56). These types of metaphors focus on the connection between members of the Balin family. In wonderment, Becky says "you know, it's like we all got on the boat together to come in or something" (Becky_5). Other living things, such as the flower bush or aspen tree, are used metaphorically to describe how individuals are connected to "the Source" through their "roots." Metaphors that compare dying to familiar family celebrations and kinship rituals are also common. Death is graduation day, explains Gigi. Or, dying is like receiving a baby on the other side. It's a cause to celebrate because the spirit is returning "home."

The Balin family also uses metaphors to explain the similarity and proximity of the spiritual and physical worlds. Place terms, or physical locations, such as "the other side," "spirit side," and "home" coupled with actions such as "passing over," "crossing over," and "it's like walking from one room right into the other room" signify the ease with which a person can move between the two "dimensions." They use the term "thin veil" or "overlay" to describe how the spiritual world is separated from the physical. Another metaphor describes people as radios "you can tune in clearer without static the more you advance, the more you see things" (Gigi_1_18), explains that with time and practice it is possible to become more aware of the spiritual dimension. Gigi uses a helicopter metaphor to explain differences in people's physical-spiritual awareness. When there is no power, she explains, anyone can count the individual blades, but add the power and it becomes impossible to count individual blades. Because the spirit world works on a different "vibration" than the physical world, many people are unable to perceive the spirit side, much like they are unable to perceive the individual helicopter blades at the higher vibration.

Discussion

The approach that the Balin family takes toward understanding life transitions may be unique, but seeking connection and spiritual guidance towards the end-of-life is not. In fact, there is much evidence to suggest that many people sensing the end-of-life seek spiritual or religious means of making sense of their life (Moremen, 2004-05). Women in particular, argues Scheitle (2004-05), are likely to seek comfort in spirituality and spiritualism toward the end-of-life as Gigi has. Spiritual experiences toward the end-of-life, such as pre-death dreams and visitations from the other side, can offer a sense of peace for the dying individual and prepare them for their journey (Bulkeley & Bulkeley, 2005). The reasons, perhaps, lie in sociohistorical contexts in which women have held significant roles in (birthing and) raising children, nursing the sick, caring for the elderly, and maintaining family ties (Scheitle). Historically, women have been emotionally attached to those just entering the world and those about to exit.

Moremen (2004-05) suggests that spirituality in later life helps women to find their own place in the world and secure a sense of connectedness with themselves, others, and a higher power. Being universally connected includes an acceptance of the process of dying—something Gigi's family establishes intergenerationally through open talk and disclosure. Moreover, spiritual connectedness, like the Balin family experiences, often includes a perception of enhanced intuition about life events, a strong sense of connection with the deceased, vivid, prophetic end-of-life dreams, perceived ability to contact the dead, and visits from the deceased who serve as guides into the next life (Betty, 2006; Bulkeley & Bulkeley, 2005; Moreman; Scheitle, 2004-05). Regardless of the *matter* of those experiences (real or imagined), many people who have near-death experiences or experience nearing-death awareness (Callanan, 1994) report being able to communicate with both worlds (living and dead) at the same time and feeling comforted by those experiences (Betty). Women like those in Gigi's family who feel a strong connection with the "other side" also experience less fear and anxiety about dying (Betty; Bulkeley & Bulkeley).

Briller (2005) applies Turner's (1969) notion of *liminality* by arguing that people transitioning into death (like other rites of passage) may experience, "a finite time of limbo in which people are between states of being—having left one state but not yet entered or joined the next" (p. 84). Although liminality often brings with it confusion and perhaps anxiety over social roles and expectations, it is also a space of creativity wherein people can actively co-construct an experience. Social conventions and everyday behaviors might become inverted as "liminality provides a social space for individuals to behave very differently than at other times in community life" (Briller, p. 86). As in the case with Gigi's family, the liminal space opens opportunities for greater acceptance, tolerance, nurturance, and openness to spiritual experiences.

Although the Balin family is perhaps not unique in their desire for spiritual connection and meaning when it comes to managing end-of-life transitions, the process by which they communicate and share expectations and experiences with each other is unique. Earlier research suggests that when the dying process is gradual, at the natural aging pace, women have more time to seek answers to the meaning of life and prepare for their end-of-life journey as is the case for the Balin family. When a gradual dying process is coupled with open communication about dying, women feel more positive and experience less death-related anxiety (Moremen, 2004-05). Gigi's family is preparing for her eventual transition through open discussions about the meaning of living and dying across generations and over time. The daughters are emphatic when they say there will be a lot of crying and it will hurt.

> We're all crying now, I mean—(pause) that's just the human nature. But I don't think any of us are fearful of it [Gigi's death]. . . And maybe that's the difference with all of us. (pause) We're not afraid of it [death]. (pause) We know we're going to pass through it, we know we're gonna cry. We know we're gonna have feelings. But we're not afraid of it. (pause) Maybe that's what the difference is. (pause) That fear is gone. (pause) and the only—only because we've been interested enough in seeking it out, (pause) and with the experiences that we've had then. (pause) We know there's something (pause) that carries on, so—(pause) I think that's part of it (softens voice), just we're not afraid. (Becky_23)

The daughters in this family believe that their parents will always be with them in spirit form. This belief and embracing a philosophy that death is a form of spiritual graduation makes the transition into death a positive one. Open communication, sharing spiritual experiences with each other, and creating shared understanding about dying through frequent use of metaphor provides a firm foundation of beliefs. Gigi's family is successful in constructing the process of dying as a positive experience by maintaining it as a family belief across the lifespan and across generations.

Significance and Contributions of This Case

There is sometimes a tendency to question the authenticity, quality, and usefulness of case study research, especially that which is done within an interpretive paradigm. In my writing, I am mindful to align this text with standards of quality for qualitative research, and case studies in particular, presented by Lincoln and Guba (2002). The final case study report is marked not only by the quality of the product, but the quality of the process throughout the investigation. Authenticity is not only found in the final document, but in the careful ways that the researcher captures extraordinary and mundane elements of a specific case. Both the process and the product, then, are influenced by *resonance, rhetoric, empowerment,* and *applicability* (Lincoln & Guba).

Resonance refers to the degree of fit between the methodological paradigm guiding the research and the way that paradigm is expressed in the writing. Reflexivity and presence of the researcher's voice in the final product contribute to the authenticity of the text. Gigi's presence is unmistakable in this final report. Her narrative style resonates throughout the text in my effort to emphasize participants' meaning-making and to honor those experiences. But, my presence in the field and established family rapport are also subtle features of this text. The Balin family invited me to receive their family narratives. Thus, my role of story keeper is maintained in this text.

The *rhetorical* form of the text encompasses the internal organization and elegance of the text itself. One way this report honors participants' experiences, privileges their familial meaning-making structures, and maximizes the authenticity of the text is by presenting thick description of the Balin family, writing in *their* voices, and optimizing the organizational flow of the text in a way that folds scholarly literature and research into the real experiences of the Balin family.

Empowerment criteria assess the potential for the text to move the audience to action or to raise their awareness of an issue. This case study emphasizes the importance of death talk and dying as part of living; making it a natural topic of family discussion and normalizing and privileging end-of-life transitions. Talking about end-of-life experiences and expectations is an important step in creating the potential for a meaningful transition. The Balin family discourse makes evident the possibilities of constructing a meaningful experience for all involved through everyday talk and family rituals. The case study has potential to empower readers by illustrating how important and how natural it can be to embrace their own unique end-of-life experiences and communicate to create a meaningful transition. Conversations at the end-of-life, such as those shared with and by Gigi, can be particularly empowering because they produce opportunities for "authentic" talk that not only addresses pragmatic concerns that arise toward the end-of-life, but also helps the dying person and her loved ones find meaning in the process of living and dying (Keeley, 2007; McQuellon & Cowan, 2000).

Applicability is what makes a case study useful—does the case provide an experience or vicarious experience that readers can connect to their lives? Beyond the in-depth exploration into the ways in which one family has created positive expectations about death, this case study also connects the Balin family experience to relevant research and theories on end-of-life communication and dying.

This study is important for two reasons. First, it provides evidence of positivity in the construction of the dying experience. Second, it illustrates how powerful everyday talk across the lifespan is in creating experiences and expectations about the end-of-life. Although death cannot come without grief, it also has moments of joy that should be celebrated. The positive aspects of death and dying are important to communicate broadly. People play various death and dying roles across the lifetime, sometimes as mourner, sometimes as caretaker. The grand moment comes when individuals play their final role as dying person. Like other life roles, there is at least some creative freedom that comes with enacting that role. Unfortunately, individuals do not talk about death and dying enough within their families and among their loved ones to open that creative freedom. As Gelfand et al. (2005) note, "people experience dying as they experience living—through stories" (p. xxiii). The most important thing to be learned from the story of Gigi's family is not their unique spiritual take on death and dying; rather, it is that their open communication, the development of family narratives and metaphor, and sharing these across generations have helped this family to prepare for a successful end-of-life journey for Gigi.

References

Berger, C., & Calabrese, R. (1975). Some explorations in initial interaction and beyond. *Human Communication Research, 1,* 99-112.

Betty, S. (2006). Are they hallucinations or are they real? The spirituality of deathbed and near-death visions. *Omega, 53,* 37-49.

Bulkeley, K., & Bulkeley, P. (2005). *Dreaming beyond death: A guide to pre-death dreams and visions.* Boston: Beacon Press.

Book, P. L. (1996). How does the family narrative influence the individual's ability to communicate about death? *Omega, 33,* 323-341.

Briller, S. H. (2005). Stories of Avery: Living and dying well (Cultural response). In D. E. Gelfand, R. Raspa, S. H. Briller, & S. Myers Schim (Eds.), *End-of-life stories: Crossing disciplinary boundaries* (pp. 84-88). New York: Springer.

Callanan, M. (1994). Dealing with death: Farewell messages. *The American Journal of Nursing, 94* (5), 19-20.

Carstensen, L. L. (1992). Social and emotional patterns in adulthood: Support for socioemotional selectivity theory. *Psychology and Aging, 7,* 331-338.

Coffman, V. T., & Coffman, S. L. (1995-96). Behavioral rehearsal: A way of talking about the dying process. *Omega, 32,* 63-76.

Costello, J. (2006). Dying well: Nurses' experiences of 'good and bad' deaths in hospital. *Journal of Advanced Nursing, 54,* 594-601.

Emanuel, L., Bennett, K., & Richardson, V. (2007). The dying role. *Journal of Palliative Medicine, 10,* 159-168.

Emanuel, E. J., & Emanuel, L. L. (1998). The promise of a good death. *The Lancet, 351,* S21-S29.

FitzSimmons, E. (1994-95). One man's death: His family's ethnography. *Omega, 30,* 23-39.

Foster, E. (2007). *Communicating at the end-of-life: Finding magic in the mundane.* Mahwah, NJ: Lawrence Erlbaum.

Gelfand, D. E., Raspa, R., Briller, S. H., & Myers Schim, S. (2005) (Eds.). *End-of-life stories: Crossing disciplinary boundaries.* New York: Springer.

Gudykunst, W. B., & Kim, Y. Y. (1997). *Communicating with strangers: An approach to intercultural communication* (3rd ed.). New York: McGraw-Hill.

Kastenbaum, R. (2004). *On our way: The final passage through life and death.* Los Angeles: University of California Press.

Keeley, M. P. (2007). "Turning toward death together": The functions of messages during final conversations in close relationships. *Journal of Social and Personal Relationships, 24,* 225-253.

Keeley, M. P., & Kellas, J. K. (2005). Constructing life and death through final conversation narratives. In L. M. Harter, P. M. Japp, & C. S. Beck (Eds.), *Narratives, health and healing: Communication theory, research and practice* (pp. 365-390). Mahwah, NJ: Lawrence Erlbaum.

Keeley, M. P., & Yingling, J. M. (2007). *Final conversations: Helping the living and the dying talk to each other.* Acton, MA: Vander Wyk & Burnham.

Leichtentritt, R. D., & Rettig, K. D. (2001). The construction of a good death: A dramaturgy approach. *Journal of Aging Studies, 15,* 85-103.

Lincoln, Y. S., & Guba, E. G. (2002). Judging the quality of case study reports. In A. M. Huberman & M. B. Miles (Eds.) *The qualitative researcher's companion* (pp. 205-215). Thousand Oaks, CA: Sage.

Lynch, T. (1997). *The undertaking: Life studies from the dismal trade.* New York: Penguin Books.

McQuellon, R. P., & Cowan, M. A. (2000). Turning toward death together: Conversation in mortal time. *American Journal of Hospice and Palliative Care, 17,* 312-318.

Mitchell, D. R. (1997). The "good" death: Three promises to make at the bedside. *Geriatrics, 52,* 91-92.

Moremen, R. D. (2004-2005). What is the meaning of life? Women's spirituality at the end of the lifespan. *Omega, 50,* 309-330.

Nakashima, M., & Canda, E. R. (2005). Positive dying and resiliency in later life: A qualitative study. *Journal of Aging Studies, 19,* 109-125.

Nuland, S. B. (1993). *How we die: Reflections on life's final chapter.* New York: Vintage Books.

Nussbaum, J. F., Pecchioni, L. L., Robinson, J. D., & Thompson, T. L. (2000). *Communication and aging* (2nd ed.). Mahwah, NJ: Lawrence Erlbaum Associates.

Olson, D. H., Sprenkle, D. H., & Russell, C. S. (1979). Circumplex model of marital and family systems: I. Cohesion and adaptability dimensions, family types, and clinical applications. *Family Process, 18,* 3-28.

Reinard, J. C. (2008). *Introduction to communication research* (4th ed.). Boston: McGraw-Hill.

Scheitle, C. P. (2004-2005). Bringing out the dead: Gender and historical cycles of spiritualism. *Omega, 50,* 237-253.

Sedney, M. A., Baker, J. E., & Gross, E. (1994). "The story" of a death: Therapeutic considerations with bereaved families. *Journal of Marital and Family Therapy, 20,* 287-296.

Servaty, H. L., & Hayslip, B. Jr. (1996-97). Death education and communication apprehension regarding dying persons. *Omega, 34,* 139-148.

Stake, R. E. (1995). *The art of case study research.* Thousand Oaks, CA: Sage.

Stake, R. E. (1998). Case studies. In N. K. Denzin & Y. S. Lincoln (Eds.), *Stages of qualitative inquiry* (pp. 86-109). Thousand Oaks, CA: Sage.

The Course in Miracles. (2008). Retrieved from http://www.thecourseinmiracles.com

Turner, V. W. (1969). *The ritual process: Structure and Anti-structure.* Chicago: Aldine Publishing Company.

Yin, R. K. (2003). *Case study research.* Thousand Oaks, CA: Sage.

CHAPTER 15

"Uv Ü": Communicating at the End-of-Life

Leah Vande Berg and Nick Trujillo

SACRAMENTO STATE UNIVERSITY

Editor's note: This chapter was originally published in L. Vande Berg and N. Trujillo, *Cancer and Death: A Love Story in Two Voices,"*© 2008 Hampton Press, Inc. Reprinted with permission of the publisher.

This chapter is an honest and compelling description of how one married couple—Nick and Leah—navigated an end-of-life transition. This story embodies the notion of "going through this together" and is, ultimately, a tribute to their love.

Nick

Leah is barely hanging on. She went to bed at 8 pm on Sunday night and didn't wake up until 2 pm on Monday. She had a bit to eat and then slept the rest of the day and into the night. Yesterday she slept for the entire day and did not eat, just drank a little juice. The hospice people said it could be very soon. They come again today at 1 pm.

She is not feeling any pain, just mild discomfort when she wakes up. She is in and out of consciousness throughout the day and night. I whispered in her ear that the boys (the dogs) and I will be fine, that everything is all right, and that it is okay for her to go. I cancelled my last week of school this week to be with her (colleagues have taken over for me).

The wind has been blowing fiercely for the last few days during an intense winter storm. Knowing Leah, it sounds like there is a heated debate going on at the gates of heaven. I think it will be peaceful very soon.

Leah

It is so hard to leave the people that I love so much, especially Nick and the boys. On the other hand, every day I wake up and ask myself, what am I still doing here? I get up and feel good for about an hour, and then I go lie down on the couch and sleep my life away. Right now I am having a hard time swallowing. It takes longer and longer for me to do simple things. I get tired walking from the bedroom to the bathroom. If I am just going to be a vegetable on the couch, I might as well be a vegetable on the couch for a short time.

Nick and I had a fight this week. Not unpredictable, I suppose. But this is part of loving through cancer too. The argument was about my unwillingness to recognize my situation. I am trying to realize how frail and fragile I am becoming, how very little I actually can do, and how dangerous it is for me to do many things. Nick expressed concern that I walked over to my roll-top desk and stepped over a wooden box to get some papers. That would not normally seem like a particularly onerous or dangerous thing, but given the hospice nurse's discussion of the dangers during this phase, it was very timely. She talked about how the biggest danger that I face right now is not recognizing all of the places where I could fall down and be hurt and have no way of helping myself. Of course I pooh-poohed it.

Nick reminded me that it was the second time in two days that I had put myself in danger. Yesterday after dinner I was trying to carry a smorgasbord of six different kinds of dressings back to the kitchen on a tray in my shaky and fragile condition.

That is the crux of the problem: my unwillingness to recognize that I am dying and that I cannot do everything I want to do. I have to say I cannot do some things and ask Nick to do them for me. He said he would no longer be able to trust me not to do something stupid, like step over boxes with sharp edges. He needs for me to acknowledge that I am dying. I do not seem to be facing this reality terribly well.

Bill (a friend)

In the bed she will die in, my good friend's body contorted, limbs limp and intertwined, cheeks sunken as if puckering like we did when sharing a brew, me vowing to plant my own vines, crush my own grapes, make my own wine, we laughed thinking of the purple feet I'd have, but not caring. I hold her hand this last time, gently because she bruises easily, the color of wine.

winter sky

the contrail stretches

horizon to horizon

("Horizons," from a book of haibun by our friend Bill)

Nick

I was certain that Leah would die the night of Sunday, December 5th. As was typical of previous nights, she took a gasping breath once every twenty or so seconds and experienced brief convulsive tremors with her hands and body every twenty or so minutes. But that night she lay in bed calmly. When she finally fell asleep, she reached for someone or something with her arms. She also seemed to talk to someone, though I couldn't understand what she was mouthing.

During research for a book I wrote about my grandmother's life and death, I read about people with near-death experiences who say their spirits floated above their bodies and that deceased family members served as escorts to guide them. As Leah reached up, I looked around the room, searching for God, an angel, the spirit of Leah's mother, a beam of light, for any sign that she was being called.

"Do you see your Mom?" I whispered in Leah's ear. "Do you see God?"

Leah didn't respond.

At one point when I thought she was about to die, I gazed at the ceiling and actually waved.

"Goodbye, Miss Leah," I said. "Can you see us down here?"

Again, no response.

I stayed awake for most of the night watching Leah. I held her hand and whispered to her that the boys and I would be okay and that it was time for her to go.

I fell asleep around four o'clock and woke up a few hours later surprised that Leah was still breathing. I got up and fed the dogs and let them outside. I also telephoned the office receptionist and said I was calling in sick for the week—the last week of the semester-and I had arranged for colleagues to take over. For the next two days Leah did not get out of bed except to go to the bathroom, though she only peed twice each day and hadn't had a bowel movement for almost a week. She no longer reached up with her arms or talked while she slept. When she woke up for a few minutes every five or six hours, I offered her food and liquids. She ate a few crumbs one day, but otherwise just drank sips of orange juice.

During those two days a winter storm hit northern California with fierce winds that knocked down part of our fence in the backyard. The following week I would joke with Leah's Pastor that God had indeed called Leah on Sunday, debated with her at the gates of heaven, and then told her that HE needed a few more days to prepare for her.

The winds let up on Wednesday morning. Leah slept the entire morning and then, to my amazement, she got out of bed and walked into the living room. She ate a small salad and nearly tripped as she carried a tray of dressings.

I told her that hospice officials were coming to the house that afternoon. Despite my objections, she insisted on taking a shower before they arrived. I placed the shower chair in the tub and helped her undress. I had seen Leah without her top whenever I placed a new pain patch on her back, and without her bottoms every night when I helped her change into her pajamas. But I hadn't seen her completely naked for several weeks.

I nearly collapsed at the sight. Her arms and legs were rail-thin, her entire ribcage protruded, and her stomach was severely bloated. She looked like a starving woman in a picture from the Holocaust or from a plague-ridden country in Africa. I maintained my composure, barely, and helped her wash herself and get dressed. At one o'clock, hospice officials arrived to finish processing Leah's case. Leah stayed awake for the two-hour meeting as the nurse and social worker went over details, ranging from her various medications to the funeral arrangements. The nurse emphasized the risk of falling, though Leah seemed defensive about that topic, probably because she knew she was losing control of even the most basic activities. I ordered an adjustable hospital bed with railings to be delivered the following week and set up a tentative schedule for the nurse.

As I walked the hospice officials to their car after our meeting, the nurse said that Leah could die at any moment and likely would do so within a week. She said Leah would probably fall asleep and not wake up.

That possibility sounded pretty good, at least when compared to a painful death in a conscious state.

When I returned to the house, Leah had already walked to the bedroom and was asleep.

On Thursday, the sun came out on a peaceful day, but Leah woke up uncomfortable and restless.

"I don't know why I'm so tired," she said, kicking the covers off the bed.

She got up and lay on the couch for a few hours. At one point, she pulled herself up and hobbled to the roll-top desk.

"Can I get something for you, Miss Leah?" I asked.

"I'm not an invalid," she snapped, and then nearly fell over a box.

I rushed to assist her and helped her back to the couch. I told her sternly that she could not put herself in danger of falling. She argued, but I interrupted her.

"This isn't open for debate," I said, raising my voice.

I reiterated what the hospice nurse told her about falling and warned that I wouldn't be able to leave her alone if she put herself at risk.

Leah continued to disagree, but I cut her off again.

"God damn it, stop arguing with me!" I shouted and left the room.

I took the dogs outside and sat on the patio. I cried, feeling anger, sadness, and guilt. As I petted the boys, I realized that for Leah to stop debating with me would be a sign that she had given up.

I returned to the living room and apologized. We hugged, and I helped her to the bedroom where she slept for the rest of the day.

Leah didn't suffer any significant pain during the week, just moderate discomfort when she woke up. She took her oral pain pills and every few days I placed a new pain patch on her back. But everything changed on Friday.

Leah

I don't know why Nick thinks I'm going to die. . . . I'll feel better if I just lie down.

Jillian
(Nick and Leah's Former Graduate Student)

On Friday afternoon Nick called and asked me to buy some food and bring it over to their house. Leah had requested organic chicken, but Nick said not to worry about it. When I arrived, Leah called me into the living room and asked if the chicken was organic. I told her it wasn't, and she said that it needed to be organic. "It's not that difficult," she said. "I do it all the time."

Nick took the dogs for a walk and I stayed with Leah. "I don't know why Nick thinks I'm going to die," she said, out of nowhere. I paused, not knowing what to say. Then I told her that Nick was concerned because she was sleeping so much. It was pretty clear that she was not accepting of the fact that she was dying.

Nick

Our plan was for Leah to die at home, but as we learned throughout this ordeal, plans don't always work out.

Leah slept most of Friday morning, but when she woke up and staggered onto the couch in the living room, she was more agitated than the day before. She expressed uncharacteristic frustration with me, even at the dogs.

She said she was hungry for a chicken salad, but I had not shopped for several days and the refrigerator was bare. I called Jillian and asked her to buy some food.

I hung up the phone and returned to the living room. Leah asked if the chicken was organic, as we had eaten more organic food during the past few years. I should have told her that it was organic, but I said I didn't know. She became upset and insisted that she would only eat organic chicken.

Jillian arrived with the food, and I asked her to stay with Leah while I took the dogs for a walk. I needed to clear my head and calm down. I didn't want to fight with Leah again, even though she seemed determined to win one last argument.

When I returned, Jillian told me that Leah was really upset about the chicken and about the fact that I thought she was going to die.

Leah's aggravation continued into the evening. She sighed loudly and tossed and turned in bed.

At one point she stood up and stumbled toward the bathroom. I guided her to the toilet and helped pull down her pajama bottoms. Before she sat down, two mushy globs of feces dropped to the floor. I stared at the sight for a moment, startled by the image and surprised that anything could come out of her after she ate so little. When she finished, I helped her up and wiped her.

She also threw up several times. I called hospice, and a nurse said to give Leah oral anti-nausea medication. A few minutes later Leah threw up the medicine and I called hospice again.

The nurse asked if Leah's vomit looked like coffee grounds.

I said it appeared to be mucous.

She told me that was a good sign and instructed me to go to the emergency pharmacy and get new anti-nausea medication that would dissolve in Leah's mouth.

I called my friend Kimo and asked him to get the drugs, as I was not about to leave Leah. Kimo agreed to pick up the meds, but then he called a half hour later and said there was a mix-up at the pharmacy and it would take another forty-five minutes. I called hospice again and they apologized for the delay. They told me to hold on for the medicine.

While we waited, Leah's pain intensified. She threw up several times and moaned in obvious pain. Every second was excruciating.

I could clean up her vomit and wipe her butt, but I couldn't stop her suffering with the medication we had at home. And the anti-nausea medication Kimo was getting would not relieve the pain she was experiencing at that point. I told Leah she needed to go to the hospital, but she resisted.

"I'll feel better if I just lie down," she said, dropping onto the bed after another messy trip to the bathroom.

I finally couldn't watch her suffer any longer. I called hospice one last time and they agreed that Leah needed to be admitted to emergency. Kimo arrived with the meds a few minutes before the paramedics took her to the hospital.

Kimo
(Nick and Leah's Friend and Colleague)

That Friday night about 11 pm, Nick called and said Miss Leah wasn't doing well and asked me to get some medicine for her. I got to their house about 1:30 in the morning, and it was obvious that the medication wasn't going to help her. She was in a lot of pain. The ambulance came to transport her, and they put her on a gurney. She had her eyes closed and I walked over and held her hand. She did not even know I was there and had no energy at this point.

Nick said, "Miss Leah, Kimo's here. He's holding your hand."

Like she got power from some mystical force, she opened her eyes, turned and looked at me, somehow managed to lift herself slightly up off the gurney, reached out for me, and gave me the biggest hug that I've ever had. At that moment, I knew it was no longer about her; it was about her telling me that things were going to be okay.

Nick

Leah was admitted to emergency around two o'clock in the morning on Saturday. Ironically, or perhaps fittingly, she was placed in the same cubicle where she received the initial diagnosis the year before. They hooked her up to a morphine drip, which relieved the pain but made her more nauseous. She threw up mucous, blood, tissue, and other gunk that did indeed look like coffee grounds and smelled like Hawkeye with a really bad yeast infection. I stood vigil over her with a small plastic container, catching whatever I could of the bile that spewed from her mouth.

When a new shift came on duty near dawn, a doctor came in to check on Leah. He looked at her, and then at me.

"I'm sorry about your mother," he said.

"She's my wife," I told him.

He apologized profusely, explaining that he did not have time to read the chart.

"Don't worry about it," I said. "She looks like my grandmother."

In actuality, she barely looked human.

Leah was admitted to a private room in the ward for terminally-ill patients at four in the afternoon, over twelve hours after she entered the ER. I went home to feed the dogs, though my neighbor Dee-Dee took care of them from that point on as I stayed at the hospital.

Several friends visited Leah that evening and night. I told her whenever someone came into the room. She struggled to open her eyes, though she could not keep them open for more than a split second.

That night, Juliane pointed out that I was wearing my favorite Rasputin stout tee shirt from the North Coast Brewing Company. The "Never Say Die" motto on the back struck her as ironic, as I was coaching my wife to actually die. The next time I went home, I took off that shirt and vowed to never wear it again.

Leah gasped loudly throughout the night, and the duration between breaths became longer and longer, up to thirty-five seconds. I held her hand, stroked her hair, and said everything I could to help her die. I told her that I loved her, that I'd take care of the boys, that there wasn't anything left for her to do, that it wasn't her fault, that it was okay to go, to look for her mom.

But somehow she hung on.

On Sunday, Leah's condition deteriorated further. She barely acknowledged visitors, although Kimo takes pride that Leah opened her eyes briefly and partially mouthed a goodbye to him when he left.

Our friend Sylvia visited that afternoon and suggested that I bring in a CD player and play holiday music for Leah. I rushed home and returned with our portable CD player and several Christmas and choir CDs. Leah responded the most when I played choir music, especially a Sacramento Choral Society CD recorded in 2000 when Leah was a member of the choir. A soprano, Leah twitched her eyes and moved her mouth whenever the female sopranos sang. Even in a seemingly unconscious state, she somehow heard the music and sang along.

I stayed next to her all night long, unable to sleep as her gasping intensified and her tremors became more frequent. I said everything I could to help her to die. I even lied to her at midnight on December 13th and told her that it was my birthday. She had said that she would try to hang on for that date, which was the next day.

I continued to play her CDs, but then I wondered if that music was keeping her alive. Late that night I decided to play my music. I whispered in her ear that I was getting a CD from the car and asked her not to die in the next thirty seconds. I sprinted to the parking lot and retrieved "The Essential Bob Dylan." When I returned I serenaded her for the rest of the night, especially during the song "Not Dark Yet," which had become my theme song of the previous month because of the refrain, "It's not dark yet, but it's getting there." I played that song over and over, and Leah continued to hang on.

During one period of sleep-deprived delirium, I considered smothering Leah with a pillow. I yelled at God for not taking her sooner, but then the dark vestiges of my Catholic upbringing resurfaced and I realized it was Satan who was tormenting me with the ultimate paradox: the only way I could relieve my wife's suffering was to kill her, but then I'd be haunted with that memory for the rest of my life. I prayed, I cried, I swore, I sang, and I even laughed, fueled by adrenaline and feeling every possible emotion.

In the wee hours of Monday morning, I felt a moment of calm. Even though Leah gasped for breath and smelled horribly, the scene was eerily serene, even elegant. I did not feel a greater spiritual presence, but the moment itself was profound in its own right. I gazed around the room for several minutes and then summoned Leah's attention.

"Leah?" I said, and repeated her name several times until she partially responded. "I have to tell you something. I want you to know that I love you. I love you so much."

Leah twitched her eyes. "Uv ü," she whispered, barely audible.

I kissed her forehead and wept.

Dave
(Nick and Leah's Friend and Colleague)

By the time I got to the hospital it was probably after eleven at night. Nick was by Leah's bedside, and he told her that I was there. She stirred a little, but didn't say anything. At that point, she was heavily medicated on morphine and coughing up a lot of blood and tissue. I spoke to her a little, but mostly spent my time trying to give what comfort I could to her and to Nick.

We talked about the irony—I guess that's the right word—of Nick being the first person to visit my wife and newborn daughter in the very same hospital just months before. One tries to say something comforting and wise in such circumstances, but what can be said at that point? My wife tells me that when her father died, the best thing that anyone said to her was that they can't possibly know how she must feel. I said that, and brought Nick some food so that he could have some strength as he sat with Leah. After a while, I whispered some words of peace to her and then left.

Nick

At six o'clock in the morning, Sylvia returned. She took one look at me and told me to go home and take a shower. I resisted, knowing that Leah could die at any moment, but then she could have died at any time during the previous week. I thought Leah might hang on for another day or two, so I decided to go home for a quick shower.

As I gathered my belongings, two nurses came in and said they wanted to turn Leah again to prevent bedsores. They started to move her and she became very distressed. She opened her eyes widely and craned her neck. In her withered condition and with bulging eyes and a stretched neck, she did not appear to be human. As ghastly and surreal as this might sound, she looked like E.T. from the Steven Spielberg movie.

I held her hand and told her it was okay, but she remained agitated even after the nurses left the room. Her breathing changed dramatically, shifting to what sounded like a higher octave but in a minor chord.

"Something is different," I said.

Sylvia backed off and let me have privacy with Leah as I stroked her hair and coached her to die. I told her that it wasn't her fault, that I was so proud of her, and that she could do this. Her breathing slowed and her gasps shortened, until I could see only faint reflexes in her mouth and throat.

A few minutes past seven o'clock, Leah took one last micro-gasp, and then became completely calm.

Sylvia approached and asked, "Is she gone?"

"I don't know," I said. "I've never done this before."

I put my finger on Leah's neck to feel for a pulse, and her throat quivered ever so slightly. We let her lie in peace for several additional minutes. She probably was dead for five minutes before I went to get a nurse.

I walked to the nurses' station and asked for help.

"Be right with you, honey," the nurse said as she filled out some paperwork.

"Take your time," I said calmly. "My wife just died and she's not going anywhere."

The nurse dropped her pen, stood up, and gave me her full attention.

"Are you okay?" she asked.

I told her I was fine and that I had been expecting Leah to die at any time for the last week. The nurse checked on Leah and called for a doctor.

Sylvia
(Nick and Leah's friend and colleague)

Some nurses' aides came in to move Leah, to avoid bedsores—in more lucid moments later I realized the absurdity of needing to move someone so close to death—and it distressed Leah a lot. Her blue, blue eyes opened up wide, panicked, and she turned, not seeing anything in the room. Nick rushed to her other side, soothing her through words, stroking her hair, her arm, her hands, telling her how much he loved her, that it was okay to let go, reminding her that they had talked about everything, that "the boys" were okay.

I stepped back by then, not wanting to intrude, but not wanting to abandon Nick if he needed me. Each silence between breaths took longer, longer, with Nick softly talking to her the whole time, a murmur of loving words. Finally, there were long silences between the harsh, hard sounds of those last, final breaths. When she took her last breath, we just sat with her for a while, quiet, waiting.

Nick

Kimo arrived shortly after Leah died and sat with me as I continued to hold Leah's hand.

He said he would always remember Leah's clear blue eyes.

I told him her eyes were still crystal clear, a condition I never understood given what her body went through. I stood up and moved over Leah's body. I told Kimo to approach, and I propped open Leah's left eyelid with my finger and thumb.

"Look at how clear they still are," I said.

Kimo took a quick look at her and sat back down. I closed her eyelid, and then he looked up at me. "And you wouldn't look at your grandmother's body?" he said and smiled, a reference to when my paternal grandmother died and I refused to look at her body in the casket because I do not like the last memory of a loved one to be of their stiff cadaver in a box.

"Things have changed a little," I said and smiled.

A doctor came in around eight o'clock to make the pronouncement of death. Kimo and I stayed with Leah until nearly nine o'clock, when the man from the crematorium came to take her body. He looked like a character from "The Sopranos."

"I'm sorry for your loss," he said softly.

Kimo helped me to my car and gave me one last long hug. I cried in his arms and then managed to drive home. I couldn't believe that she was actually gone.

ABOUT THE EDITOR AND CONTRIBUTORS

Michelle Miller-Day (Ph.D., Arizona State University, 1995) (*editor*) is an Associate Professor in the Department of Communication Arts and Sciences at Pennsylvania State University and a faculty affiliate with the Center for Diverse Families and Communities and the Center for Health Care and Policy Research. The Pennsylvania State University's Qualitative Research Group is organized under the direction of Dr. Miller-Day. She is currently the Principle Qualitative Investigator on a National Institute on Drug Abuse [NIDA/NIH] funded project and has served as the primary qualitative methodologist for this line of research funded by NIDA for the past 20 years. This work has developed one of the most successful evidence-based substance use prevention programs in the United States. Dr. Miller-Day has published three books, numerous refereed articles in scholarly journals and chapters in books, and has served on the editorial boards of several scholarly journals such as the *Journal of Family Communication* and *Health Communication*. She also served as a past President of the Family Communication Division of the National Communication Association and is currently Chair of the Applied Communication Division.

LaKesha Anderson Dearman (M.A., East Tennessee State University) is an Assistant Professor in the Department of Communication at Indiana State University where she teaches courses in persuasion, health communication, and research methods. She completed her Ph.D. in Communication with an emphasis in Health at George Mason University. She received her MA from East Tennessee State University and her BS from the University of Virginia at Wise. Before joining ISU, she taught public relations, persuasion, rhetoric, and public speaking at George Mason University for six years. She has an extensive research agenda which focuses primarily on health communication. Her dissertation focused on the ways in which women seek and receive social support when experiencing postpartum depression. Her research has also explored media representations, campaign development, and interpersonal dynamics most particurarly in familial and organizational health settings. Dr. Anderson has presented at international, national, and regional communication conferences.

Terry A. Badger (Ph.D., University of Texas at Austin) is a Professor and Division Director at the University of Arizona, College of Nursing. Her research interests lie at the intersection of psychological distress and chronic illness. Her most recent research focuses on the psychological distress and interdependence in psychological distress of cancer survivors and their partners. She has authored numerous articles in such journals as *Nursing Research, Psycho-Oncology, Research in Nursing and Health, and Journal of Social and Personal Relationships.* She is a member of the Arizona Cancer Center and Fellow in the American Academy of Nursing.

Erica D. Bauer (Ph.D., University of Illinois at Champaign-Urbana) earned a bachelor's degree in communication from the University of Dayton in 2003. She also received a master's degree in communication from the University of Dayton in 2005. She went on to complete a doctoral degree in communication at the University of Illinois in Urbana-Champaign. In the fall of 2010, Bauer will begin her postdoctoral work at the Center for Management of Complex Chronic Care in Health Services Research at the Hines VA hospital near Chicago, Illinois.

Emily Bowlby (M.A., Penn State University) studies disability communication—specifically invisible disabilities (IDs) and invisible chronic illnesses (ICIs)—using the method of autoethnography. She is an educational consultant in the area of disabilities for post-secondary and university institutions and applies her knowledge of health communication in her professional career as a Pharmaceutical Sales Representative for GlaxoSmithKline.

J Lynne Brown (PhD, MIT) is Professor in the Department of Food Science at The Pennsylvania State University. Her research interests include examining how family interaction patterns affect foods served at family meals. This work focuses on mid-life families where the emergence of chronic disease risk factors or diagnosis may evoke renegotiation of meal patterns. She has found that gender role expectations can affect how the initial meal patterns are established early in a relationship and how any subsequent adjustment is handled. Her other research interest is determining the basis for consumer reactions to products of new technologies entering the food system. As an extension specialist, she has developed educational materials for consumers addressing nutrition, food irradiation, genetic engineering and more recently nanotechnology. She serves on the Board of Editors for the *Journal of Nutrition Education and Behavior* and reviews articles regularly for *Risk Analysis and Social Science and Medicine.*

Danielle Catona (M.A., Pennsylvania State University) is a doctoral student. She investigates intergenerational communication and older-adult health outcomes. Her research focuses specifically on the impact of age-adapted speech in formal care settings. Her professional affiliations include the National Communication Association and the International Communication Association.

Joanne Cohen-Katz (Ph.D., University of Florida) is a clinical psychologist who has been training Family Medicine physicians for over 20 years. She received her Ph.D. in Psychology and completed an internship at the Philadelphia Child Guidance Center, a renowned family therapy training center. One of her professional passions is in helping physicians to view patients within the context of their family systems, so that the family becomes a resource for the care of the patient. She also is passionate about training physicians in self-reflection and mindfulness techniques, so that they can bring their best selves to the highly challenging work of being a healer. Dr. Cohen-Katz is blessed with a very supportive husband and two beautiful children! She is a longtime practitioner and teacher of mindfulness meditation and also a certified yoga instructor.

Carla L. Fisher (Ph.D., Pennsylvania State University) is an Assistant Professor of Communication Studies at Arizona State University. Her research focuses on the centrality of family communication to wellness using a life-span developmental perspective, particularly how families communicatively adapt to aging and health transitions, therapeutic implications of intergenerational interaction, and associations between kin communication and long-term health outcomes. She has explored this in the contexts of cancer, genetic counseling, geriatric caregiving, and eating disorders. Her research on mother-daughter communication and breast cancer was awarded the 2009 Sandra Petronio Dissertation Award and will be published in Hampton Press's health communication book series. Currently, she is collaborating with Mayo Clinic to extend this research. A National Institute on Aging Predoctoral Fellow and Juran Fellow, she serves on the editorial board of the *Journal of Family Communication* and as Chair of NCA's Communication and Aging Division. She has co-authored one book and multiple publications including recent articles in *Health Communication* and *Journal of Language and Social Psychology*.

Elissa Foster (Ph.D., University of South Florida) is a Medical Educator in the Department of Family Medicine at Lehigh Valley Health Network, where she supports the development of graduate medical education through research and faculty development initiatives. Her principal areas of research are health communication and interpersonal relationships with a specialization in end-of-life communication and ethnographic research methods. Her book, *Communicating at the End-of-Life: Finding Magic in the Mundane* (Erlbaum, 2007), won the 2009 Distinguished Scholarly Book Award from the Applied Communication Division of NCA. She has also published book chapters and peer-reviewed articles on a variety of topics including marital conflict, motherhood, and spirituality in health care; examples of her research can be found in *Qualitative Inquiry, Journal of Ageing and Identity, Journal of Cancer Integrative Medicine, Women's Studies in Communication,* and the *Southern Communication Journal*. She was the 2007 recipient of the Janice Hocker Rushing Early Career Research Award from the Southern States Communication Association.

Thomas J. Hipper (B.A., The College of New Jersey) is a M.A. candidate at The Pennsylvania State University and is currently completing his thesis on the role of social support messages on adolescent substance use. Concurrently, he is an M.H.S. candidate in the Health, Behavior & Society Department at The Johns Hopkins Bloomberg School of Public Health. His research interests are grounded in a number of areas including health communication, disaster communication, and public health preparedness. Thomas has attended the Invitational Masters Student Institute at Rutgers University, co-authored an article in *Health Communication,* and served as the National President of Lambda Pi Eta, the Communication Studies Honor Society.

Barbara L. Jones (PhD, MSW, University at Albany) is an Assistant Professor and Co-Director of The Institute for Grief, Loss and Family Survival at the UT Austin School of Social Work. Dr. Jones is the Immediate Past President of the Association of Pediatric Oncology Social Workers (APOSW) and a member of the Children's Oncology Group. Dr. Jones is a Steering Committee Member of the LiveSTRONG Survivorship Center of Excellence Network and a Board Member of the Social Work Hospice/ Palliative Care Network. Dr. Jones is also a Project on Death in America Social Work Scholar and serves on the editorial board of the *Journal of Social Work in Palliative and End-of-Life Care.* Dr. Jones' clinical experience has been primarily in the field of pediatric oncology, children's grief and loss, pediatric palliative and end-of-life care, grief, trauma, and survival. Dr. Jones conducts research on pediatric palliative care, mindfulness meditation interventions for children with cancer, Hispanic/Latino adolescent cancer survivors and on the health promotion needs of childhood cancer survivors. In 2009, Dr. Jones received the Social Work in Hospice and Palliative Care Network PDIA Social Work Leadership Award.

Jon Nussbaum (Ph.D. Purdue, 1981) is a Professor of Communication Arts & Sciences and Human Development & Family Studies at Penn State University. He is the Past President of the International Communication Association, former editor of the *Journal of Communication,* a Fulbright Research Fellow in the UK (1991-92) and a Fellow within the Adult Development and Aging Division of APA. Nussbaum has a well established publication record (10 books and over 70 journal articles and book chapters) studying communication behaviors and patterns across the life span including research on family, friendship and professional relationships with well and frail older adults. He has served as major professor and has directed 25 dissertations and currently has seven doctoral students completing their dissertations at Penn State.

Sandra Petronio (Ph.D., University of Michigan) is a Professor in the Department of Communication Studies at Indiana University-Purdue University, Indianapolis, a Core faculty in the Indiana University Center for Bioethics, and an Adjunct faculty member in the IU School of Nursing and the School of Informatics. Specializing in communication, Professor Petronio's areas of research are in the ethics of privacy, disclosure, and confidentiality. Recently she was invited by the Consortium of Social Science Associations to give a Congressional Briefing in Washington, DC on protecting privacy. During the last 25 years, she has developed the "Communication Privacy Management" (CPM) theory, completing a book detailing the theory in 2002 published by State University of New York Press entitled, *Boundaries of Privacy: Dialectics of Disclosure,* which won the Gerald R. Miller Award from the National Communication Association in 2003 and the 2004 book award from the International Association of Relationship Research. Professor Petronio has published five books, numerous refereed articles in scholarly journals and chapters in books, served as a journal editor for the Western Journal of Communication as well as editor for several special issues in Communication Research on group boundaries, and the *Journal of Applied Communication Research* on "translating scholarship into practice." She is currently the Vice President for the International Association for Relationship Research and a Past President of the Western States Communication Association.

Jonathan Pettigrew (M.A., Indiana University Purdue University Indianapolis) is A.B.D at Penn State University in the department of Communication Arts and Sciences. He was named a 2008 DeKruyter Graduate Scholar in Communication by the Gainey Institute for Faith and Communication and has been a licensed Christian minister since 2001. Both his academic and personal interests center on family formation, family processes, and family communication.

Breanne Pettigrew (B.A., Indiana University Purdue University Indianapolis). In fall 2006 she was awarded the prodigious Witherspoon Fellowship and inaugurated into its academic fraternity. She has also worked as a research assistant for the Family Research Council in Washington D.C., where she investigated public policy issues concerning embryology.

Margaret J. Pitts (Ph.D., Pennsylvania State University) is an assistant professor of communication in the Department of Communication and Theatre Arts at Old Dominion University. She conducts naturalistic research in the areas of communication and identity across the lifespan. Specifically, she is interested in how people use everyday talk to manage interpersonal and intergroup relationships during transitions across the lifespan. To achieve this end, Dr. Pitts has investigated identity and U.S. American sojourners, family health decision making regarding issues such as organ donation and the HPV vaccine, and issues related to retirement, successful aging, and end-of-life communication. She has also authored or co-authored scholarship on qualitative research methods. She is actively involved with the International Association of Language and Social Psychology and the International Communication Association, among other professional associations.

Kelly R. Rossetto (Ph.D., University of Texas at Austin) is an Assistant Professor in the Department of Communication at Boston College. Her research focuses on the communication processes (e.g., social support, disclosure, coping) that aid in or influence family relationships and resilience during stressful events. She is interested in how families individually and collectively cope with stressful events including illness, death, separation, and deployment.

Chris Segrin (Ph.D., University of Wisconsin) is a behavioral scientist whose specialty is interpersonal relationships and mental health. His research focuses on social skills, relationship development and satisfaction, and such problems as depression, anxiety, loneliness, and marital distress. He is author of the books *Interpersonal Processes in Psychological Problems* (2001, Guilford Press) and *Family Communication* (2005, Lawrence Erlbaum Publishers). Professor Segrin was also the editor of the journal *Communication Theory* from 2003 to 2005. In addition to his appointment in the Department of Communication, Professor Segrin is an Adjunct Professor in the departments of Psychology and Family Studies, and a member of the University of Arizona's Graduate Interdisciplinary Program in Statistics. Prior to joining the faculty at the University of Arizona, Professor Segrin was on the faculty of the University of Kansas and the University of Wisconsin-Milwaukee.

Rachel A. Smith (Ph.D., Michigan State University) is an Assistant Professor at the Pennsylvania State University. She investigates social influences in health communication. Her research focuses specifically on the impact of social phenomena (e.g., social networks, social support, social cognition, and stigma) on message diffusion and behavioral adoption in both domestic and international contexts.

Denise Solomon (Ph.D., Northwestern University) is a Professor of Communication Arts and Sciences at Pennsylvania State University. Professor Solomon's research focuses generally on the causes and consequences of turbulence in romantic associations, as well as how communication participates in those experiences. In more than 40 refereed articles in scholarly journals, Professor Solomon has examined how relationship qualities, including interpersonal power, relational uncertainty, and interdependence, shape people's perceptions of and communication about relational irritations, problematic events or *faux pas*, uncertainty-provoking events, changes in sexual intimacy, jealousy experiences, hurtful messages, and sexually harassing statements. This work has culminated in the relational turbulence model, which is a theory describing how transitions in romantic relationships promote relationship qualities that polarize cognitive, emotional, and communicative reactions to both ordinary and extraordinary experiences. Professor Solomon also serves on the editorial boards of four journals, and she was an associate editor for *Personal Relationships* from 2005-2009.

Keli Ryan Steuber (Ph.D., Penn State) is an Assistant Professor in the Department of Communication Studies at The University of Iowa. Her research examines how married partners negotiate relational transitions across the lifespan, specifically focusing on how transitions influence communication between spouses and how partners share private information with individuals outside their marriage. Her most recent work incorporates the medical, social, and marital stressors that accompany infertility by examining how social networks can facilitate or complicate a couple's efforts to cope with and treat infertility. Keli has co-authored articles in the *Journal of Social and Personal Relationships, Communication Monographs,* and *Human Communication Research.*

Shannon Sweeney Lewis (B.S., Taylor University) is an Adjunct Professor at Taylor University and Indiana Wesleyan University. She is finishing her Master's in Applied Communication at Indiana University Purdue University Indianapolis. She has worked as a research assistant for the Communication Studies Department at Indiana University Purdue University Indianapolis and as a research assistant for the Charles Warren Fairbanks Center for Medical Ethics. Her personal and professional interests focus on how family communication influences interactions in other interpersonal relationships and family communication in health contexts.

Nick Trujillo (Ph.D., University of Utah) is Professor of Communication Studies at Sacramento State University. He has published many scholarly and trade articles as well as four books, including *Organizational Life on Television* (Ablex, 1989, with Leah Vande Berg), *The Meaning of Nolan Ryan* (Texas A&M University Press, 1994), *In Search of Naunny's Grave: Age, Class, Gender, and Ethnicity in an American Family* (AltaMira, 2004), and *Cancer and Death: A Love Story in Two Voices* (Hampton, 2008, with Leah Vande Berg). His Internet alter ego, Gory Bateson, is lead singer of the mythical band The Ethnogs, whose music videos can be found by doing a Google search of the singer's name.

Leah Vande Berg (Ph.D., University of Iowa) was a Professor of Communication Studies at Sacramento State University until her death from ovarian cancer in December 2004. She published many scholarly articles as well as five books, including *Organizational Life on Television* (Ablex, 1989, with Nick Trujillo), *Television Criticism: Approaches and Applications* (Longman, 1991, with Lawrence Wenner and Bruce Gronbeck), *Critical Approaches to Television* (Allyn & Bacon, 2003, with Lawrence Wenner and Bruce Gronbeck), *Cancer and Death: A Love Story in Two Voices* (Hampton, 2008, with Nick Trujillo), and *Bad Girls: Cultural Politics and Media Representations of Transgressive Women* (Peter Lang, 2007, with A. Susan Owen and Sarah Stein).

Kirsten M. Weber (Ph.D., Pennsylvania State University) is an Assistant Professor at the University of Georgia. Her research interests lie at the intersection of interpersonal and health communication. Specifically, she is interested in understanding how interpersonal relationships both influence and are an influence on illness experiences.

Kirsten's most recent work explores how social and medical network members influence treatment decision making for breast cancer patients. Her work has been published in *Human Communication Research* and *Health Communication,* and she has co-authored a number of book chapters.

AUTHOR INDEX

SUBJECT INDEX

Health Communication

Gary L. Kreps, Series Editor

This series examines the powerful influences of human and mediated communication in delivering care and promoting health.

Books analyze the ways that strategic communication humanizes and increases access to quality care as well as examining the use of communication to encourage proactive health promotion. The books describe strategies for addressing major health issues, such as reducing health disparities, minimizing health risks, responding to health crises, encouraging early detection and care, facilitating informed health decisionmaking, promoting coordination within and across health teams, overcoming health literacy challenges, designing responsive health information technologies, and delivering sensitive end-of-life care.

All books in the series are grounded in broad evidence-based scholarship and are vivid, compelling, and accessible to broad audiences of scholars, students, professionals, and laypersons.

For additional information about this series or for the submission of manuscripts, please contact:

Gary L. Kreps
University Distinguished Professor and Chair, Department of Communication
Director, Center for Health and Risk Communication
George Mason University Science & Technology 2, Suite 230, MS 3D6
Fairfax, VA 22030-4444
gkreps@gmu.edu

To order other books in this series, please contact our Customer Service Department:

(800) 770-LANG (within the U.S.)
(212) 647-7706 (outside the U.S.)
(212) 647-7707 FAX

Or browse online by series:
www.peterlang.com